Perinatal Pharmacology

Editors

JONATHAN M. DAVIS
ERROL R. NORWITZ

CLINICS IN PERINATOLOGY

www.perinatology.theclinics.com

Consulting Editor
LUCKY JAIN

June 2019 • Volume 46 • Number 2

ELSEVIER

1600 John F. Kennedy Boulevard • Suite 1800 • Philadelphia, Pennsylvania, 19103-2899

http://www.theclinics.com

CLINICS IN PERINATOLOGY Volume 46, Number 2
June 2019 ISSN 0095-5108, ISBN-13: 978-0-323-68229-9

Editor: Kerry Holland
Developmental Editor: Casey Potter

Clinics in Perinatology (ISSN 0095-5108) is published quarterly by Elsevier Inc., 360 Park Avenue South, New York, NY 10010-1710. Months of issue are March, June, September, and December. Business and Editorial Offices: 1600 John F. Kennedy Blvd., Ste. 1800, Philadelphia, PA 19103-2899. Customer Service Office: 3251 Riverport Lane, Maryland Heights, MO 63043. Periodicals postage paid at New York, NY and additional mailing offices. Subscription prices are $309.00 per year (US individuals), $578.00 per year (US institutions), $365.00 per year (Canadian individuals), $708.00 per year (Canadian institutions), $435.00 per year (international individuals), $708.00 per year (international institutions), $100.00 per year (US students), and $195.00 per year (Canadian and international students). International air speed delivery is included in all Clinics subscription prices. All prices are subject to change without notice. **POSTMASTER:** Send address changes to *Clinics in Perinatology*, Elsevier Health Sciences Division, Subscription Customer Service, 3251 Riverport Lane, Maryland Heights, MO 63043. **Customer Service: Telephone: 1-800-654-2452** (U.S. and Canada); **1-314-447-8871** (outside U.S. and Canada). **Fax: 1-314-447-8029. E-mail: journalscustomerservice-usa@elsevier.com** (for print support); **journalsonlinesupport-usa@elsevier.com** (for online support).

Reprints. For copies of 100 or more, of articles in this publication, please contact the Commercial Reprints Department, Elsevier Inc., 360 Park Avenue South, New York, NY 10010-1710. Tel. 212-633-3874; Fax: 212-633-3820; E-mail: reprints@elsevier.com.

Clinics in Perinatology is also published in Spanish by McGraw-Hill Interamericana Editores S.A., P.O. Box 5-237, 06500 Mexico D.F., Mexico.

Clinics in Perinatology is covered in *MEDLINE/PubMed (Index Medicus) Current Contents, Excepta Medica, BIOSIS and ISI/BIOMED.*

Contributors

CONSULTING EDITOR

LUCKY JAIN, MD, MBA
George W. Brumley Jr Professor and Chair, Emory University School of Medicine, Department of Pediatrics, Chief Academic Officer, Children's Healthcare of Atlanta, Executive Director, Emory and Children's Pediatric Institute, Atlanta, Georgia, USA

EDITORS

JONATHAN M. DAVIS, MD
Vice-Chair of Pediatrics, Chief of Newborn Medicine, Floating Hospital for Children at Tufts Medical Center, Boston, Massachusetts, USA

ERROL R. NORWITZ, MD, PhD, MBA
Louis E. Phaneuf Professor of Obstetrics and Gynecology, Tufts University School of Medicine, Chief Scientific Officer, Chairman, Department of Obstetrics and Gynecology, Tufts Medical Center, Boston, Massachusetts, USA

AUTHORS

STEVEN H. ABMAN, MD
Director, Pediatric Heart Lung Center, Section of Neonatology, Professor, Department of Pediatrics, University of Colorado Denver, Anschutz Medical Center, Children's Hospital Colorado, Aurora, Colorado, USA

ZARKO ALFIREVIC, MD, FRCOG
Professor of Fetal and Maternal Medicine, Institute of Translational Medicine, University of Liverpool a member of Liverpool Health Partners, Centre for Women's Health Research, Liverpool Women's Hospital, Liverpool, United Kingdom

TERESA BAKER, MD
Associate Professor, Department of Obstetrics and Gynecology, Texas Tech University Health Sciences Center, Amarillo, Texas, USA

RICHARD H. BEIGI, MD, MSc
Professor and Vice Chair of Operations, Department of Obstetrics, Gynecology, and Reproductive Sciences, University of Pittsburgh School of Medicine, Chief Medical Officer and Vice President of Medical Affairs, University of Pittsburgh Medical Center Magee-Womens Hospital, Pittsburgh, Pennsylvania, USA

HELENE B. BERNSTEIN, MD, PhD
Associate Professor of Obstetrics and Gynecology, Microbiology and Immunology, The State University of New York Upstate Medical University, Syracuse, New York, USA

PATRICK M. CATALANO, MD
Maternal Infant Research Institute, Vice Chair, Obstetrics and Gynecology Research, Professor of Obstetrics and Gynecology, Tufts University School of Medicine, Friedman School of Nutrition Science and Policy, Boston, Massachusetts, USA

LEE S. COHEN, MD
Perinatal and Reproductive Psychiatry Program, Director, Massachusetts General Hospital Center for Women's Mental Health, Professor of Psychiatry, Harvard Medical School, Boston, Massachusetts, USA

PALIKA DATTA, PhD
Senior Research Associate, Department of Pediatrics, Texas Tech University Health Sciences Center, Amarillo, Texas, USA

EUGENE DEMPSEY, MD
Professor, Department of Paediatrics and Child Health, Neonatal Intensive Care Unit, Irish Centre for Fetal and Neonatal Translational Research (INFANT), University College Cork, Cork, Ireland

MAISA N. FEGHALI, MD
Assistant Professor, Department of Obstetrics, Gynecology and Reproductive Sciences, Magee Women's Research Institute, University of Pittsburgh School of Medicine, Pittsburgh, Pennsylvania, USA

THOMAS W. HALE, PhD
Professor, Department of Pediatrics, Texas Tech University Health Sciences Center, Amarillo, Texas, USA

REBECCA A. JAMESON, MD, MPH
PGY4, Department of Obstetrics and Gynecology, The State University of New York Upstate Medical University, Syracuse, New York, USA

HENDRÉE E. JONES, PhD
Professor, Department of Obstetrics and Gynecology, University of North Carolina at Chapel Hill, Executive Director, UNC Horizons, Chapel Hill, North Carolina, USA; Adjunct Professor, Departments of Psychiatry and Behavioral Sciences, and Obstetrics and Gynecology, School of Medicine, Johns Hopkins University, Baltimore, Maryland, USA

KENNETH L. JONES, MD
Professor, Department of Pediatrics, University of California, San Diego, La Jolla, California, USA

LOUISE KENNY, MBChB (Hons), PhD, MRCOG
Executive Pro-Vice-Chancellor, Vice Chancellor's Office, University of Liverpool a member of Liverpool Health Partners, Centre for Women's Health Research, Liverpool Women's Hospital, Liverpool, United Kingdom

ELIZABETH KIERNAN, MPH
Teratogen Information Specialist, Department of Pediatrics, University of California, San Diego, La Jolla, California, USA

WALTER K. KRAFT, MD
Professor of Pharmacology, Medicine and Surgery, Director, Clinical Research Unit, Department of Pharmacology and Experimental Therapeutics, Thomas Jefferson University, Philadelphia, Pennsylvania, USA

PANAGIOTIS KRATIMENOS, MD, PhD
Neonatology and Hospital Based Specialties, Children's National Medical Center, Assistant Professor of Pediatrics, George Washington University, Washington, DC, USA

KARLA LEAVITT, MD, MPH
Department of Obstetrics and Gynecology, Fellow, Division of Maternal-Fetal Medicine, University of South Florida, Morsani College of Medicine, Tampa, Florida, USA

JACK LUDMIR, MD
Department of Obstetrics and Gynecology, Division of Maternal-Fetal Medicine, Thomas Jefferson University, Philadelphia, Pennsylvania, USA

ERICA W. MANDELL, DO
Assistant Professor of Pediatrics, Pediatric Heart Lung Center, Sections of Neonatology and Pulmonary Medicine, University of Colorado Denver, Anschutz Medical Center, Children's Hospital Colorado, Aurora, Colorado, USA

MELANIE A. McNALLY, MD
Neonatal Neurology Fellow, Department of Neurology, Boston Children's Hospital, Boston, Massachusetts, USA

SAGORI MUKHOPADHYAY, MD, MMSc
Assistant Professor of Pediatrics, University of Pennsylvania Perelman School of Medicine, Section on Newborn Medicine, Pennsylvania Hospital and Division of Neonatology, Children's Hospital of Philadelphia, Philadelphia, Pennsylvania, USA

RUTA NONACS, MD, PhD
Perinatal and Reproductive Psychiatrist, Perinatal and Reproductive Psychiatry Program, Massachusetts General Hospital Center for Women's Mental Health, Instructor in Psychiatry, Harvard Medical School, Boston, Massachusetts, USA

SARAH OBIČAN, MD
Assistant Professor, Department of Obstetrics and Gynecology, Division of Maternal-Fetal Medicine, University of South Florida, Morsani College of Medicine, Tampa, Florida, USA

SOHA S. PATEL, MD, MS, MSPH
Department of Obstetrics and Gynecology, Division of Maternal-Fetal Medicine, Vanderbilt University Medical Center, Nashville, Tennessee, USA

KAREN M. PUOPOLO, MD, PhD
Associate Professor of Pediatrics, University of Pennsylvania Perelman School of Medicine, Section on Newborn Medicine, Pennsylvania Hospital and Division of Neonatology, Children's Hospital of Philadelphia, Philadelphia, Pennsylvania, USA

HEIKE RABE, MD
Brighton and Sussex Medical School, University of Sussex, Department of Neonatology, Brighton and Sussex University Hospitals NHS Trust, Brighton, United Kingdom

EDWIN R. RAFFI, MD, MPH
Perinatal and Reproductive Psychiatrist, Perinatal and Reproductive Psychiatry Program, Massachusetts General Hospital Center for Women's Mental Health, Instructor in Psychiatry, Harvard Medical School, Boston, Massachusetts, USA

SARAH C. ROGAN, MD, PhD
Fellow, Maternal and Fetal Medicine Division, Department of Obstetrics, Gynecology, and Reproductive Sciences, University of Pittsburgh School of Medicine, Pittsburgh, Pennsylvania, USA

JANET S. SOUL, MDCM, FRCPC
Director, Fetal-Neonatal Neurology Program, Department of Neurology, Boston Children's Hospital, Associate Professor of Neurology, Harvard Medical School, Boston, Massachusetts, USA

ROBIN H. STEINHORN, MD
Neonatology and Hospital Based Specialties, Children's National Medical Center, Professor of Pediatrics, George Washington University, Washington, DC, USA

MARK A. TURNER, BSc, PhD, MBChB (Hons), MRCP (UK), MRCPCH, DRCOG, FFPM (Hon)
Professor of Neonatology and Research Delivery, Institute of Translational Medicine, University of Liverpool a member of Liverpool Health Partners, Centre for Women's Health Research, Liverpool Women's Hospital, Liverpool, United Kingdom

JASON G. UMANS, MD
Associate Professor, Departments of Medicine, and Obstetrics and Gynecology, Georgetown-Howard Universities Center for Clinical and Translational Science, Georgetown University, Washington, DC, USA

MICHAEL W. VARNER, MD
Professor, Department of Obstetrics and Gynecology, University of Utah, Salt Lake City, Utah, USA

KELLY C. WADE, MD, PhD, MSCE
Associate Professor of Clinical Pediatrics, University of Pennsylvania Perelman School of Medicine, Section on Newborn Medicine, Pennsylvania Hospital and Division of Neonatology, Children's Hospital of Philadelphia, Philadelphia, Pennsylvania, USA

ROBERT M. WARD, MD, FAAP, FCP
Professor Emeritus, Pediatrics, Pediatric Clinical Pharmacology, University of Utah, University of Utah School of Medicine, Salt Lake City, Utah, USA

JEROME YANKOWITZ, MD
James M. Ingram Professor and Chair, Department of Obstetrics and Gynecology, Division of Maternal-Fetal Medicine, University of South Florida, Morsani College of Medicine, Tampa, Florida, USA

Contents

Preterm birth can be medically-indicated or spontaneous. Almost half of spontaneous preterm deliveries are preceded by preterm labor. Preterm labor is a clinical diagnosis characterized by regular uterine contractions (painful or painless) with concomitant cervical change. This article discusses the prevention and treatment of spontaneous preterm labor utilizing progesterone and tocolytic agents and provides management recommendations in patients with and without a history of prior spontaneous preterm birth.

This article reviews the pharmacology of the most commonly used antihypertensive medications during pregnancy; their mechanism of action; and the effects on the mother, the fetus, and lactation. Each class of antihypertensive pharmacologic agents have specific mechanisms of action by which they exert their antihypertensive effect. β-Adrenoreceptor antagonists block these receptors in the peripheral circulation. Calcium channel blockers result in arterial vasodilation. α-Agonists inhibit vasoconstriction. Methyldopa is a centrally acting adrenoreceptor antagonist. Vasodilators have a direct effect on vascular smooth muscle. Diuretics decrease intravascular volume. Medications acting on the angiotensin pathway are avoided during pregnancy because of fetotoxic effects.

Cerebral palsy occurs more often in preterm than in term deliveries and is one of the major neurologic injuries seen in preterm infants. Magnesium sulfate has been found to reduce the risk of cerebral palsy in patients at risk of delivery before 32 weeks' gestational age. Multiple large clinical trials have shown this effect. The authors recommend magnesium sulfate bolus followed by continuous dosing of magnesium sulfate in those at risk of delivery before 32 weeks' gestation until delivery occurs or is no longer imminent. This article also discusses novel and emerging therapies for the prevention of cerebral palsy.

Dopamine remains the most commonly studied and prescribed cardiotonic drug in the neonatal intensive care unit (NICU), but evidence of its effect on endorgan perfusion still remains. Unlike adult and pediatric critical care, there are significant gaps in our knowledge on the use of various cardiotonic drugs in various forms of circulatory failure in the NICU.

Rates of bronchopulmonary dysplasia (BPD) are increasing. After preterm birth, there are important developmental periods in which neonates are more vulnerable to stressful events. These periods are opportunities for pharmacologic interventions. Many drugs remain inadequately tested and no new drugs have been approved in more than 25 years for BPD prevention or therapy. More progress is needed in defining appropriate end points based on the pathophysiology of BPD and postdischarge chronic pulmonary insufficiency of prematurity and to develop effective new drugs. In addition, much work is needed to better define perinatal factors, early postnatal findings, and physiologic phenotypes or endotypes.

Neonatal brain injury (NBI) remains a major contributor to neonatal mortality and long-term neurodevelopmental morbidity. Although therapeutic hypothermia is the only proven treatment to minimize brain injury caused by neonatal encephalopathy in term neonates, it provides incomplete neuroprotection. There are no specific drugs yet proven to prevent NBI in preterm neonates. This review discusses the scientific and emerging clinical trial data for several neuroprotective drugs in development, examining potential efficacy and safety concerns. Drugs with the highest likelihood of success and closest to clinical application include erythropoietin for term and preterm neonates and antenatal magnesium for preterm neonates.

Antimicrobial medications are the most commonly used medications in the neonatal intensive care unit. Antibiotics are used for infection prophylaxis, empiric treatment, and definitive treatment of confirmed infection. The choice of medication should be informed by the epidemiology and microbiology of infection in specific clinical scenarios and by the clinical condition of the infant. Understanding evolving pathogen susceptibility to antimicrobials and key pharmacotherapy determinants in neonates can inform optimal antibiotic use.

When opioid misuse rises in the United States, pregnant women and their neonates are affected. This article summarizes the use of Food and Drug

Administration–approved products, including methadone, buprenorphine, and the combination formulation of buprenorphine and naloxone to treat adult opioid use disorder during the perinatal period. All labels include pregnancy, neonatal, and lactation information and note the accepted use of these medications during the perinatal period if the benefits outweigh the risks. A summary of the neonatal abstinence syndrome definition, its assessment tools, treatment approaches, and future genetic directions are provided.

Breast milk is the most beneficial nutrition a mother can give her infant. Fortunately, the dose of most drugs transferred into milk is small and does not lead to clinically significant effects on the infant. In almost all instances, the mother should be advised to continue breastfeeding. Certain medications are absolutely contraindicated, including anticancer agents, radioactive drugs, and those that inhibit milk production. However, most medications can be used safely. An improved understanding of the relationship between maternal and infant exposure to medications would provide a more enlightened understanding of the risk and benefit analysis for individual drugs.

Pregnancy profoundly alters a woman's physiology. These changes alter drug absorption, distribution, metabolism, and elimination and emphasize the pharmacologic complexity of pregnancy. They also emphasize the dangers of extrapolating pharmacologic expectations from nonpregnant populations to pregnant women and their fetuses. Although concerns about fetal safety have historically limited pharmacokinetic studies during pregnancy, it is important to recognize that many medications are clinically indicated for various maternal or fetal conditions, and it is particularly important that these therapies be evidence-based with appropriate study, including short-term and long-term outcomes data.

The need for new drugs in pregnancy is widely recognized. This review identifies several unique challenges and describes some solutions. Specific studies and drug development programs need careful planning that accounts for the needs of regulatory agencies. The perinatal (obstetric/pediatric) community needs to establish collaborations to develop methodologies, to facilitate data sharing, and to lobby for research and access to medicines. There is a need to gather and present information that promotes proportionate judgments of the balance between potential benefits and risks. This will require researchers to look beyond their traditional ways of working.

PROGRAM OBJECTIVE
The goal of *Clinics in Perinatology* is to keep practicing perinatologists, neonatologists, obstetricians, practicing physicians and residents up to date with current clinical practice in perinatology by providing timely articles reviewing the state of the art in patient care.

TARGET AUDIENCE
Perinatologists, neonatologists, obstetricians, practicing physicians, residents and healthcare professionals who provide patient care utilizing findings from *Clinics in Perinatology*.

LEARNING OBJECTIVES
Upon completion of this activity, participants will be able to:
1. Review the use of medications to treat common pregnancy-related conditions such as preterm labor, preeclampsia, depression, and diabetes.
2. Discuss potential risks and benefits of drugs on fetal structural and neurological development.
3. Recognize challenges of caring for complex medical and surgical issues in the NICU.

ACCREDITATION
The Elsevier Office of Continuing Medical Education (EOCME) is accredited by the Accreditation Council for Continuing Medical Education (ACCME) to provide continuing medical education for physicians.

The EOCME designates this enduring material for a maximum of 15 *AMA PRA Category 1 Credit*(s)™. Physicians should claim only the credit commensurate with the extent of their participation in the activity.

All other health care professionals requesting continuing education credit for this enduring material will be issued a certificate of participation.

DISCLOSURE OF CONFLICTS OF INTEREST
The EOCME assesses conflict of interest with its instructors, faculty, planners, and other individuals who are in a position to control the content of CME activities. All relevant conflicts of interest that are identified are thoroughly vetted by EOCME for fair balance, scientific objectivity, and patient care recommendations. EOCME is committed to providing its learners with CME activities that promote improvements or quality in healthcare and not a specific proprietary business or a commercial interest.

The planning committee, staff, authors and editors listed below have identified no financial relationships or relationships to products or devices they or their spouse/life partner have with commercial interest related to the content of this CME activity:
Steven H. Abman, MD; Zarko Alfirevic, MD; Teresa Baker, MD; Richard H. Beigi, MD, MSc; Helene B. Bernstein, MD, PhD; Patrick M. Catalano, MD; Palika Datta, PhD; Jonathan M. Davis, MD; Eugene Dempsey, MD; Maisa N. Feghali, MD; Thomas W. Hale, PhD; Kerry Holland; Lucky Jain, MD, MBA; Rebecca A. Jameson, MD, MPH; Hendrée E. Jones, PhD; Kenneth L. Jones, MD; Alison Kemp; Louise Kenny, PhD; Elizabeth Kiernan, MPH; Panagiotis Kratimenos, MD, PhD; Karla Leavitt, MD, MPH; Jack Ludmir, MD; Erica W. Mandell, DO; Melanie A. McNally, MD; Sagori Mukhopadhyay, MD, MMSc; Swaminathan Nagarajan; Errol R. Norwitz, MD, PHD, MBA; Sarah Običan, MD; Soha S. Patel, MD, MS, MSPH; Karen M. Puopolo, MD, PhD; Heike Rabe, MD; Edwin R. Raffi, MD, MPH; Sarah C. Rogan, MD, PhD; Janet S. Soul, MD; Robin H. Steinhorn, MD; Mark A. Turner, BSc, PhD; Jason G. Umans, MD; Michael W. Varner, MD; Kelly C. Wade, MD, PhD, MSCE; Robert M. Ward, MD; Jerome Yankowitz, MD.

The planning committee, staff, authors and editors listed below have identified financial relationships or relationships to products or devices they or their spouse/life partner have with commercial interest related to the content of this CME activity:
Lee S. Cohen, MD: is a consultant/advisor for and receives research support from Alkermes and receives research support from Teva Pharmaceutical Industries Ltd, Otsuka Pharmaceutical Co., Ltd., Sunovion Pharmaceuticals Inc., JAYMAC Pharmaceuticals, LLC, and Sage Therapeutics, Inc.
Walter K. Kraft, MD: receives research support from CHIESI USA, Inc.
Ruta Nonacs, MD, PhD: receives royalties from Simon & Schuster, Inc.

UNAPPROVED/OFF-LABEL USE DISCLOSURE
The EOCME requires CME faculty to disclose to the participants:
1. When products or procedures being discussed are off-label, unlabelled, experimental, and/or investigational (not US Food and Drug Administration [FDA] approved); and

2. Any limitations on the information presented, such as data that are preliminary or that represent ongoing research, interim analyses, and/or unsupported opinions. Faculty may discuss information about pharmaceutical agents that is outside of FDA-approved labelling. This information is intended solely for CME and is not intended to promote off-label use of these medications. If you have any questions, contact the medical affairs department of the manufacturer for the most recent prescribing information.

TO ENROLL
To enroll in the *Clinics in Perinatology* Continuing Medical Education program, call customer service at 1-800-654-2452 or sign up online at http://www.theclinics.com/home/cme. The CME program is available to subscribers for an additional annual fee of 244.40 USD.

METHOD OF PARTICIPATION
In order to claim credit, participants must complete the following:
1. Complete enrolment as indicated above.
2. Read the activity.
3. Complete the CME Test and Evaluation. Participants must achieve a score of 70% on the test. All CME Tests and Evaluations must be completed online.

CME INQUIRIES/SPECIAL NEEDS
For all CME inquiries or special needs, please contact elsevierCME@elsevier.com.

CLINICS IN PERINATOLOGY

SERIES OF RELATED INTEREST

Pediatric Clinics
https://www.pediatric.theclinics.com/

THE CLINICS ARE AVAILABLE ONLINE!
Access your subscription at:
www.theclinics.com

Foreword
Perinatal Pharmacology at Crossroads

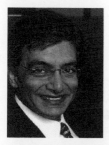

Lucky Jain, MD, MBA
Consulting Editor

Drug development for newborns and young children has never been a huge priority for the pharmaceutical industry. It should come as no surprise then that more than 90% of drugs used in newborns and infants are either off-label or unlicensed.[1,2] Many reasons account for this gap: logistical and ethical challenges in conducting clinical trials in newborns, complexities in pathophysiology of the disease process, and market size of products when they finally get commercialized. Add to this the burden of unknown long-term effects of drugs in a growing child. Child advocacy and legislative efforts have sought to overcome these impediments and have begun to make inroads, but we have a long way to go!

Several promising approaches to drug development are on the horizon, but their potential has yet to be realized. The emergence of cell-based assay technologies (induced pluripotent stem cells, three-dimensional models, coculture, and organ on a chip systems) along with other advances, such as gene editing, has the potential to transform the field (**Fig. 1**).[3] Similarly, machine learning and image-based profiling can greatly enhance drug discovery and address questions related to efficacy, toxicity, and mechanism of action.[4]

Drs Davis and Norwitz have covered a vast array of topics related to perinatal pharmacology in this issue of the *Clinics in Perinatology*. As always, I am grateful to Kerry Holland and Casey Potter at Elsevier for their support in bringing this high-quality publication to you.

Clin Perinatol 46 (2019) xv–xvi
https://doi.org/10.1016/j.clp.2019.03.002
0095-5108/19/© 2019 Published by Elsevier Inc.

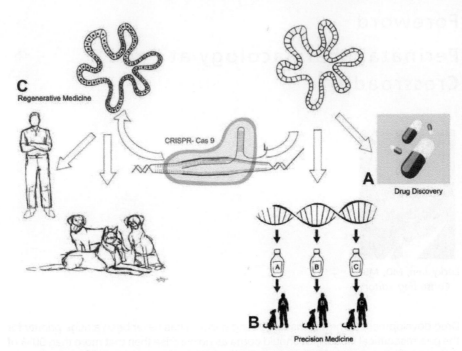

Fig. 1. Organoids: a promising in vitro system for drug discovery, precision, and regenerative medicine in human and veterinary medicine. (*A*) Organoids can be used as a preclinical model to evaluate the efficacy and safety of candidate drugs prior to live studies in animals and humans. (*B*) In addition, because they are derived from individuals with different genotypes, organoids are a relevant screening system for precision medicine. (*C*) Finally, transplantation of genetically engineered organoids has the potential to repair and/or replace damaged tissue. (*Adapted from* Mochel JP, Jergens AE, Kingsbury D, et al. Intestinal stem cells to advance drug development, precision, and regenerative medicine: a paradigm shift in translational research. AAPS J 2018;20(1):15.)

Lucky Jain, MD, MBA
Emory University School of Medicine
and Children's Healthcare of Atlanta
1760 Haygood Drive, W409, Atlanta, GA 30322, USA

E-mail address:
ljain@emory.edu

REFERENCES

1. Coppini R, Simons SHP, Mugeli A, et al. Clinical research in neonates and infants: challenges and perspectives. Pharmacol Res 2016;108:80–7.
2. Smith AM, Davis JM. Challenges and opportunities to enhance global drug development in neonates. Curr Opin Pediatr 2017;29:149–52.
3. Mochel JP, Jergens AE, Kingsbury D, et al. Intestinal stem cells to advance drug development, precision, and regenerative medicine: a paradigm shift in translational research. AAPS J 2018;20(1):1–17.
4. Scheeder C, Heigwer F, Boutros M. Machine learning and image-based profiling in drug industry. Curr Opin Syst Biol 2018;10:43–52.

Preface

Current Understanding of Medication Use in Pregnancy/ Lactation and Neonates: What Are the Key Knowledge Gaps?

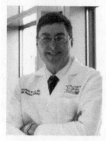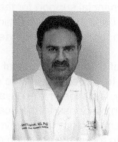

Jonathan M. Davis, MD   Errol R. Norwitz, MD, PhD, MBA
Editors

Of the 6 million women who are pregnant in the United States each year, an estimated 90% are prescribed at least one medication while pregnant or lactating, and many receive multiple concomitant medications with significant potential for adverse drug-drug interactions. In addition to potential harmful effects on the developing fetus, the physiologic changes that accompany pregnancy may affect the way drugs are absorbed, distributed, and metabolized in the mother, resulting in standard doses being too high or too low. Despite these concerns, relatively few drugs have been approved by the Food and Drug Administration (FDA) as safe and effective in pregnancy/lactation, and most medications prescribed to pregnant women are done so "off-label." Neonates too can be considered "therapeutic orphans." More than 90% of drugs used routinely in the neonatal intensive care unit (NICU) are not FDA approved and are used "off-label," and very preterm neonates can be exposed to up to 60 drugs during their NICU stay. The last drug approved by the FDA to improve survival in preterm neonates was pulmonary surfactant in 1991, over 27 years ago.

The pharmaceutical industry and US regulatory agencies have been reluctant to include pregnant/lactating women and neonates in their clinical trials, citing concerns about safety, liability, finances, and ethics. In addition, a number of regulatory barriers make it difficult to include these populations in research studies. One such example is the Common Rule, the federal policy designed to protect human subjects in biomedical research, which requires consent from both the pregnant woman and the father to participate in studies designed to benefit the fetus and neonate. Congress recently authorized a federal task force to conduct a series of public meetings to address these

Clin Perinatol 46 (2019) xvii–xviii
https://doi.org/10.1016/j.clp.2019.03.001
0095-5108/19/© 2019 Published by Elsevier Inc.

concerns. The report, which includes a number of specific recommendations (https://www.nichd.nih.gov/sites/default/files/2018-09/PRGLAC_Report.pdf), was sent to US Department of Health and Human Services Secretary Alex Azar in September 2018.

Most drug development for pregnant/lactating women and neonates is being driven by government regulations. In the United States, the FDA Safety and Innovation Act of 2012 mandated that these vulnerable populations be included in drug trials. However, there are no requirements for companies to develop new drugs specifically for these populations. The FDA recently released recommendations urging pharmaceutical companies to gather more data "through judicious inclusion of pregnant women in clinical trials and careful attention to potential fetal risk" (https://www.fda.gov/ucm/groups/fdagov-public/@fdagov-drugs-gen/documents/document/ucm603873.pdf). The FDA also provides significant financial support for the International Neonatal Consortium and Institute for Advanced Clinical Trials for Children, two burgeoning organizations established specifically to accelerate drug development efforts in these populations.

We applaud the recent actions of Congress, National Institute of Child Health and Human Development, and the FDA to improve the public's understanding of the safety and efficacy of drugs for pregnancy, lactation, the fetus, and neonates. It is in the spirit of these efforts, and in particular in response to their call to educate the public and improve research in the area of pharmacology in these vulnerable and highly complex populations, that we have chosen to focus the attention of this issue of *Clinics in Perinatology* on "Perinatal Pharmacology." This issue summarizes the current state-of-the-science around the effect of pregnancy and breast feeding on pharmacokinetics, potential risks and benefits of drugs (including illicit drugs and opioids) on fetal structural and neurologic development, and the use of medications to treat common pregnancy-related conditions (such as preterm labor, preeclampsia, depression, and diabetes). Other articles address the challenges of caring for complex medical and surgical issues in the NICU, ranging from extreme prematurity at the limit of viability to neonates who can remain in the NICU for up to 1 year of age with underlying structural or metabolic disorders. We will define the limits of our current understanding regarding medication use in pregnancy/lactation and neonates as well as identify areas most in need of additional research.

Jonathan M. Davis, MD
The Floating Hospital for Children at Tufts Medical Center
800 Washington Street
Boston, MA 02111, USA

Errol R. Norwitz, MD, PhD, MBA
Tufts University School of Medicine
Department of Obstetrics & Gynecology
Tufts Medical Center
800 Washington Street
Boston, MA 02111, USA

E-mail addresses:
jdavis@tuftsmedicalcenter.org (J.M. Davis)
enorwitz@tuftsmedicalcenter.org (E.R. Norwitz)

Drugs for the Treatment and Prevention of Preterm Labor

Soha S. Patel, MD, MS, MSPH[a],*, Jack Ludmir, MD[b]

KEYWORDS

- Preterm labor • Treatment • Prevention • Tocolytics • Progesterone

KEY POINTS

- Approximately 50% of spontaneous preterm deliveries are preceded by preterm labor.
- The mainstay of tocolysis is to delay delivery for 48 hours for the administration of antenatal corticosteroids proven to enhance fetal lung maturity.
- Progesterone supplementation is effective in prevention of preterm delivery in patients with short cervical length or in patients with history of preterm delivery.

DEFINITION OF PRETERM LABOR AND BIRTH

Preterm birth (PTB) refers to the delivery of a fetus between $20^{0/7}$ and $36^{6/7}$ weeks' gestation. Approximately 50% of spontaneous preterm deliveries are preceded by preterm labor.[1] Preterm labor is a clinical diagnosis characterized by regular uterine contractions (painful or painless) with concomitant cervical change.

PTB is estimated to occur in 9.6% of all births in the United States in 2016[2] and 10% worldwide.[1] Prematurity caused by PTB is the main cause of perinatal mortality in developed countries and is associated with an annual rate of one million deaths worldwide.[2] PTB can be medically-indicated or spontaneous. In this article, we refer to spontaneous PTB (sPTB) only.

PHYSIOLOGY OF PRETERM BIRTH

Uterine contractions involve the interaction of actin and myosin (specifically myosin light-chain phosphorylation) with myometrial cells.[3] This interaction is directed by myosin light-chain kinase. The mechanism of action of tocolytic agents involves the regulation of the myosin light-chain kinase activity, specifically, calcium and cyclic AMP.[3] In order for the myometrium to contract effectively for labor, individual smooth

Financial Disclosures: None.
[a] Department of Obstetrics and Gynecology, Division of Maternal-Fetal Medicine, Vanderbilt University Medical Center, 1161 21st Avenue South, B-1100 Medical Center North, Nashville, TN 37232-2519, USA; [b] Department of Obstetrics and Gynecology, Division of Maternal-Fetal Medicine, Thomas Jefferson University, 1020 Walnut Street, Philadelphia, PA 19107, USA
* Corresponding author.
E-mail address: Soha.S.Patel@vumc.org

muscle cells function in an interlinked manner and communicate with nearby smooth muscle cells.[3]

TREATMENT OF PRETERM LABOR: TOCOLYTICS

Tocolytics are a class of medications used to inhibit myometrial contractions of the uterus, and subsequently, preterm labor and birth. The mainstay of tocolysis is to delay delivery for 48 hours to give adequate timing for the administration of antenatal corticosteroids that are proven to enhance fetal lung maturity. Tocolytics were initially characterized 60 years ago and are generally administered when a diagnosis of preterm labor is confirmed between $23^{0/7}$ and $33^{6/7}$ weeks' gestation.[4]

Maternal contraindications to tocolytics include: severe preeclampsia, hemorrhage, and significant cardiac disease as these medications create a greater risk for maternal hemodynamic compromise and collapse.[3] Fetal contraindications to tocolysis include: gestational age greater than or equal to 34 weeks, lethal fetal anomalies, intrauterine fetal demise, chorioamnionitis, and fetal compromise that may necessitate immediate delivery.[3]

Selection of the appropriate tocolytic is determined by the efficacy, maternal and fetal risks, and the side effect profile of each medication. Although no class of medications is specifically approved by the US Food and Drug Administration (FDA) as a tocolytic, various classes of medications have been administered as off-label use in the setting of preterm labor, including calcium channel blockers, nonsteroidal anti-inflammatory drugs, and betamimetics.[3] Based on the existing literature, the most effective tocolytics include: cyclooxygenase (COX) inhibitors, betamimetics, and calcium channel blockers. The least effective tocolytics include: magnesium sulfate, oxytocin receptor antagonists, and nitric oxide (NO) donors.

In multiple gestations, there is insufficient evidence to demonstrate a decrease in the risk of sPTB or an improvement in neonatal outcomes with the use of tocolytics in the management of acute preterm labor.[4] In fact, the use of tocolytics in multiple gestations has been correlated with an increased risk of maternal pulmonary edema.[4] However, because of the proven benefit of tocolytics in delaying delivery by 48 hours in singleton gestations, many clinicians recommend their use in multiple gestations complicated by preterm labor.[4]

CLASSES OF TOCOLYTICS
Cyclooxygenase Inhibitors

Pharmacokinetics

- Mechanism of action: COX (also known as prostaglandin synthase) is an enzyme that converts arachidonic acid to prostaglandins, which constitutes the final common pathway in the parturition cascade. COX inhibitors block prostaglandin synthesis, and therefore, inhibit myometrial contractions. There are two COX isoforms: COX-1 and COX-2. COX-1 is constitutively expressed in most gestational tissues. COX-2 is located in the decidua and myometrium and is significantly increased during labor. Indomethacin, which is a nonselective COX-1 and COX-2 inhibitor, is the most commonly used tocolytic in this specific class.[5–9] Selective COX-2 inhibitors (eg, sulindac) are not well-studied in human pregnancy and significant adverse cardiovascular outcomes have been associated with its use.
- Contraindication: Indomethacin is not recommended after 32 weeks gestation because of severe fetal adverse risks (discussed later). Maternal

contraindications to COX inhibitors include: gastrointestinal ulcerative disease, renal and hepatic dysfunction, platelet dysfunction, and asthma.
- Dosing: The dose of indomethacin is 50- to 100-mg loading dose (orally or rectally), followed by 25 mg orally every 4 to 6 hours for 48 hours.
- Half-life: In the fetal circulation, concentrations of indomethacin are 50% greater than in the maternal circulation. The half-life of indomethacin in a neonate is longer than that in the mother (15 hours vs 2.2 hours, respectively).
- Monitoring: If indomethacin is administered for greater than 48 hours, regular ultrasound assessments should be performed to evaluate the fetus for oligohydramnios and potential narrowing of the fetal ductus arteriosus.[10,11]

Efficacy

A 2015 systematic review including two randomized controlled trials compared indomethacin with placebo in the treatment of preterm labor. Indomethacin seemed to decreased the risk of preterm delivery within 48 hours, but this did not achieve statistical significance with wide confidence intervals (CIs; relative risk [RR], 0.20; 95% CI, 0.03–1.28).[12] Additionally, there were no differences between the groups with regards to adverse neonatal outcomes.

In comparative trials, indomethacin significantly decreased the risk of PTB less than 37 weeks within 48 hours of beginning tocolytic treatment compared with any betamimetic agents (RR, 0.27; 95% CI, 0.08–0.96), and seemed to be as effective as nifedipine in this regard (RR, 1.08; 95% CI, 0.58–2.01).[13] However, no benefit was shown with regards to neonatal morbidity or mortality between these various tocolytic agents.

Maternal side effects

COX inhibitors are associated with less maternal adverse outcomes when compared with betamimetics, but no differences were noted when comparing COX inhibitors with other tocolytic classes, such as calcium channel blockers or magnesium sulfate.[12] The most common maternal side effects of indomethacin include platelet dysfunction, nausea, emesis, gastroesophageal reflux, and gastritis.

Fetal side effects

The use of indomethacin for greater than 48 hours at greater than or equal to 32 weeks is associated with significant fetal adverse outcomes, such as premature closure or constriction of the fetal ductus arteriosus (eventually leading to the development of fetal pulmonary hypertension and/or tricuspid regurgitation), oligohydramnios, and fetal renal insufficiency.[14–16] Whether the use of indomethacin is associated with neonatal complications[17–22] and/or long-term development effects is still controversial.[23–25]

Betamimetics

Pharmacokinetics

- Mechanism of action: Betamimetics (ie, β-adrenergic receptor agonists) act on β_2 receptors in smooth muscles. They affect myometrial relaxation by signaling through β_2 adrenergic receptors and increasing intracellular adenyl cyclase. This results in activation of protein kinase, which phosphorylates target proteins within the cytoplasm. The overall decrease in intracellular free calcium interrupts the activity of myosin light-chain kinase, which alters the interaction between myosin and actin. This then leads to a decrease in myometrial contractility.[26] Examples of this class of tocolytics include: ritodrine hydrochloride and terbutaline.

- Contraindications: Betamimetics are contraindicated in women with tachycardia because of their positively chronotropic effects. It is generally recommended to withhold the drug if the maternal heart rate is greater than or equal to 120 beats/min.[4] They should also be used with caution in women at risk for hemorrhage because the cardiovascular effects of the medication may interfere with maternal response to hemorrhage. For many years, betamimetics were the tocolytic drug of choice, but are now rarely used because there are other classes of medications that are equally effective with fewer maternal side effects. Of note, ritodrine hydrochloride is no longer available in the United States. Additionally, the FDA recommends that injectable terbutaline not be used in the management of prolonged preterm labor (defined as 48–72 hours) because of potential serious maternal side effects, specifically cardiac events and death.[27]
- Dosing: In the United States, despite the FDA warning, terbutaline is the most commonly used betamimetic agent for the inhibition of uterine contractions. The dose is variable, but generally, 0.25 mg terbutaline is administered subcutaneously every 20 to 30 minutes, for up to four doses or until tocolysis has occurred. It can also be administered as a continuous intravenous infusion at a rate of 2.5 to 5 µg/min, increasing by 2.5 to 5 µg/min every 20 to 30 minutes to a maximum of 25 µg/min or until the contractions have quiesced. The infusion can then be maintained at the lowest possible dose to maintain uterine quiescence, although maintenance tocolytics has not been shown to delay PTB.
- Half-life: The half-life of terbutaline is about 3 to 4 hours.

Efficacy

Betamimetics have been studied in numerous randomized controlled trials, mostly using ritodrine. A 2014 meta-analysis showed that betamimetics decreased the number of women who delivered within 48 hours (RR, 0.68; 95% CI, 0.53–0.88) and within 7 days (RR, 0.80; 95% CI, 0.65–0.98), but did not affect deliveries before 37 weeks of gestation (RR, 0.95; 95% CI, 0.88–1.03). Betamimetics did not improve overall perinatal morbidity or mortality (RR, 0.90; 95% CI, 0.27–3.00), but were associated with a significant reduction in respiratory distress syndrome (RR, 0.87; 95% CI, 0.71–1.08), likely because it delayed delivery long enough to allow for the administration of a course of antenatal corticosteroids.[28]

Maternal side effects

Maternal side effects result from the stimulation of β_1-adrenergic receptors (which increase maternal heart rate) and β_2-adrenergic receptors (which cause peripheral vasodilation, bronchial relaxation, and hypotension). Side effects are common and include: nausea and vomiting, palpitations, tachycardia, tremor, headaches, dyspnea, and nonspecific chest pain.[29]

Fetal side effects

Betamimetics readily cross the placenta resulting in fetal side effects that are similar to that seen in the mother, most commonly, fetal tachycardia. However, this does not seem to adversely affect the fetal acid-base status and overall neonatal outcome.[30]

Calcium Channel Blockers

Pharmacokinetics

- Mechanism of action: Calcium channel blockers inhibit voltage-dependent calcium channels, thereby, inhibiting calcium influx into smooth muscle cells.[3]

They also work by inhibiting the release of intracellular calcium stores from the sarcoplasmic reticulum, which leads to a reduction in cytoplasmic calcium concentration and an increase in calcium efflux from the cell. This interferes with actin-myosin interactions, thus, inhibiting myometrial contractions and leading to myometrial relaxation. Nifedipine is the most common calcium channel blocker used for tocolysis.

- Contraindications: Calcium channel blockers are contraindicated in women with known allergies to these drugs, hypotension, or preload-dependent cardiac lesions.[4]
- Dosing: The optimal dosing regimen for nifedipine is still unknown. However, the American College of Obstetricians and Gynecologists (ACOG) recommends a 30-mg loading dose followed by 10 to 20 mg every 4 to 6 hours with a maximum dose of 180 mg/d.[4] Adverse side effects generally occur only with dosages greater than 60 mg/d.[3]
- Half-life: The half-life of nifedipine is 2 to 3 hours. Maternal plasma concentrations peak in 30 to 60 minutes, and the duration of action of a single dose of nifedipine is approximately 6 hours.
- Excretion: Nifedipine is mostly metabolized in the liver and excreted by the kidneys.

Efficacy

In a 2014 meta-analysis of randomized controlled trials of calcium channel blockers versus no treatment or placebo for preterm labor, the use of a calcium channel blocker decreased the risk of PTB within 48 hours (RR, 0.30; 95% CI, 0.21–0.43).[31] However, there was no statistically significant decrease in this outcome when calcium channel blockers were compared with the other classes of tocolytics (RR, 0.86; 95% CI, 0.67–1.10).[31] When compared with betamimetics, calcium channel blockers showed statistical benefits with regards to prolongation of pregnancy (mean difference, 4.38 days; 95% CI, 0.25–8.52), serious neonatal morbidities, and maternal adverse effects.[31] In general, calcium channel blockers have a more favorable safety profile, maternal tolerance, side effect profile, and ease of administration when compared with betamimetics for the treatment of preterm labor.

Maternal side effects

Calcium channel blockers, specifically nifedipine, are known to act as peripheral vasodilators, and can therefore, cause nausea, flushing, dizziness, and lower extremity edema. The most common side effects are hypotension-related symptoms (eg, supine hypotension) and headache.

Fetal side effects

Earlier studies in animals showed a decreased in blood flow to the uterus and subsequent reduction in fetal oxygen saturation with the use of nifedipine; however, these findings could not be replicated in human studies. Additionally, evaluation using Doppler velocimetry of fetal middle cerebral arteries, renal arteries, umbilical arteries, ductus arteriosus, or maternal vessels revealed no significant changes in blood flow.[32–35]

Magnesium Sulfate

Pharmacokinetics

- Mechanism of action: Despite many years of research, the precise mechanism of action of magnesium is not completely understood. It is postulated to work, at least in part, as an intracellular calcium antagonist at the voltage-gated channels in the plasma membrane by inhibiting myosin light-chain kinase activity, and thereby, competing with intracellular calcium (ie, as a physiologic calcium antagonist). This then decreases myometrial contractions.[36–38]

- Contraindications: Magnesium sulfate is contraindicated in women with a diagnosis of myasthenia gravis and in those with myocardial compromise. It should be used with caution in women with renal impairment because magnesium toxicity can develop even with standard doses.
- Dosing: Magnesium sulfate is administered as a 4- to 6-g intravenous bolus administered over 20 to 30 minutes, followed by a continuous intravenous infusion of 1 to 2 g/h.[39] The infusion rate is titrated based on assessment of contraction frequency and maternal toxicity. The optimum regimen has not been determined.[40]
- Half-life: The half-life of magnesium sulfate is unknown.
- Excretion: Magnesium sulfate is excreted by the kidneys. Therefore, in women with renal insufficiency, dosing should be adjusted accordingly. These women should receive the standard loading dose (because the volume of distribution does not change) but with a decreased or even no maintenance dose. Such patients should have their clinical status and urine output closely monitored, and consideration should be given to following serum magnesium concentrations every 6 to 8 hours.
- Monitoring: In women with normal renal function, signs and symptoms of magnesium toxicity are assessed by history and physical examination. Routine serum magnesium levels are not routinely indicated. If life-threatening symptoms of magnesium toxicity occur, intravenous calcium gluconate (1 g over 5–10 minutes) should be emergently administered.

Efficacy

When compared with placebo, there is a no consistent evidence that magnesium sulfate decreases the incidence of PTB or reduces perinatal morbidity and mortality. In a 2014 systematic review that compared magnesium sulfate with no treatment or placebo, magnesium sulfate did not statistically decrease the rate of PTB less than 48 hours after initial presentation (RR, 0.56; 95% CI, 0.27–1.14).[41] In addition, it did not improve neonatal and maternal outcomes, and the incidence of PTB 48 hours after initial presentation and less than 37 weeks' gestation was similar between the magnesium treated and untreated groups.[41] This was consistent regardless of the dose of magnesium sulfate administered.[42] ACOG and the Society for Maternal-Fetal Medicine (SMFM) consider magnesium sulfate a reasonable option for prolongation of pregnancy in the setting of preterm labor of up to 48 hours to give adequate timing for administration of antenatal corticosteroids.[43]

Maternal side effects

The most common maternal side effects of magnesium sulfate include: excessive diaphoresis and flushing. Magnesium toxicity is directly related to serum concentrations and can, at high serum levels, lead to pulmonary edema and cardiac arrest.

Fetal side effects

Fetal side effects include: neonatal lethargy and respiratory distress. Prior retrospective studies have showed a significant increase in bone abnormalities on radiographic imaging in neonates who were exposed to magnesium sulfate in utero for more than 7 days. In this cohort, there was also a significant difference in the neonatal serum values of calcium, magnesium, phosphorous, and osteocalcin at birth.[44,45] Although these findings are thought to be transient,[46] additional data are needed to confirm the absence of long-term sequelae. Based on these findings, it is recommended that magnesium sulfate be used for no longer than 48 hours and only in women between 24 and 34 weeks' gestation with a clinical diagnosis of preterm labor.[43]

Oxytocin Receptor Antagonists

Pharmacokinetics

- Mechanism of action: Oxytocin receptor antagonists compete with the peptide hormone, oxytocin, at binding sites (oxytocin receptors) located in the myometrium and decidua. This prevents the increase in intracellular unbound calcium that occurs when oxytocin binds to its receptor.[47,48] Atosiban is an example of a selective oxytocin receptor antagonist. Although commonly used in Europe as a tocolytic, it has not been approved by the FDA and is not available in the United States in part because of the potential fetal effects shown in one clinical trial.[49]
- Contraindications: There are no absolute contraindications to the use of atosiban in pregnancy.
- Dosing: Atosiban is administered intravenously starting with a bolus of 6.75 mg followed by a 300 µg/min infusion for 3 hours, followed by 100 µg/min infusion for up to 45 hours.[50]
- Half-life: The half-life of atosiban is 18 minutes.

Efficacy

In a 2014 meta-analysis of randomized trials comparing oxytocin receptor antagonists (atosiban, barusiban) with placebo as tocolytic agents in patients with preterm labor, the use of this class of drugs did not reduce the risk of PTB within 48 hours of treatment (RR, 1.05; 95% CI, 0.15–7.43), the risk of PTB less than 28 weeks' gestation (RR, 3.11; 95% CI, 1.02–9.51), or the risk of PTB less than 37 weeks' gestation (RR, 1.17; 95% CI, 0.99–1.37).[51] Moreover, neonatal morbidity and mortality outcomes were statistically similar in both groups. The same systematic review found that atosiban was as effective as betamimetics for reducing PTB within 48 hours of treatment (RR, 0.89; 95% CI, 0.66–1.22).[51] Use of atosiban was associated with a significantly lower risk of maternal side effects when compared with betamimetics (RR, 0.05; 95% CI, 0.02–0.11).[51]

A subsequent trial (APOSTEL III) randomized women with preterm labor to oral nifedipine versus intravenous atosiban for 48 hours. The results showed that both medications resulted in similar overall composite perinatal outcomes and an equal number of pregnancies in which delivery was delayed more than 48 hours; of note, there was no placebo control group.[52]

Maternal side effects

The most common maternal side effects associated with use of atosiban are hypersensitivity and injection site reactions. The overall frequency of side effects was significantly less than that for any other drug used for tocolysis, which makes it a popular tocolytic in Europe.[29,53]

Fetal side effects

Atosiban readily crosses the placenta. One trial showed a possible association between atosiban and fetal/neonatal deaths.[49] Although these deaths were attributed primarily to infection and extreme prematurity, a causal relationship to atosiban treatment could not be excluded. One of the weaknesses of this study was that the randomization was not stratified based on gestational age; as such, most very preterm infants were assigned to the atosiban group.

Nitric Oxide Donors

Pharmacokinetics

- Mechanism of action: NO is produced by many different cell types and is critical for the preservation of normal smooth muscle tone. The interaction of NO and guanylyl cyclase demonstrates a signal transduction mechanism that couples the formation of NO to cGMP synthesis. The increase in cGMP in smooth muscle cells leads to the activation of myosin light chain kinases, which results in smooth muscle relaxation.[54] The most common NO donor used as a tocolytic is glyceryl trinitrate.
- Contraindications: NO donors should not be used in women with hypotension or preload-dependent cardiac lesions, such as aortic stenosis or hypertrophic obstructive cardiomyopathy.
- Dosing: NO donors are administered via transdermal patches or intravenously. The optimum dose is unknown. Generally, the dose and interval should be titrated to the cessation of contractions while maintaining an appropriate blood pressure. Commonly, a 10-mg glyceryl trinitrate patch is applied transdermally to the abdomen. If there is no reduction in contraction frequency and/or intensity over the course of 1 hour, a second patch can be applied and left in place for 24 hours. An alternative method of administration involves an intravenous infusion at a rate of 20 μg/min until contractions cease.

Efficacy

In a 2014 meta-analysis of several randomized controlled trials, NO donors were compared with placebo, betamimetics, and nifedipine. When compared with other tocolytics, NO donors did not significantly prolong pregnancy greater than 48 hours, reduce the incidence of PTB, or improve perinatal or neonatal outcomes.[55]

Maternal side effects

NO causes dilation of arterial smooth muscle throughout the body, which can lead to headache, dizziness, nausea, vomiting, flushing, palpitations, and may result in maternal hypotension.

Fetal side effects

There are limited studies evaluating the fetal effects of NO.

PREVENTION OF PRETERM LABOR: PROGESTERONE SUPPLEMENTATION

Progesterone was first discovered in 1934, and its ability to cause uterine quiescence was first reported in 1954. Between 2003 and 2011, several randomized trials were published that evaluated the effect of progesterone in its various forms (intramuscular 17-α-hydroxyprogesterone caproate [17P] versus vaginal progesterone versus oral progesterone) in the prevention of PTB, with variable results.[1] It should be clarified that this refers to progesterone supplementation in patients at high risk starting in the second trimester of pregnancy and not in the treatment of patients presenting in acute preterm labor.

Although the precise mechanism of action of progesterone in preventing PTB is unclear, several theories have been postulated. Current evidence favors two possible mechanisms: an anti-inflammatory effect that reduces the intrauterine inflammatory process causing PTB and a mechanism that affects the isolated decrease in progesterone levels within specific tissues of the uterus (a so-called functional with-drawal of progesterone activity within the uterus) that leads to preterm labor and birth.[1] The safety profile of progesterone supplementation is overall favorable. There are now several studies looking at the long-term developmental outcome of infants exposed to progesterone in utero, including exposure in the first trimester, which have, thus far, failed to show any significant adverse effects.[56]

MANAGEMENT RECOMMENDATIONS: NO HISTORY OF PRIOR SPONTANEOUS PRETERM BIRTH

In women with singleton pregnancies, no history of prior sPTB, and a short cervical length on transvaginal ultrasound at the time of the fetal anatomical survey, adminis-tration of vaginal progesterone has been associated with a reduction in PTB and com-posite perinatal morbidity and mortality (**Fig. 1**).[1] Therefore, if a cervical length less than or equal to 20 mm is diagnosed between 18 0/7 and 23 6/7 weeks' gestation, vaginal progesterone is recommended for the prevention of PTB.

The two major studies supporting the use of vaginal progesterone each used different preparations and dosages of progesterone. In the 2003 double-blinded ran-domized controlled trial of women at high risk for PTB, da Fonseca and colleagues[57] studied whether vaginal progesterone 200-mg versus placebo for cervical lengths less than or equal to 15 mm showed a difference in rates of PTB. The study showed that there was a decreased incidence of PTB less than 34 weeks' gestation (18.6% to 2.7%; $P = .002$) and less than 37 weeks' gestation (28.5% to 13.8%; $P = .03$).[57] In a 2011 randomized controlled trial, Hassan and colleagues[58] compared vaginal pro-gesterone gel 90-mg with placebo for women with singleton pregnancies and cervical lengths of 10 to 20 mm. This study showed that, in women with no history of a prior sPTB, vaginal progesterone gel was associated with a reduction in sPTB less than 33 weeks' gestation (15.3% to 7.6%; RR, 0.50; 95% CI, 0.27–0.90; $P = .02$).[58] How-ever, when a subgroup analysis was performed in women with a history of sPTB

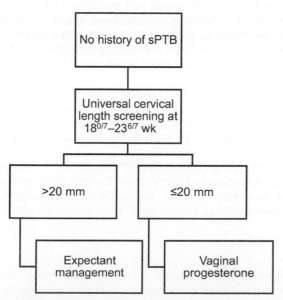

Fig. 1. Prevention of sPTB in women with no history of sPTB.

(20–35 weeks), there was no statistically significant difference in the rate of subsequent sPTB (15.8% vs 20.6%; RR, 0.77; 95% CI, 0.29–2.06; $P = .60$).[58]

Additionally, the OPPTIMUM study was published in 2016, a large multicenter, double-blinded randomized controlled trial comparing 200 mg of vaginal progesterone with placebo in women at high risk for sPTB (defined as a history of prior sPTB <34 weeks, a cervical length ≤25 mm, and/or a positive cervicovaginal fetal fibronectin biomarker test).[59] Results showed no significant differences in the rate of sPTB or perinatal morbidity or mortality between the two groups.[59]

Overall, in women with no prior history of sPTB, there is insufficient evidence regarding the superiority of either preparation or dose of vaginal progesterone because they have not been compared head-to-head in a clinical trial. Therefore, cost, availability of the preparation, patient preference, and other factors may influence the preferred type and dosing of progesterone.

Society for Maternal-Fetal Medicine supports using vaginal progesterone to prevent sPTB in women with a shortened cervical length of less than or equal to 20 mm on transvaginal ultrasound without a history of a prior sPTB.[1] Conversely, in women with a history of a prior sPTB, vaginal progesterone has not been proven to reduce the rate of subsequent sPTB in multiple trials and should, therefore, not be routinely recommended in this setting. It should further be noted that vaginal progesterone is not approved by the FDA to prevent sPTB in any cohort.

MANAGEMENT RECOMMENDATIONS: HISTORY OF PRIOR SPONTANEOUS PRETERM BIRTH

In 2003, Meis and colleagues[60] published a multicenter, double-blinded, randomized controlled trial that involved women with a singleton pregnancy and a prior sPTB. These women were randomized to 17P or placebo. Results showed a statistically significant decrease in the incidence of recurrent sPTB less than 37 weeks with 17P prophylaxis (from 54.9% to 36.3%).[60] This study was discontinued early because the planned interim analysis showed significant reductions in the overall rate of PTB less than 37 weeks, less than 35 weeks, and less than 32 weeks, which translated into significant reductions in neonatal complications (including necrotizing enterocolitis, intraventricular hemorrhage, and need for supplemental oxygen) in those women who received 17P.[60] In February 2011, the FDA approved the use of 17P supplementation for the prevention of recurrent sPTB in patients with a singleton pregnancy at risk by virtue of a prior sPTB.

Therefore, in women with a singleton gestation and a history of a prior sPTB, 17P supplementation is recommended. The dosing is 250 mg given by weekly intramuscular injection starting at 16 to 20 weeks until 36 weeks of gestation. Furthermore, vaginal progesterone should not be regarded as an adequate substitute for 17P in these patients.

Follow-up studies of children exposed to 17P in utero for the prevention of recurrent sPTB have been conducted up to 4 years of age. These studies showed no differences in overall physical examination, health status, mental development, or skill performance (motor, problem solving, interpersonal) when compared with children exposed to placebo.[61]

REFERENCES

1. Society for Maternal-Fetal Medicine Publications Committee, with assistance of Vincenzo Berghella. Progesterone and preterm birth prevention: translating clinical trials data into clinical practice. Am J Obstet Gynecol 2012;206:376–86.

2. March of Dimes. 2017 Premature birth report cards. Available at: https://www.marchofdimes.org/mission/prematurity-reportcard.aspx. Accessed August 10, 2018.
3. Creasy RK, Resnik R, Iams JD, et al. Creasy & Resnik's maternal-fetal medicine: principles and practice. Philadelphia: Elsevier Saunders; 2014. p. 624–53.
4. Practice bulletin no. 159: management of preterm labor. Obstet Gynecol 2016; 127:e29.
5. Gross G, Imamura T, Vogt SK, et al. Inhibition of cyclooxygenase-2 prevents inflammation-mediated preterm labor in the mouse. Am J Physiol Regul Integr Comp Physiol 2000;278:R1415.
6. Doret M, Mellier G, Benchaib M, et al. In vitro study of tocolytic effect of rofecoxib, a specific cyclo-oxygenase 2 inhibitor. Comparison and combination with other tocolytic agents. BJOG 2002;109:983.
7. Yousif MH, Thulesius O. Tocolytic effect of the cyclooxygenase-2 inhibitor, meloxicam: studies on uterine contractions in the rat. J Pharm Pharmacol 1998;50:681.
8. Slattery MM, Friel AM, Healy DG, et al. Uterine relaxant effects of cyclooxygenase-2 inhibitors in vitro. Obstet Gynecol 2001;98:563.
9. Sadovsky Y, Nelson DM, Muglia LJ, et al. Effective diminution of amniotic prostaglandin production by selective inhibitors of cyclooxygenase type 2. Am J Obstet Gynecol 2000;182:370.
10. Niebyl JR, Blake DA, White RD, et al. The inhibition of premature labor with indomethacin. Am J Obstet Gynecol 1980;136:1014.
11. Van den Veyver IB, Moise KJ Jr. Prostaglandin synthetase inhibitors in pregnancy. Obstet Gynecol Surv 1993;48:493.
12. Reinebrant HE, Pileggi-Castro C, Romero CL, et al. Cyclooxygenase (COX) inhibitors for treating preterm labour. Cochrane Database Syst Rev 2015;(6):CD001992.
13. Zuckerman H, Shalev E, Gilad G, et al. Further study of the inhibition of premature labor by indomethacin. Part II double-blind study. J Perinat Med 1984;12(1):25–9.
14. Moise KJ Jr. Effect of advancing gestational age on the frequency of fetal ductal constriction in association with maternal indomethacin use. Am J Obstet Gynecol 1993;168:1350.
15. Moise KJ Jr, Huhta JC, Sharif DS, et al. Indomethacin in the treatment of premature labor. Effects on the fetal ductus arteriosus. N Engl J Med 1988;319:327.
16. Vermillion ST, Scardo JA, Lashus AG, et al. The effect of indomethacin tocolysis on fetal ductus arteriosus constriction with advancing gestational age. Am J Obstet Gynecol 1997;177:256.
17. Norton ME, Merrill J, Cooper BA, et al. Neonatal complications after the administration of indomethacin for preterm labor. N Engl J Med 1993;329:1602.
18. Souter D, Harding J, McCowan L, et al. Antenatal indomethacin: adverse fetal effects confirmed. Aust N Z J Obstet Gynaecol 1998;38:11.
19. Major CA, Lewis DF, Harding JA, et al. Tocolysis with indomethacin increases the incidence of necrotizing enterocolitis in the low-birth-weight neonate. Am J Obstet Gynecol 1994;170:102.
20. Doyle NM, Gardner MO, Wells L, et al. Outcome of very low birth weight infants exposed to antenatal indomethacin for tocolysis. J Perinatol 2005;25:336.
21. Sood BG, Lulic-Botica M, Holzhausen KA, et al. The risk of necrotizing enterocolitis after indomethacin tocolysis. Pediatrics 2011;128:e54.
22. Hammers AL, Sanchez-Ramos L, Kaunitz AM. Antenatal exposure to indomethacin increases the risk of severe intraventricular hemorrhage, necrotizing enterocolitis, and periventricular leukomalacia: a systematic review with meta-analysis. Am J Obstet Gynecol 2015;212:505.e1.

23. Amin SB, Kamaluddeen M, Sangem M. Neurodevelopmental outcome of premature infants after exposure to antenatal indomethacin. Am J Obstet Gynecol 2008; 199:41.e1.
24. Salokorpi T, Eronen M, von Wendt L. Growth and development until 18 months of children exposed to tocolytics indomethacin or nylidrin. Neuropediatrics 1996;27: 174.
25. al-Alaiyan S, Seshia MM, Casiro OG. Neurodevelopmental outcome of infants exposed to indomethacin antenatally. J Perinat Med 1996;24:405.
26. Gary CF, Gant N, Leveno K, et al. Williams obstetrics. New York: McGraw-Hill; 2005. p. 823–9.
27. US Food and Drug Administration. FDA drug safety communication: new warnings against use of terbutaline to treat preterm labor. Available at: http://www.fda.gov/Drugs/DrugSafety/ucm243539.htm#ds. Accessed August 10, 2018.
28. Neilson JP, West HM, Dowswell T. Betamimetics for inhibiting preterm labour. Cochrane Database Syst Rev 2014;(2):CD004352.
29. Gyetvai K, Hannah ME, Hodnett ED, et al. Tocolytics for preterm labor: a systematic review. Obstet Gynecol 1999;94(5 Pt 2):869–77.
30. Golichowski AM, Hathaway DR, Fineberg N, et al. Tocolytic and hemodynamic effects of nifedipine in the Ewe. Am J Obstet Gynecol 1985;151:1134.
31. Flenady V, Wojcieszek AM, Papatsonis DN, et al. Calcium channel blockers for inhibiting preterm labour and birth. Cochrane Database Syst Rev 2014;(6):CD002255.
32. Cornette J, Duvekot JJ, Roos-Hesselink JW, et al. Maternal and fetal haemodynamic effects of nifedipine in normotensive pregnant women. BJOG 2011; 118:510.
33. Ray D, Dyson D. Calcium channel blockers. Clin Obstet Gynecol 1995;38:713.
34. Guclu S, Saygili U, Dogan E, et al. The short-term effect of nifedipine tocolysis on placental, fetal cerebral and atrioventricular Doppler waveforms. Ultrasound Obstet Gynecol 2004;24:761.
35. Mari G, Kirshon B, Moise KJ Jr, et al. Doppler assessment of the fetal and uteroplacental circulation during nifedipine therapy for preterm labor. Am J Obstet Gynecol 1989;161:1514.
36. Cunze T, Rath W, Osmers R, et al. Magnesium and calcium concentration in the pregnant and non-pregnant myometrium. Int J Gynaecol Obstet 1995;48:9.
37. Lemancewicz A, Laudańska H, Laudański T, et al. Permeability of fetal membranes to calcium and magnesium: possible role in preterm labour. Hum Reprod 2000;15:2018.
38. Mizuki J, Tasaka K, Masumoto N, et al. Magnesium sulfate inhibits oxytocin-induced calcium mobilization in human puerperal myometrial cells: possible involvement of intracellular free magnesium concentration. Am J Obstet Gynecol 1993;169:134.
39. Elliott JP, Lewis DF, Morrison JC, et al. In defense of magnesium sulfate. Obstet Gynecol 2009;113:1341.
40. McNamara HC, Crowther CA, Brown J. Different treatment regimens of magnesium sulphate for tocolysis in women in preterm labour. Cochrane Database Syst Rev 2015;(12):CD011200.
41. Crowther CA, Brown J, McKinlay CJ, et al. Magnesium sulphate for preventing preterm birth in threatened preterm labour. Cochrane Database Syst Rev 2014;(8):CD001060.
42. Terrone DA, Rinehart BK, Kimmel ES, et al. A prospective, randomized, controlled trial of high and low maintenance doses of magnesium sulfate for acute tocolysis. Am J Obstet Gynecol 2000;182(6):1477–82.

43. American College of Obstetricians and Gynecologists Committee on Obstetric Practice Society for Maternal-Fetal Medicine. Committee opinion no. 573: magnesium sulfate use in obstetrics. Obstet Gynecol 2013;122:727.
44. Holcomb WL Jr, Shackelford GD, Petrie RH. Magnesium tocolysis and neonatal bone abnormalities: a controlled study. Obstet Gynecol 1991;78:611.
45. Schanler RJ, Smith LG Jr, Burns PA. Effects of long-term maternal intravenous magnesium sulfate therapy on neonatal calcium metabolism and bone mineral content. Gynecol Obstet Invest 1997;43:236.
46. Matsuda Y, Maeda Y, Ito M, et al. Effect of magnesium sulfate treatment on neonatal bone abnormalities. Gynecol Obstet Invest 1997;44:82.
47. Goodwin TM, Valenzuela G, Silver H, et al. Treatment of preterm labor with the oxytocin antagonist atosiban. Am J Perinatol 1996;13:143.
48. Phaneuf S, Asbóth G, MacKenzie IZ, et al. Effect of oxytocin antagonists on the activation of human myometrium in vitro: atosiban prevents oxytocin-induced desensitization. Am J Obstet Gynecol 1994;171:1627.
49. Romero R, Sibai BM, Sanchez-Ramos L, et al. An oxytocin receptor antagonist (atosiban) in the treatment of preterm labor: a randomized, double-blind, placebo-controlled trial with tocolytic rescue. Am J Obstet Gynecol 2000;182:1173.
50. Worldwide Atosiban versus Beta-agonists Study Group. Effectiveness and safety of the oxytocin antagonist atosiban versus beta-adrenergic agonists in the treatment of preterm labour. The Worldwide Atosiban versus Beta-agonists Study Group. BJOG 2001;108:133.
51. Flenady V, Reinebrant HE, Liley HG, et al. Oxytocin receptor antagonists for inhibiting preterm labour. Cochrane Database Syst Rev 2014;(6):CD004452.
52. van Vliet EO, Nijman TA, Schuit E, et al. Nifedipine versus atosiban for threatened preterm birth (APOSTEL III): a multicentre, randomised controlled trial. Lancet 2016;387:2117.
53. de Heus R, Mol BW, Erwich JJ, et al. Adverse drug reactions to tocolytic treatment for preterm labour: prospective cohort study. BMJ 2009;338:b744.
54. Yallampalli C, Dong YL, Gangula PR, et al. Role and regulation of nitric oxide in the uterus during pregnancy and parturition. J Soc Gynecol Investig 1998;5:58.
55. Duckitt K, Thornton S, O'Donovan OP, et al. Nitric oxide donors for treating preterm labour. Cochrane Database Syst Rev 2014;(5):CD002860.
56. Resseguie LJ, Hick JF, Bruen JA, et al. Congenital malformations among offspring exposed in utero to progestins, Olmsted County, Minnesota, 1936-1974. Fertil Steril 1985;43:514–9. Level II-2.
57. da Fonseca EB, Bittar RE, Carvalho MH, et al. Prophylactic administration of progesterone by vaginal suppository to reduce the incidence of spontaneous preterm birth in women at increased risk: a randomized placebo-controlled double-blind study. Am J Obstet Gynecol 2003;188:419–24.
58. Hassan SS, Romero R, Vidyadhari D, et al. PREGNANT Trial. Vaginal progesterone reduces the rate of preterm birth in women with a sonographic short cervix: a multicenter, randomized, double-blind, placebo- controlled trial. Ultrasound Obstet Gynecol 2011;38:18–31.
59. Norman JE, Marlow N, Messow CM, et al, OPPTIMUM Study Group. Vaginal progesterone prophylaxis for preterm birth (the OPPTIMUM study): a multicentre, randomised, double-blind trial. Lancet 2016;387:2106–16.
60. Meis PJ, Klebanoff M, Thom E, et al, National Institute of Child Health and Human Development Maternal-Fetal Medicine Units Network. Prevention of recurrent preterm delivery by 17 alpha-hydroxyprogesterone caproate. N Engl J Med 2003; 348:2379–85.

61. Northen AT, Norman GS, Anderson K, et al, for the National Institute of Child Health and Human Development (NICHD) Maternal-Fetal Medicine Units (MFMU) Network. Follow-up of children exposed in utero to 17 alpha-hydroxyprogesterone caproate compared with placebo. Obstet Gynecol 2007; 110:865–72.

Treatment and Prevention of Hypertensive Disorders During Pregnancy

Karla Leavitt, MD, MPH*, Sarah Običan, MD, Jerome Yankowitz, MD

KEYWORDS

- Hypertension during pregnancy • Hypertensive disorders of pregnancy
- Maternal hypertension • Treatment of hypertension during pregnancy
- Hypertensive disorders during pregnancy
- Hypertension medications during pregnancy
- Pharmacologic therapy of hypertension during pregnancy

KEY POINTS

- Hypertensive disorders are one of the most common complications of pregnancy.
- Obstetric management guidelines have been developed with the goal of reducing maternal morbidity, long-term disability, and death.
- The exact mechanism of gestational hypertension and preeclampsia is still not well elucidated.
- Early detection and treatment with safe and effective pharmacologic therapies is effective in optimizing outcome for mother and fetus.
- Aspirin or acetylsalicylic acid (ASA) has been proposed to be a safe pharmacologic agent for the secondary prevention of preeclampsia.

INTRODUCTION

Blood volume expansion begins between the sixth and eighth week of gestation and increases to 50% over baseline by 32 weeks of pregnancy. Although blood pressure and vascular resistance decreases in midpregnancy, cardiac stroke volume and heart rate increase resulting in an overall increase in cardiac output of 30% to 50% at term. During parturition, cardiac output and blood pressure rise further with normalization to prepregnancy levels over days to weeks postpartum.[1]

Hypertensive disorders are one of the most common complications of pregnancy. According to the Centers for Disease Control and Prevention, hypertensive disorders

Disclosure Statement: The authors have nothing to disclose.
Department of Obstetrics and Gynecology, Division of Maternal Fetal Medicine, University of South Florida, Morsani College of Medicine, 2 Tampa General Circle, 6th Floor, Tampa, FL 33606, USA
* Corresponding author.
E-mail address: kleavitt@health.usf.edu

affect 900 per 10,000 hospitalizations for delivery in the United States. Worldwide, hypertensive disorders contribute significantly to maternal morbidity, accounting for 10% of all maternal deaths in Asia and Africa and 25% of all maternal deaths in Latin America.[2] Hence, obstetric management guidelines have been developed with the goal of reducing maternal morbidity, long-term disability, and death.

Of concern with the treatment of hypertensive disorders of pregnancy is the safety of antihypertensive medications. Some antihypertensive medications have been extensively evaluated for teratogenicity, whereas others have not. Some antihypertensive medications continue to be used commonly in obstetric practice and are considered safe, whereas other classes are contraindicated because of teratogenic or fetotoxic concerns. This article reviews the pharmacology of the most commonly used antihypertensive medications during pregnancy; their mechanism of action; and the effects on the mother, the fetus, and lactation.

DIAGNOSIS

According to the report by the American College of Obstetricians and Gynecologists (ACOG) task force on hypertension in pregnancy, hypertensive disorders of pregnancy are classified into the following four categories: (1) chronic hypertension, (2) gestational hypertension, (3) preeclampsia, and (4) chronic hypertension with superimposed preeclampsia.[3]

Chronic hypertension is defined as hypertension that predates the pregnancy or develops before 20 weeks of gestational age. ACOG guidelines state that a diagnosis of chronic hypertension is established by two or more episodes of high blood pressure, defined as systolic blood pressure equal or greater than 140 mm Hg and/or diastolic pressure equal or greater than 90 mm Hg at least 4 hours apart diagnosed prepregnancy or before 20 weeks of gestational age. Gestational hypertension, formerly known as pregnancy-induced hypertension, is defined by hypertension that develops after 20 weeks of gestation in the absence of proteinuria and systemic findings consistent with preeclampsia.[3]

Preeclampsia refers to hypertension with significant proteinuria, defined as excretion of 300 mg or more of protein in a 24-hour urine collection or a protein/creatinine ratio of greater or equal to 0.3 mg/dL. Gestational hypertension with severe features, even in the absence of proteinuria, can also define preeclampsia, including[3]:

- Significant blood pressure elevation: systolic greater than 160 mm Hg and/or diastolic greater than 110 mm Hg.
- Thrombocytopenia: platelet count less than 100,000/μL.
- Impaired liver functions: elevated liver transaminases to twice the normal concentration.
- New-onset renal insufficiency: elevated serum creatinine greater than 1.1 mg/dL or doubling of serum creatinine in the absence of other renal disease.
- End organ damage including pulmonary edema or new-onset cerebral or visual disturbances.

Importantly, chronic hypertension is a significant risk factor for preeclampsia, so-called superimposed preeclampsia. This distinction is challenging to diagnose and manage, and often depends on the presence of severe features.

PATHOPHYSIOLOGY OF PREECLAMPSIA

Although preeclampsia is one of the most common complications in obstetrics, the pathogenesis and underlying mechanism of disease have not been clearly elucidated.

Box 1 shows the risk factors associated with the development of preeclampsia. Recognized pathophysiologic findings related to preeclampsia include disturbances in placentation early in pregnancy, generalized inflammation, and progressive endothelial damage throughout the mother's body.[4] One of the prevailing disease models is that inadequate remodeling of the maternal spiral arteries by the invading cytotrophoblast cells causes a physiologic hypoxic environment within the tissues of the placenta and generates a complex cascade that leads to abnormal endothelial function throughout the mother's body, which is characterized by increased vascular resistance and permeability.[5] A generalized inflammatory reaction within the maternal circulation causes vasoconstriction, reduction of intravascular volume, and activation of the coagulation cascade. This generalized inflammatory reaction is powered by activation of monocytes, granulocytes, and proinflammatory cytokines, such as interleukin-6 and tumor necrosis factor-α. Physiologically, a normal placenta would produce a reduction on adrenergic activity, increasing the production of prostacyclin and nitric oxide by endothelial cells, which has a vasodilation effect and enables the development of a low-resistance high-volume system, with release of angiogenic factors and their receptors.[6] In addition, recent studies have suggested a role of the natural killer cells, which secrete a higher concentration of some cytokines and angiogenic factors, such as soluble interleukin-2, endostatin, and placental growth factor,[7] which may lead to the development of preeclampsia.

TREATMENT OVERVIEW

The early diagnosis of and treatment of hypertension during pregnancy is the cornerstone for the prevention of severe morbidity, long-term sequelae, and death. Most of these complications are considered preventable, which has prompted the publication of management and safety guidelines.[14] Important factors to consider for the treatment of hypertensive disorders of pregnancy include timing of diagnosis, whether it is chronic or gestational hypertension, when to treat, and what medications to recommend. According to ACOG, treatment with antihypertensive medications is

---

Box 1
Risk factors for preeclampsia

- Maternal age extremes (<20 or >35 years of age)
- Nulliparity
- Infertility
- Obesity
- History of preeclampsia
- Multifetal gestation
- Family history of preeclampsia (mother or sister)
- Underlying medical conditions: chronic hypertension, diabetes mellitus, autoimmune disorders (ie, systemic lupus erythematosus, antiphospholipid antibody syndrome), renal disease
- Limited exposure to sperm
- Paternal genetics
- Urinary tract infection

Data from Refs.[8–13]

recommended when blood pressure measurements reach the severe range (defined as >160 mm Hg systolic and/or >110 mm Hg diastolic) in the absence of chronic hypertension. There is currently a paucity of data on the benefit of treating mild-range hypertension to prevent adverse pregnancy outcomes and future maternal long-term health. Prospective studies are ongoing to help answer this important question, such as the Chronic Hypertension and Pregnancy Project (NCT02299414).

SUMMARY OF ANTIHYPERTENSIVE AGENTS

Each of the classes of antihypertensive pharmacologic agents have specific mechanisms of action by which they exert their antihypertensive effect. β-Adrenoreceptor antagonists work by blocking these receptors in the peripheral circulation, heart, airways, liver, and pancreas.[15] Within this family, labetalol, one of the most commonly used antihypertensive medications in pregnancy, has vasodilatory effects at the arteriolar level, which reduces systemic vascular resistance. Calcium channel blockers, with nifedipine being the most widely studied, impede the influx of calcium into smooth muscle cells, resulting in arterial vasodilation.[16] α-Agonists act as central antiadrenergic agents that inhibit vasoconstriction. Methyldopa has been available since 1963 and is still the centrally acting adrenoreceptor antagonist that is most widely used in pregnancy. Vasodilators, such as hydralazine, have a direct effect on the vascular smooth muscle, especially the arterioles. Diuretics are not used as often in pregnancy because they are in the treatment of essential hypertension outside of pregnancy, but are still relevant in obstetrics and act directly on the renal transport of sodium with the aim of decreasing intravascular volume. Lastly, medications acting on the angiotensin pathway are usually avoided during pregnancy because of well-recognized fetotoxic effects.

All of these classes of antihypertensive medications are reviewed in detail next, classified based on their mechanism of action: peripheral, central, direct vasodilators, diuretics, and those affecting angiotensin pathways.

PERIPHERAL-ACTING ANTIADRENERGIC AGENTS

The first group of antihypertensive medications is the peripheral-acting antiadrenergic agents, including β-adrenergic, α-adrenergic, and calcium channel blockers. β-Adrenergic antagonists (β-blockers) decrease blood pressure by reducing myocardial contractility, blocking the receptors of the juxtaglomerular complex, and decreasing the secretion of renin, thus reducing the secretion of angiotensin II. β-blockers also change baroreceptor sensitivity, thereby modifying the function of the peripheral adrenergic neurons and increasing the synthesis of prostacyclin. Adverse effects may be predicted as consequence of receptor blockade, such as fatigue, lethargy, and exercise intolerance caused by their effects on skeletal muscle vasculature and peripheral vasoconstriction.[17] These medications should be avoided in patients with significant pulmonary bronchoconstriction, such as asthma, and in patients with long-standing diabetes mellitus with microvascular disease.

β-Blockers have been extensively studied and used during pregnancy without evidence of significant teratogenicity.[18] Theoretically, β-blockers could decrease placental perfusion and contribute to fetal growth restriction and low birthweight.[19] However, most studies refute these risks, with labetalol being the most widely studied. Some reports associate the use of parenteral β-blockers with temporary neonatal signs of β-blockade, including bradycardia, hypoglycemia, and tachypnea,[20] although systematic reviews have refuted a significant effect of this class of drug on fetal and neonatal cardiac function.[21]

Labetalol has and α- and β-receptor blocking activity, and is therefore referred to as a nonselective β-blocker. It is one of the most widely used and accepted treatments for hypertension during pregnancy. Studies have shown a similar safety profile with less side effects and higher effectiveness when compared with methyldopa.[18] It has additional arteriolar vasodilatory effects that reduce peripheral vascular resistance. Labetalol is rapidly absorbed, achieving a peak concentration 20 minutes after ingestion with a half-life of 1.7 hours. As with most medications, labetalol crosses the placenta and has been measured in cord blood at up to 50% of the maternal concentration.[22] It is transferred into human milk, but in extremely small concentrations at 0.004% to 0.07% of maternal levels.[23]

Calcium-channel blockers are another type of peripheral-acting adrenoreceptor blockers that are widely used in obstetrics. Physiologically, calcium enters the cell through ion channels located on the myocardium, atrioventricular node, and smooth muscle throughout the body. Calcium channel blockers act predominantly on the slow channels leading to coronary and peripheral arterial vasodilation, resulting in turn to a decrease in vascular peripheral resistance. Common side effects include tachycardia, headache, and facial flushing.[24]

The dihydropyridine nifedipine has been the most studied calcium channel blocker in pregnancy, with no evidence of teratogenicity or adverse neonatal effects in the best available studies, including no association with reduced uterine perfusion.[25,26] Its effects on the myocardium are less than in the vasculature and it lacks antiarrhythmic activity; and its negatively ionotropic effect is compensated by a reduction in left ventricular exertion.[27] Consequently, short-acting nifedipine has been associated with myocardial infarction and death in nonpregnant patients with preexisting coronary artery disease and to maternal hypotension and fetal bradycardia in case studies. As such, it is not recommended for the acute treatment of hypertensive crisis.[28,29] However, long-acting nifedipine preparations are considered safe for the treatment of severe range hypertension.[30] Of note, although older reports suggested that concomitant use of nifedipine and magnesium could precipitate neuromuscular blockade and circulatory collapse,[31–33] this interaction has been refuted by more recent studies.[34,35] In terms of lactation, its excretion into breast milk is minimal, its composition is not altered, and no adverse effects have been observed in exposed infants.[36]

α-Adrenergic antagonists are another subgroup of peripherally active adrenoreceptors. The use of prazosin and phenoxybenzamine during pregnancy is largely limited to use in conjunction with β-blockers as adjuvant therapy for patients with pheochromocytoma.[37]

CENTRAL-ACTING ANTIADRENERGIC AGENTS

The second group of antihypertensive medications under review based on mechanism of action are the central-acting antiadrenergic agents. Methyldopa was first used in obstetrics in 1963, and is still widely used today because of its perceived safety and efficacy. This agent is an α_2-adrenergic agonist that has central nervous system (CNS) and peripheral nervous system effects.[38,39]

Methyldopa inhibits the enzyme dopa decarboxylase, and causes depletion of norepinephrine, with no direct effect on cardiac function, glomerular filtration rate, renal blood flow, or filtration fraction. Although the mechanism of action has yet to be conclusively demonstrated, the resultant hypotensive effect is most likely caused by the drug's action on the CNS. Methyldopa is converted into the active metabolite, α-methylnorepinephrine, which stimulates the central inhibitory α-adrenergic receptors in the CNS, leading to a reduction in sympathetic tone, total peripheral resistance, and blood pressure. Methyldopa is still an accepted agent for the treatment of hypertension during pregnancy based on its effectiveness and safety, although it has been largely displaced by labetalol as the first-line agent of choice for most patients.[18] Its adverse effects on the cardiovascular system are related to a reduction of sympathetic tone and include bradycardia, orthostatic hypotension, sedation, and a possible association with postpartum depression.[40] In addition, cases of elevated liver enzymes, hepatic necrosis, antinuclear antigens, and hemolytic anemia have been reported.[41]

Within this group of centrally acting adrenoreceptors, clonidine is an α_2-adrenergic receptor agonist that acts on the CNS to cause a reduction in the sympathetic response, leading to a decrease in peripheral resistance, renovascular resistance, heart rate, and blood pressure. Clonidine is indicated as a treatment of hypertension, migraine prophylaxis, and alcohol and opioid abstinence syndrome.[42] For an oral regimen, the maximum plasma concentration is achieved in 3 to 4 hours. Its physiologic effects start 1 to 2 hours after administration and last for 8 hours. As a precaution, clonidine should be tapered slowly to avoid rebound hypertension and Raynaud phenomenon, and is not recommended for patients with history of depression or sinoatrial disease. Other side effects include somnolence, dizziness, fatigue, insomnia, nightmares, and dry eyes. Clonidine is compatible with lactation, although it may hinder the production of prolactin and thus impair breast milk production.[36] Overall, the data do not support an increase in birth defects with the use of clonidine and methyldopa in pregnancy.

DIRECT VASODILATORS

Direct vasodilators also have a role in the treatment of hypertension during pregnancy, which is mediated by a baroreceptor reflex mechanism located specifically on arterioles. This vasodilatory effect generates a sympathomimetic stimulus leading to an increase in cardiac function, contractility, and plasma renin levels.

Hydralazine, a commonly used vasodilator, is rarely used as monotherapy, and is usually added when other agents fail to effectively treat severe hypertension. It is also used parenterally for acute hypertensive episodes. The most common side effects include palpitations, tachycardia, headache, and hypotension. In patients with preexisting coronary artery disease, it may cause myocardial ischemia or infarction. Neonatal effects may include an association with abnormal fetal heart rate and Apgar score at 1 minute.[43] Other studies have reported neonatal effects of drug-induced lupus with thrombocytopenia being the most common finding.[44] Hydralazine use has been largely supplanted by β-blockers and calcium channel blockers because of their more favorable safety profiles, although it is still widely used in the acute management of severe hypertension.[45,46] Overall, the data do not indicate there are teratogenic effects with the use of hydralazine.

DIURETICS

Diuretics comprise another group of antihypertensive medications used in pregnancy, although not typically used as a first-line agent. Diuretics stimulate renal excretion of water and electrolytes by altering the transport of ions through the cell membrane of the nephrons. The main goal of this treatment is to obtain a negative water balance by acting directly on sodium transport channels and have vasodilatory effects on the arterioles. Diuretics are commonly used in the setting of pulmonary edema.

Thiazides are the most commonly used diuretic during pregnancy, usually added when other treatments fail. Although the mechanism of action is to cause volume contraction, there is no consistent evidence that it is associated with fetal growth restriction or worsening intravascular depletion in patients with preeclampsia. Hence, patients with chronic hypertension on treatment with hydrochlorothiazide may continue a low-dose regimen during pregnancy.[47] Adverse effects include postural hypotension and electrolyte imbalances. In the neonate, thiazides have been associated with thrombocytopenia, hypokalemia, and jaundice.[47]

Furosemide is a diuretic that works at the loop of Henle in the kidney, reducing the reabsorption of sodium and chloride. It is particularly useful when used in the first 24 hours postpartum in patients with pulmonary edema, showing a faster recovery and less antihypertensive medication requirements compared with other medication classes.[48]

As expected, given the mechanism of action of intravascular volume reduction, diuretics may decrease breast milk production and volume, although it is considered safe for lactation. Overall, these two diuretics have not been associated to an increased risk of birth defects.

Spironolactone is contraindicated during the preconception period and throughout pregnancy because of its antiandrogenic effect that can lead to fetal feminization.[49] It is recommended that all women who are being treated with spironolactone for polycystic ovarian syndrome should have a reliable contraceptive method.

ANGIOTENSIN PATHWAY INHIBITORS

Although no longer recommended during pregnancy, angiotensin-converting enzyme inhibitors (ACE-I), have been widely studied during pregnancy. ACE-I are used for the treatment of hypertension, congestive heart failure, coronary disease, and diabetic nephropathy. They are an effective treatment of hypertension because they suppress the plasma renin-angiotensin-aldosterone system.

Although some studies show a small increase in fetal malformations, especially skeletal malformations, in association with use of ACE-I, the available data do not consistently show that ACE-I are teratogenic in the first trimester.[50,51] However, ACE-I do seem to be fetotoxic. ACE-I do cross the placenta and their use in the second and third trimester has been associated with reduced placental circulation, decreased fetal urine production, hypotension, fetal growth restriction, pulmonary hypoplasia, and fetal death.[52–54] Since 1992, the US Food and Drug Administration has required a warning statement on all ACE-I regarding their potential fetotoxic effects when used during the second and third trimesters of pregnancy.

Some small studies have measured ACE-I in breast milk at small doses. For example, after a maternal dose of 20 mg of enalapril, the infant is expected to be exposed to less than 2 μg.[55]

Angiotensin II receptor blockers (ARBs) are an effective treatment of hypertension and heart failure. ARBs are also helpful in diabetic nephropathy to reduce proteinuria and increase the glomerular filtration rate. They selectively and competitively block the angiotensin-I receptor thereby inhibiting angiotensin II formation. Similar to ACE-I, they have not been shown to be overtly teratogenic in the first trimester, but may have similar fetotoxic effects.[56] The use of ARBs in the second and third trimester has been associated with anhydramnios, fetal renal dysfunction, skull and skeletal deformities, pulmonary hypoplasia, and fetal death.[57–59] In some reports, the discontinuation of the ARB reversed the compromised renal function and oligohydramnios.[60–62]

A systematic review by Bullo and colleagues[63] compared neonatal outcomes between fetuses exposed to an ACE-I or ARB and found that those exposed to ARBs had worse outcomes, including higher rates of oligohydramnios, fetal growth restriction, respiratory distress, skeletal defects, and fetal/neonatal death.

PREVENTION

Given the significant morbidity associated with hypertensive disorders of pregnancy, much attention has been focused on prevention in high-risk women. Since 1978, aspirin or acetylsalicylic acid (ASA) has been proposed to be a safe pharmacologic agent for the secondary prevention of preeclampsia and other adverse perinatal outcomes, such as preterm birth, fetal growth restriction, and stillbirth.[64]

ASA inhibits the enzyme cyclooxygenase within platelets and endothelial cells, thereby inhibiting the synthesis of thromboxane A_2. Multiple studies have shown that low-dose aspirin is able to affect the thromboxane-prostacyclin equilibrium, favoring prostacyclin and its vasodilatory effects and inhibition of platelet aggregation. This is hypothesized to improve implantation, placentation, and vascular remodeling when administered early in pregnancy.[65,66]

In 2014, the US Preventive Services Task Force recommended the use of low-dose aspirin (81 mg daily) for patients with one or more major risk factors, including a history of preeclampsia; multiple gestation; chronic hypertension; diabetes mellitus; renal disease; and/or autoimmune disorders, such as systemic lupus erythematosus. The risk reduction was estimated at 24% for preeclampsia, 20% for growth restriction, and 14% in preterm birth.[64] Moreover, based on a recent study published in the *New England Journal of Medicine* in 2017, the benefit of ASA may be dose-dependent, suggesting that a dose of 150 mg may have a greater risk reduction (up to 82%) for early preeclampsia (before 34 weeks) for select patients when started between 11 and 14 weeks of gestational age versus placebo control.[67]

In addition to such medications as ASA, nutritional supplements have also been studied for the prevention of preeclampsia. Given the putative role of oxidative stress in the pathophysiology of preeclampsia, nutritional supplementation with antioxidants (eg, vitamin C and vitamin E) has biologic plausibility, and yet multiple large randomized controlled trials have shown no statistically significant reduction in the rate of preeclampsia using these antioxidants.[68] Similarly, supplementation with calcium in a large cohort in the United States also failed to reduce the incidence of preeclampsia, whereas other studies suggest a small benefit in patients in underdeveloped countries with preexisting calcium deficiency (relative risk, 0.36). Based on these data, the World Health Organization recommends supplementation with 1.5 to 2 g daily of calcium for the prevention of preeclampsia.[69]

SUMMARY

Hypertensive disorders are one of the most common complications of pregnancy and pose a significant increase in maternal, fetal, and neonatal mortality and morbidity worldwide. Although the exact mechanism of gestational hypertension and preeclampsia is still not well elucidated, early detection and treatment with safe and effective pharmacologic therapies is effective in optimizing outcome for mother and fetus. Prevention of hypertensive disorders of pregnancy has been a more elusive target, but data suggest that ASA prophylaxis may have some benefit.

> **Best practices**
>
> *What is the current practice?*
>
> Treatment of hypertensive disorders during pregnancy
>
> Best practice/guideline/care path objectives:
>
> - Early detection of hypertension
> - Prompt treatment with safe and effective pharmacologic therapies
> - Reduce maternal morbidity, long-term disability, and death
> - Increase maternal safety
>
> *What changes in current practice are likely to improve outcomes?*
>
> - Adequate treatment of hypertensive disorders during pregnancy
> - Understand the mechanism of action, indications, contraindications, and side effects of some antihypertensive agents
> - Prevention of preeclampsia
>
> *Major Recommendations*
>
> - Screen for hypertension during pregnancy (two episodes of systolic blood pressure ≥140 mm Hg and/or diastolic blood pressure ≥90 mm Hg at least 4 hours apart)
> - Ask specifically about history of hypertension before pregnancy or prior pregnancies affected by hypertension
> - For women of reproductive age with history of chronic hypertension on medications and interested in childbearing or not on a reliable contraceptive method, preconceptional counseling is advised to ensure that the patient is on treatment medications that are safe and effective during pregnancy
> - Classify as: chronic hypertension, gestational hypertension, preeclampsia, and chronic hypertension with superimposed preeclampsia based on current guidelines
> - Start low-dose aspirin ideally at 12 weeks of gestation and before 16 weeks of gestational age in patients with chronic hypertension and/or other risk factors for preeclampsia
> - Start antihypertensive medications or adjust the dose or agent for severe or near-severe range blood pressure
> - The most commonly used and safe first-line agents include labetalol (β-blocker), nifedipine (Ca^{+2} channel blocker), and methyldopa (central antiadrenergic)
> - Hydralazine (direct vasodilator) and diuretics (except spironolactone) are considered safe but rarely used as monotherapy
> - Medications that act on the angiotensin pathways, such as ACE-I and ARBs, are considered fetotoxic and are not generally recommended during pregnancy
> - Start prompt treatment of acute hypertensive crisis with intravenous labetalol or intravenous hydralazine if systolic blood pressure ≥160 and/or diastolic blood pressure ≥110
>
> *Summary Statement*
>
> Early diagnosis, classification, and treatment of hypertension with safe and effective pharmacologic agents during pregnancy is critical for the reduction of preventable complications of severe maternal morbidity, long-term sequelae, and mortality.
>
> *Data from Refs.*[3,14,15,46,67]

REFERENCES

1. Creasy RK, Resnik R, Iams JD. Maternal-fetal medicine: principles and practice. 5th edition. Philadelphia: W.B. Saunders Co.; 2004.

2. Khan KS, Wojdyla D, Say L, et al. WHO analysis of causes of maternal death: a systematic review. Lancet 2006;367(9516):1066–74.

3. American College of Obstetricians and Gynecologists, Task Force on Hypertension in Pregnancy. Hypertension in pregnancy. Report of the American College of Obstetricians and Gynecologists' Task Force on hypertension in pregnancy. Obstet Gynecol 2013;122(5):1122–31.

4. Redman CW, Sacks GP, Sargent IL. Preeclampsia: an excessive maternal inflammatory response to pregnancy. Am J Obstet Gynecol 1999;180(2):499–506.

5. Sacks GP, Studena K, Sargent K, et al. Normal pregnancy and preeclampsia both produce inflammatory changes in peripheral blood leukocytes akin to those of sepsis. Am J Obstet Gynecol 1998;179(1):80–6.

6. Zhou Y, Fisher SJ, Janatpour M, et al. Human cytotrophoblasts adopt a vascular phenotype as they differentiate. A strategy for successful endovascular invasion? J Clin Invest 1997;99(9):2139–51.

7. Wallace AE, Fraser R, Gurung S, et al. Increased angiogenic factor secretion by decidual natural killer cells from pregnancies with high uterine artery resistance alters trophoblast function. Hum Reprod 2014;29(4):652–60.

8. Saftlas AF, Olson DR, Franks AL, et al. Epidemiology of preeclampsia and eclampsia in the United States, 1979-1986. Am J Obstet Gynecol 1990;163(2): 460–5.

9. Zhang J, Zeisler J, Hatch MC, et al. Epidemiology of pregnancy-induced hypertension. Epidemiol Rev 1997;19(2):218–32.

10. Eskenazi B, Fenster L, Sidney S. A multivariate analysis of risk factors for preeclampsia. JAMA 1991;266(2):237–41.

11. Bodnar LM, Ness RB, Markovic N, et al. The risk of preeclampsia rises with increasing prepregnancy body mass index. Ann Epidemiol 2005;15(7):475–82.

12. Branch DW, Silver RM, Blackwell JL, et al. Outcome of treated pregnancies in women with antiphospholipid syndrome: an update of the Utah experience. Obstet Gynecol 1992;80(4):614–20.

13. Lima F, Khamashta MA, Buchanan NM, et al. A study of sixty pregnancies in patients with the antiphospholipid syndrome. Clin Exp Rheumatol 1996;14(2):131–6.

14. Bernstein PS, Martin JN Jr, Barton JR, et al. National partnership for maternal safety: consensus bundle on severe hypertension during pregnancy and the postpartum period. Obstet Gynecol 2017;130(2):347–57.

15. Abalos E, Duley L, Steyn DW. Antihypertensive drug therapy for mild to moderate hypertension during pregnancy. Cochrane Database Syst Rev 2014;(2):CD002252.

16. Frishman WH. Beta-adrenergic receptor blockers. Adverse effects and drug interactions. Hypertension 1988;11(3 Pt 2):Ii21–9.

17. Robinson BF, Dobbs RJ, Kelsey CR. Effects of nifedipine on resistance vessels, arteries and veins in man. Br J Clin Pharmacol 1980;10(5):433–8.

18. Magee LA, Duley L. Oral beta-blockers for mild to moderate hypertension during pregnancy. Cochrane Database Syst Rev 2003;(3):CD002863.

19. Butters L, Kennedy S, Rubin PC. Atenolol in essential hypertension during pregnancy. BMJ 1990;301(6752):587–9.

20. Stevens TP, Guillet R. Use of glucagon to treat neonatal low-output congestive heart failure after maternal labetalol therapy. J Pediatr 1995;127(1):151–3.

21. Waterman EJ, Magee LA, Lim KI, et al. Do commonly used oral antihypertensives alter fetal or neonatal heart rate characteristics? A systematic review. Hypertens Pregnancy 2004;23(2):155–69.

22. Rogers RC, Sibai BM, Whybrew WD. Labetalol pharmacokinetics in pregnancy-induced hypertension. Am J Obstet Gynecol 1990;162(2):362–6.
23. Atkinson HC, Begg EJ, Darlow BA. Drugs in human milk. Clinical pharmacokinetic considerations. Clin Pharmacokinet 1988;14(4):217–40.
24. Papatsonis DN, Lok CA, Bos JM, et al. Calcium channel blockers in the management of preterm labor and hypertension in pregnancy. Eur J Obstet Gynecol Reprod Biol 2001;97(2):122–40.
25. Lindow SW, Davies N, Davey DA, et al. The effect of sublingual nifedipine on uteroplacental blood flow in hypertensive pregnancy. Br J Obstet Gynaecol 1988; 95(12):1276–81.
26. Rizzo G, Arduini D, Mancuso S, et al. Effects of nifedipine on umbilical artery velocity waveforms in healthy human fetuses. Gynecol Obstet Invest 1987;24(3): 151–4.
27. Shekhar S, Sharma C, Thakur S, et al. Oral nifedipine or intravenous labetalol for hypertensive emergency in pregnancy: a randomized controlled trial. Obstet Gynecol 2013;122(5):1057–63.
28. Impey L. Severe hypotension and fetal distress following sublingual administration of nifedipine to a patient with severe pregnancy induced hypertension at 33 weeks. Br J Obstet Gynaecol 1993;100(10):959–61.
29. Puzey MS, Ackovic KL, Lindow SW, et al. The effect of nifedipine on fetal umbilical artery Doppler waveforms in pregnancies complicated by hypertension. S Afr Med J 1991;79(4):192–4.
30. Brown MA, Buddle ML, Farrell T, et al. Efficacy and safety of nifedipine tablets for the acute treatment of severe hypertension in pregnancy. Am J Obstet Gynecol 2002,187(4):1046–50.
31. Ales K. Magnesium plus nifedipine. Am J Obstet Gynecol 1990;162(1):288.
32. Ben-Ami M, Giladi Y, Shalev E. The combination of magnesium sulphate and nifedipine: a cause of neuromuscular blockade. Br J Obstet Gynaecol 1994; 101(3):262–3.
33. Waisman GD, Mayorga LM, Camera MI, et al. Magnesium plus nifedipine: potentiation of hypotensive effect in preeclampsia? Am J Obstet Gynecol 1988;159(2): 308–9.
34. Scardo JA, Vermillion ST, Hogg BB, et al. Hemodynamic effects of oral nifedipine in preeclamptic hypertensive emergencies. Am J Obstet Gynecol 1996;175(2): 336–8.
35. Magee LA, Miremadi S, Li J, et al. Therapy with both magnesium sulfate and nifedipine does not increase the risk of serious magnesium-related maternal side effects in women with preeclampsia. Am J Obstet Gynecol 2005;193(1): 153–63.
36. American Academy of Pediatrics Committee on Drugs. Transfer of drugs and other chemicals into human milk. Pediatrics 2001;108(3):776–89.
37. Freier DT, Thompson NW. Pheochromocytoma and pregnancy: the epitome of high risk. Surgery 1993;114(6):1148–52.
38. Sibai BM, Mabie WC, Shamsa F, et al. A comparison of no medication versus methyldopa or labetalol in chronic hypertension during pregnancy. Am J Obstet Gynecol 1990;162(4):960–6.
39. Leather HM, Humphreys DM, Baker P, et al. A controlled trial of hypotensive agents in hypertension in pregnancy. Lancet 1968;2(7566):488–90.
40. Ghuman N, Rheiner J, Tendler BE, et al. Hypertension in the postpartum woman: clinical update for the hypertension specialist. J Clin Hypertens 2009;11(12): 726–33.

41. Schweitzer IL, Peters RL. Acute submassive hepatic necrosis due to methyldopa. A case demonstrating possible initiation of chronic liver disease. Gastroenterology 1974;66(6):1203–11.

42. Horvath JS, Phippard A, Korda A, et al. Clonidine hydrochloride: a safe and effective antihypertensive agent in pregnancy. Obstet Gynecol 1985;66(5):634–8.

43. Vigil-De Gracia P, Ruiz E, Lopez JC, et al. Management of severe hypertension in the postpartum period with intravenous hydralazine or labetalol: a randomized clinical trial. Hypertens Pregnancy 2007;26(2):163–71.

44. Expert consensus document on management of cardiovascular diseases during pregnancy. Eur Heart J 2003;24(8):761–81.

45. Magee LA, Cham C, Waterman EJ, et al. Hydralazine for treatment of severe hypertension in pregnancy: meta-analysis. BMJ 2003;327(7421):955–60.

46. Committee on Obstetric Practice. Committee Opinion No. 623: emergent therapy for acute-onset, severe hypertension during pregnancy and the postpartum period. Obstet Gynecol 2015;125(2):521–5.

47. Collins R, Yusuf S, Peto R. Overview of randomised trials of diuretics in pregnancy. BMJ 1985;290(6461):17–23.

48. Magee L, von Dadelszen P. Prevention and treatment of postpartum hypertension. Cochrane Database Syst Rev 2013;(4):CD004351.

49. Groves TD, Corenblum B. Spironolactone therapy during human pregnancy. Am J Obstet Gynecol 1995;172(5):1655–6.

50. Lennestal R, Otterblad Olausson P, Kallen B. Maternal use of antihypertensive drugs in early pregnancy and delivery outcome, notably the presence of congenital heart defects in the infants. Eur J Clin Pharmacol 2009;65(6):615–25.

51. Moretti ME, Caprara D, Drehuta I, et al. The fetal safety of angiotensin converting enzyme inhibitors and angiotensin II receptor blockers. Obstet Gynecol Int 2012; 2012:658310.

52. Tabacova S, Little R, Tsong Y, et al. Adverse pregnancy outcomes associated with maternal enalapril antihypertensive treatment. Pharmacoepidemiol Drug Saf 2003;12(8):633–46.

53. Burrows RF, Burrows EA. Assessing the teratogenic potential of angiotensin-converting enzyme inhibitors in pregnancy. Aust N Z J Obstet Gynaecol 1998; 38(3):306–11.

54. Piper JM, Ray WA, Rosa FW. Pregnancy outcome following exposure to angiotensin-converting enzyme inhibitors. Obstet Gynecol 1992;80(3):429–32.

55. Redman CW, Kelly JG, Cooper WD. The excretion of enalapril and enalaprilat in human breast milk. Eur J Clin Pharmacol 1990;38(1):99.

56. Porta M, Hainer JW, Jansson SO, et al. Exposure to candesartan during the first trimester of pregnancy in type 1 diabetes: experience from the placebo-controlled DIabetic REtinopathy Candesartan Trials. Diabetologia 2011;54(6): 1298–303.

57. Alwan S, Polifka JE, Friedman JM. Angiotensin II receptor antagonist treatment during pregnancy. Birth Defects Res A Clin Mol Teratol 2005;73(2):123–30.

58. Oppermann M, Padberg S, Kayser A, et al. Angiotensin-II receptor 1 antagonist fetopathy: risk assessment, critical time period and vena cava thrombosis as a possible new feature. Br J Clin Pharmacol 2013;75(3):822–30.

59. Hunseler C, Paneitz A, Friedrich D, et al. Angiotensin II receptor blocker induced fetopathy: 7 cases. Klin Padiatr 2011;223(1):10–4.

60. Munk PS, von Brandis P, Larsen AI. Reversible fetal renal failure after maternal treatment with Candesartan: a case report. Reprod Toxicol 2010;29(3):381–2.

61. Bos-Thompson MA, Hillaire-Buys D, Muller F, et al. Fetal toxic effects of angiotensin II receptor antagonists: case report and follow-up after birth. Ann Pharmacother 2005;39(1):157–61.

62. Berkane N, Carlier P, Verstraete L, et al. Fetal toxicity of valsartan and possible reversible adverse side effects. Birth Defects Res A Clin Mol Teratol 2004; 70(8):547–9.

63. Bullo M, Tschumi S, Bucher BS, et al. Pregnancy outcome following exposure to angiotensin-converting enzyme inhibitors or angiotensin receptor antagonists: a systematic review. Hypertension 2012;60(2):444–50.

64. Henderson JT, Whitlock EP, O'Connor E, et al. Low-dose aspirin for prevention of morbidity and mortality from preeclampsia: a systematic evidence review for the U.S. Preventive Services Task Force. Ann Intern Med 2014;160(10):695–703.

65. Duley L, Henderson-Smart DJ, Meher S, et al. Antiplatelet agents for preventing pre-eclampsia and its complications. Cochrane Database Syst Rev 2007;(2):CD004659.

66. Askie L, Duley L, Henderson-Smart DJ, et al, PARIS Collaborative Group. Antiplatelet agents for prevention of pre-eclampsia and its consequences: a systematic review and individual patient data meta-analysis. BMC Pregnancy Childbirth 2005;5(1):7.

67. Rolnik DL, Wright D, Poon LC, et al. Aspirin versus placebo in pregnancies at high risk for preterm preeclampsia. N Engl J Med 2017;377(7):613–22.

68. Conde-Agudelo A, Romero R, Kusanovic JP, et al. Supplementation with vitamins C and E during pregnancy for the prevention of preeclampsia and other adverse maternal and perinatal outcomes: a systematic review and metaanalysis. Am J Obstet Gynecol 2011;204(6):503.e1-12.

69. WHO Guidelines Approved by the Guidelines Review Committee. WHO recommendations for prevention and treatment of pre-eclampsia and eclampsia. Geneva (Switzerland): World Health Organization. WHO; 2011.

Magnesium Sulfate and Novel Therapies to Promote Neuroprotection

Rebecca A. Jameson, MD, MPH[a], Helene B. Bernstein, MD, PhD[a,b,*]

KEYWORDS

- Magnesium sulfate • Neuroprotection • Cerebral palsy

KEY POINTS

- Magnesium sulfate has been shown to reduce the risk of moderate to severe cerebral palsy when given before delivery before 32 weeks' gestation.
- Magnesium sulfate has been long studied and has an excellent safety profile.
- The authors recommend a bolus followed by continuous dosing of magnesium in pregnancies at risk of delivery before 32 weeks' gestation until delivery occurs or is no longer imminent.
- Novel therapies for neuroprotection include therapeutic hypothermia, remote ischemic preconditioning, xenon, argon, creatine, stem cells, and other neuromodulators.

INTRODUCTION

Preterm delivery (PTD) is a major cause of neonatal morbidity and mortality, with surviving infants at risk for long-term neurologic sequelae. Although any birth occurring before the completion of 37 weeks' gestation is considered preterm, most serious harm occurs in the 16% of preterm deliveries occurring before 32 weeks' gestation.[1] Neurodevelopmental impairments can include cerebral palsy (CP), cognitive dysfunction, and sensory impairments (blindness and deafness). Cerebral palsy affects 2 per 1000 infants; however, the risk of CP is inversely proportional to gestational weight and age at delivery. Thus, the prevalence of CP is increased to 60 per 1000 infants in neonates weighing less than 1500 g[2]; and approximately one-third of new CP cases are associated with delivery before 32 weeks' gestation.[3] Within the spectrum of neurologic impairment associated with PTD, CP has been used as the primary

Disclosure: The authors have no financial interests to disclose.
[a] Department of Obstetrics and Gynecology, The State University of New York Upstate Medical University, 750 East Adams Street, 2204 Weiskotten Hall, Syracuse, NY 13210, USA;
[b] Department of Microbiology and Immunology, The State University of New York Upstate Medical University, 750 East Adams Street, 2204 Weiskotten Hall, Syracuse, NY 13210, USA
* Corresponding author.
E-mail address: heleneb825@gmail.com

measurable outcome variable in most of the clinical studies evaluating neuroprotection strategies.

The International Committee on Cerebral Palsy Classification defines CP as a group of developmental disorders of movement and posture causing activity limitations that can be attributed to nonprogressive disturbances occurring in the developing fetal or infant brain.[3] The motor disorders seen in CP are often seen with additional sequelae, such as changes in cognition, communication, perception, sensation, behavior, or seizures. Approximately one-third of cases of CP are associated with delivery before 32 weeks' gestation.[4] Although the pathophysiology of CP is complex, it is thought to be mediated by inflammation,[5–9] most often combined with impaired oxygen delivery to the fetal brain leading to decreased ATP level, increased lactic acid level, and damage to neurons, myelin, plasticity, and cell death. These intrauterine insults can lead to long-term neurologic damage.[10] Risk factors include prematurity, multiple gestation, intrauterine growth restriction, intracranial hemorrhage, infection, placental disorder, genetic syndromes, structural brain anomalies, birth asphyxia, trauma, and kernicterus. Significant overlap and confounding can occur with these variables as seen in premature infants.

The Centers for Disease Control and Prevention (CDC) estimated the direct lifetime cost of CP to exceed $2 billion dollars in 2003.[11] Indirect costs associated with CP are approximately 7-fold to 8-fold higher than direct costs. Lifetime costs to the individual consist of medical and indirect costs and productivity losses, which were estimated to be approximately $921,000 per person with CP in 2003.[11] Caregivers and family members are also strongly affected by having a child with CP, dependent on the child's behavioral issues, caregiving, demands, and family function, which can have lasting effects on their physical and mental health. These enormous economic and societal costs, direct and indirect, underscore the need for effective primary and secondary prevention measures. Moreover, economic evaluation has shown the cost-effectiveness of prevention efforts.[12,13]

This article reviews pharmacologic therapies and strategies used for neonatal neuroprotection. The capacity of magnesium sulfate ($MgSO_4$) to mediate neuroprotection has been investigated within multiple clinical trials using different protocols and inclusion criteria, and the salient differences between the cohorts, protocols, and results are considered. Using this information, this article reviews pharmacokinetic modeling that is helpful in considering refined $MgSO_4$ protocols for neuroprotection. It also discusses novel therapies in place for the prevention of CP (**Box 1**). Given the societal cost of neonatal neurologic injury, in the setting of a stable preterm birth rate, additional studies are required to identify and confirm other neuroprotective agents and to determine the most effective regimens to use.

PHARMACOLOGIC INTERVENTIONS
Magnesium Sulfate

Magnesium sulfate has been widely used in the obstetric environment for several decades. Historically used as a tocolytic agent and to prevent and treat eclampsia, magnesium was noted to potentially decrease the incidence of CP[14] and intraventricular hemorrhage in exposed infants following maternal administration.[14,15] Although $MgSO_4$ remains the treatment of choice for women with eclampsia,[16] the utility of magnesium as a tocolytic remains controversial. A 2002 Cochrane analysis concluded that $MgSO_4$ was not effective at preventing preterm birth.[17] It is relevant to note that only 3 of the 23 analyzed trials included placebo groups (99 placebo subjects in total) in which magnesium therapy was compared with

---

Box 1
Emerging therapies

- Pharmacologic
  - Erythropoietin
  - Darbepoetin
  - Bone marrow derived and mesenchymal stem cells
  - Vasopressin
  - Endocannabinoids
  - Melatonin
  - Xenon
  - Argon
  - Allopurinol
  - Topiramate
  - Creatine

- Non-pharmacologic
  - Delayed cord clamping
  - Cord milking
  - Therapeutic hypothermia
  - Remote ischemic preconditioning

---

no alternative tocolysis, with the investigators acknowledging sparse data of "generally poor quality."[17] After publication of this meta-analysis, MgSO₄ use for tocolysis in the United States declined, with at least 1 small study and published commentary suggesting magnesium was ineffective and potentially even dangerous.[18,19] The increasing use of MgSO₄ as a neuroprotective agent followed the publication of clinical trials, meta-analyses, and recommendations largely within the last decade.[20–31]

Mechanism of action
Magnesium is a micronutrient involved in a multitude of biochemical and physiologic pathways. Magnesium plays a role in energy metabolism, nucleic acid synthesis, regulation of adenylate cyclase, transmembrane ion flux, muscle contraction, vasomotor tone, cardiac excitability, neuronal activity, and neurotransmitter release. Its mechanism of action in the obstetric milieu is poorly understood. Related to its role as a tocolytic, magnesium competes with calcium at the motor end plate at the myometrial cell membrane, therefore reducing myometrial cell excitation and preventing contraction. Our laboratory has shown that magnesium reduces inflammatory cytokine production and nuclear factor kappa-B (NF-kB) activation.[32,33] Inflammation and infection are closely linked to preterm parturition, thus this activity could account in part for the utility of magnesium as a tocolytic therapy.

Magnesium is also a smooth muscle relaxant, potentially affecting cerebral endothelium forming the blood-brain barrier. Magnesium may also influence neurologic function via its role as an *N*-methyl-ᴅ-aspartate (NMDA) antagonist. Stimulation of NMDA receptors by neurotransmitters such as glutamate may lead to seizures when neuronal networks are overactivated. One hypothesis is that magnesium prevents eclamptic seizures by inhibiting NMDA receptors. NMDA inhibition may also reduce ischemia-associated neuronal damage; these proposed neuroprotective mechanisms are supported by work in preclinical animal models.[34–36] Magnesium's antiinflammatory properties may also ameliorate ischemia-associated damage and reduce seizure activity via NMDA inhibition and a reduction in NF-KB activation.[37,38]

Pharmacokinetics

Magnesium (Mg^{2+}), a divalent cation, is the fourth most common cation in humans, with SO_4^{2-} being the complementary anion moiety of the clinically used compound. Magnesium is almost exclusively intracellular, with only 1% of total body magnesium found extracellularly. Serum Mg^{2+} accounts for 0.3% of total body content, and circulating levels decrease during pregnancy from 0.75 to 0.95 mM to 0.54 to 0.90 mM secondary to physiologic hemodilution. Intrapartum magnesium is typically administered intravenously, with some hospitals using intramuscular administration. Myometrial contractility is inhibited with serum Mg^{2+} levels between 5 and 8 mg/dL. Loss of deep tendon reflexes is noted with serum levels between 9 and 13 mg/dL, although there can be individual variability and subjectivity in this assessment. Respiratory depression is seen with serum Mg^{2+} levels of 14 mg/dL or greater (**Fig. 1**).[39] Calcium gluconate is used to treat magnesium toxicity in the setting of respiratory depression. Neonatal Mg^{2+} levels correlate with cumulative received dose. Magnesium is excreted by the kidneys and has a half-life of less than 3 hours.

Confounders

Clearance rates have been studied in patients receiving $MgSO_4$ for seizure prophylaxis, preterm labor, and extreme prematurity. A recent pharmacokinetic study investigated the covariates gestational age, presence of preeclampsia, maternal weight, antepartum versus postpartum status, and maternal creatinine in $MgSO_4$ administered for neuroprotection with a 4-g loading dose followed by maintenance dose of 2 g/h. In this study, 111 maternal subjects with 687 magnesium levels and 66 umbilical cord blood levels were analyzed. Preeclampsia status and maternal weight significantly influenced magnesium pharmacokinetics (P values <.001).[40] The half-life of magnesium was 2.7 hours in nonpreeclamptic women and 3.9 hours in preeclamptic women. Steady-state calculations in women were additionally affected by preeclampsia status and were 5.1 mg/dL compared with 7.2 mg/dL in women without and with preeclampsia, respectively. Maternal weight also affected serum $MgSO_4$ levels, with increasing maternal weight associated with a longer time to steady state. Maternal body weight differences are theorized to be influenced by volume distribution alterations because most of pregnancy weight gain is extracellular body water.[41] Gestational age, antepartum versus postpartum status, and maternal creatinine did not influence $MgSO_4$ pharmacokinetics in this investigation.

Side effects

Maternal side effects, including hypotension, tachycardia, respiratory depression, discomfort, headache, dizziness, mouth dryness, and blurred vision, have been shown to double with $MgSO_4$ exposure. Other common side effects, such as nausea/vomiting, flushing, warmth, and sweating, can be increased up to 5 times the baseline rate, whereas itching, tingling, and muscle weakness are increased up to 15 times.[42] Lower dose regimens may decrease side effects, and lengthening

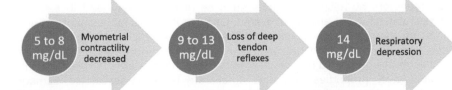

Fig. 1. Serum magnesium levels associated with effect and toxicity.

the loading dose (bolus) time can decrease flushing and feelings of warmth. Overall, maternal side effects secondary to $MgSO_4$ exposure are mild and readily tolerated. Antepartum $MgSO_4$ exposure is not associated with serious neonatal effects, including neonatal intensive care unit admission, cardiac or respiratory arrest, or death. Effects of $MgSO_4$ on the fetal/neonatal brain are not as well known. Neuroprotection is thought to be related to decreased NMDA receptor excitotoxicity, reduced proinflammatory cytokine levels, and oxidative stress.[37,38] Serious neonatal complications are uncommon with exposure of less than 48 hours and may include lethargy, hypotonia, and respiratory depression. Prolonged $MgSO_4$ administration is associated in rare instances with neonatal bone demineralization, neonatal hypermagnesemia and hypocalcemia, and maternal osteopenia. These outcomes have been shown with much longer exposure than patients typically receive, in 1 study with cumulative doses ranging from 4400 to 5500 g.[43]

Magnesium sulfate for neuroprotection
Multiple randomized controlled clinical trials using $MgSO_4$ reported long-term outcomes between 2002 and 2008.[19–22,44] Although these studies did not meet statistical significance with regard to their primary outcome (**Table 1**), they were larger and more comprehensive than previously published studies, and collectively they showed that $MgSO_4$ exposure significantly decreases the likelihood of CP.[23,24,28,29,31] The Australasian Collaborative Trial of Magnesium Sulfate (ACTOMgSO$_4$) study showed a decreased incidence of CP from 8.2% in the untreated group to 6.8% in the group receiving $MgSO_4$ for neuroprotection in patients before 30 weeks' gestation at risk of preterm delivery, although this was not statistically significant.[20] The Beneficial Effects of Antenatal Magnesium Sulfate (BEAM) trial showed a statistically significant decrease in moderate and severe CP in patients treated with $MgSO_4$, from 3.5% to 1.9%, respectively.[22] In the PREterm brain protection by MAGnesium sulfate (PREMAG) trial, the rate of combined death or gross motor dysfunction was

Table 1		
Summary of largest magnesium sulfate neuroprotection trials		
Trial	**Criteria and Characteristics**	**Outcomes**
BEAM Rouse et al,[22] 2008 n = 2336	Time to birth: median 25 h, IQR = 11–63 h Average GA = 28.3 ± 2.5 wk Inclusion criterion: GA 24-0/7 to 31-6/7 wk Exclusion criteria: >8 cm dilated or delivery expected within 2 h	1° outcome: stillbirth or infant death, moderate or severe CP at or beyond 2 y of age 2° outcome: rate of CP[a]
ACTOMgSO$_4$ Crowther et al,[20] 2003 n = 1062	Time to birth: median 3.7 h, IQR = 1.4–13.8 wk Mean GA: 27–3/7 wk, IQR 25-5/7 to 28-5/7 wk Inclusion criterion: GA ≤ 30 wk Exclusion criterion: prior magnesium exposure	1° outcome: death, CP, or death or CP at 2 y of age 2° outcome: substantial gross motor dysfunction or substantial gross motor dysfunction and death[a]
PREMAG Marret et al,[21] 2007 n = 573	Time to birth: median 1.6 h, IQR 0.08–25.08 wk Median GA: 30–1/7 wk Inclusion criterion: GA ≤ 33 wk	1° outcome: severe white matter injury or death before discharge

Abbreviations: ACTOMgSO$_4$, Australasian Collaborative Trial of Magnesium Sulfate; BEAM, Beneficial Effects of Antenatal Magnesium Sulfate; GA, gestational age; IQR, interquartile range.
[a] Statistically significant (only obtained for 2° outcome).
Data from Refs.[20–22]

decreased from 30.8% to 25.6% with $MgSO_4$ treatment of neuroprotection in children at 2 years of age.[21] Initially, PREMAG did not show any difference in mortality or severe CP at hospital discharge in infants delivered before 33 weeks' gestation. Early meta-analyses led to recommendations by the American College of Obstetricians and Gynecologists (ACOG) endorsing the use of $MgSO_4$ for neuroprotection.[23–25,31] Based on individual participant data meta-analysis, the number needed to treat (NNT) to prevent 1 case of CP in surviving infants is 46; considering only trials with neuroprotective intent, the NNT is 43. These findings are independent of preterm delivery, gestational age, or the cumulative dose amount.[29]

American College of Obstetricians and Gynecologists recommendations

The ACOG Committee on Obstetric Practice concluded in 2010 that available cumulative evidence suggests that magnesium reduces the risk of CP.[25] However, the 3 published clinical trials that the recommendations were based on used different treatment regimens (**Table 2**), so the committee recommended physicians using $MgSO_4$ for neuroprotection develop guidelines regarding inclusion criteria, treatment regimens, concurrent tocolysis, and monitoring in accordance with one of the larger clinical trials. A later ACOG practice bulletin concluded that there is level A evidence suggesting that $MgSO_4$ reduces severity and risk of CP when delivery before 32 weeks' gestation is anticipated. It further advised that hospitals electing to provide $MgSO_4$ for fetal neuroprotection should develop uniform, specific guidelines addressing inclusion criteria, treatment regimens, concurrent tocolysis, and monitoring in accordance with one of the larger clinical trials.[45] ACOG Committee Opinion No. 455 (Magnesium Sulfate Before Anticipated Preterm Birth for Neuroprotection) was reaffirmed in 2018 without refinement of the existing recommendations.

Evidence and controversies

There is no consensus on specific $MgSO_4$ dosing. Each of the previously discussed large clinical trials ($ACTOMgSO_4$, PREMAG, and BEAM) used a different protocol with unique inclusion and exclusion criteria. Moreover, query of clinicaltrials.gov does not identify registered trials investigating different dosing protocols. ACOG recommended that physicians develop specific guidelines in accordance with one of the larger published trials.[25] However, differences between the published trials' criteria and treatment regimens (see **Table 2**), combined with real-life heterogeneity in patient presentations, poses an ongoing challenge. Bain and colleagues[27] acknowledged this

---

Table 2
Dosing regimens from the largest magnesium sulfate neuroprotection trials

Study	Loading Dosage	Maintenance Dosage	Repeat Treatment
BEAM Rouse et al,[22] 2008	6 g over 20–30 min	2 g/h until birth or for 12 h	If <6 h since cessation, maintenance restarted. If >6 h, an additional loading dose was given before restarting maintenance
$ACTOMgSO_4$ Crowther et al,[20] 2003	4 g over 20 min	1 g/h until birth or for 24 h	None
PREMAG Marret et al,[21] 2007	4 g over 30 min	None	None

Data from Refs.[20–22]

conundrum and knowledge gaps in their Cochrane Intervention Review, providing 2 interim neuroprotection recommendations for regimens based on (1) published guidelines from the Australian and Canadian Medical Associations and (2) opinion articles. These recommendations (**Table 3**) are distinct from protocols used within the published clinical trials, thereby further expanding the array of endorsed neuroprotective regimens.[26,27]

Given the absence of consensus regarding optimal magnesium dosing for neuroprotection, there have been multiple secondary analyses of existing data and small follow-up studies. A recent individual participant data meta-analysis found minimal variation in outcomes related to time to birth and dosage. Unable to confirm significant benefit with longer administration or higher dosage, it stated that "it would be prudent to restrict administration of antenatal magnesium for fetal neuroprotection to close to the expected or planned birth and to use 4 g, the smallest effective dose, with or without a 1 g/hour maintenance dose."[29] This conclusion is surprising, because it is not supported by a previously published Cochrane meta-analysis performed by many of the same investigators, in which maintenance dosing was associated with reduced CP risk (relative risk [RR], 0.68; 95% confidence interval [CI], 0.51–0.91).[24] In this earlier meta-analysis, a 6-g loading dose and higher dose maintenance were also associated with reduced CP risk (RR, 0.59; 95% CI, 0.40–0.85) and retreatment (permitted only in the BEAM trial) was associated with a further decreased risk ratio of CP of 0.68 (95% CI, 0.54–0.87).[24]

Using data from the BEAM cohort,[40] a model was developed to help predict the optimal serum magnesium concentrations for neuroprotection, incorporating the influence of preeclampsia status and maternal weight. Using maternal serum and umbilical cord blood levels, simulated concentrations at delivery were modeled based on the observed pharmacokinetics and pharmacodynamics for patients receiving $MgSO_4$ or placebo within 12 hours of delivery. In this secondary analysis, there was a statistically significant difference between the two groups, with 23 cases of CP in the $MgSO_4$ group (n = 636, 3.6%) and 81 cases of CP in the placebo group (n = 1269, 6.4%).[40] In normotensive women, the lowest probability of delivering an infant with CP in the study was associated with a serum magnesium level of 4.1 mg/dL, with a target range 3.7 to 4.4 mg/dL. However, only 23 cases of CP occurred in women receiving $MgSO_4$, and there was no dose-response relationship observed when comparing $MgSO_4$ serum levels and CP rates or severity. There also seemed to be

Table 3
Recommended regimens for antenatal magnesium sulfate before very preterm birth for neuroprotection of the fetus

Recommended Regimens	Loading Dosage	Maintenance Dosage	Repeat Treatment
Australian National Practice Guidelines, Canadian Clinical Practice Guidelines	4 g over 20–30 min	1 g/h continued until birth or for 24 h	No immediate repeat doses
Reeves et al,[26] 2011	6 g over 20–30 min	2 g/h continued until birth or for 12 h	If <6 h have elapsed since cessation, restart maintenance. If at least 6 h have elapsed, give an additional loading dose before restarting maintenance

Data from Reeves SA, Gibbs RS, Clark SL. Magnesium for fetal neuroprotection. Am J Obstet Gynecol 2011;204(3):202.e1-4.

no benefit of $MgSO_4$ neuroprotection in the setting of intrapartum infection. In this model, duration of magnesium administration seems to be predictive of neuroprotection outcomes, with the greatest reduction in CP noted in those receiving greater than 18 hours of $MgSO_4$ compared with those who received 12 to 18 hours (8.8% vs 11.7%, respectively), although the primary clinical study was not sufficiently powered to determine statistical significance for this outcome. This model predicts that an average-weight woman would achieve the target serum magnesium level of 4.1 mg/dL in 5.5 hours, whereas it may take up to 3 times longer in obese women.[40]

Antibiotics

A recent Cochrane systematic review assessing antepartum and intrapartum interventions for the prevention of CP found that there was an increase in CP in children born to mothers in preterm labor with intact membranes who received prophylactic antibiotics (RR, 1.82; 95% CI, 0.99–3.32).[30] This RR was based on a single randomized controlled study including 3173 children. Based on the calculated RR, they concluded that prophylactic antibiotics given to women with intact membranes in preterm labor is probably an ineffective intervention with moderate-quality evidence of harm.[30]

CLINICAL MANAGEMENT RECOMMENDATION

Differing protocols for $MgSO_4$ administration used by the recently published studies, combined with a plethora of secondary analyses, have left obstetrics without an evidence-based standard approach to provide intrapartum magnesium for neuroprotection. Based on our opinion, following careful review of published cohort studies using $MgSO_4$, the most effective neuroprotection strategy is to provide women in preterm labor (or anticipated to deliver within 12 hours) an $MgSO_4$ bolus followed by continuous dosing until delivery or until the potential for imminent delivery has dissipated. This load (bolus) and maintenance strategy has been used for multiple decades to provide tocolysis and prevent and treat eclampsia, and has been shown to be safe. Furthermore, women receiving $MgSO_4$ in these earlier trials were also noted to have higher levels of neuroprotection, although this was not statistically significant in the BEAM cohort. Therefore, a continuous dose until delivery or until arrest of preterm labor may be more beneficial in preventing CP. The authors recommend provision of bolus and maintenance-dose $MgSO_4$ to all woman with a pregnancy less than 32 weeks' gestation at risk for imminent delivery, in the absence of absolute maternal contraindications. Although clinical trials excluded women in the second stage of labor (ACTOMgSO4) or those expected to deliver within 2 hours (BEAM), the authors think that $MgSO_4$ for neuroprotection should be offered to all women at risk, given its recognized maternal safety profile, acknowledging that reduced exposure time could limit neuroprotection.

Continuous magnesium infusion is supported by studies showing that cellular magnesium levels equilibrate rapidly.[32] Therefore, effectiveness could be limited if magnesium is not present at levels associated with protection at the time of parturition. The rapid clearance rate in normotensive women also supports the concept and safety of retreatment, as does the finding that retreatment was associated with a decreased risk ratio of CP (RR, 0.68; 95% CI, 0.54–0.87).[24] Pharmacokinetic modeling suggesting it can take between 5.5 and 18 hours for maternal serum magnesium to reach the theoretic optimal levels also supports the concept of dosing by continuous infusion.

Although the literature also does not reflect consensus regarding the dosing of $MgSO_4$ for neuroprotection, personal experience, research, and review of the literature describing MgSO$_4$ use, pharmacokinetics, and patient outcome, including the prevention of neonatal neurologic injury, prompts our proposal of clinical management recommendations. For normotensive women, we recommend MgSO$_4$ administration consistent with the higher end of the published neuroprotection protocols, a 6-g loading dose followed by a 2 g/h maintenance dose, based on published predictive models (**Fig. 2**). This recommendation is grounded on the demonstrated safety of magnesium and on evidence showing that women receiving MgSO$_4$ for neuroprotection have higher clearance rates than women receiving magnesium in the setting of preeclampsia. It follows that this higher dose would also achieve optimal serum magnesium levels more rapidly in the obese population. An abundance of data show an absence of serious side effects, including maternal intensive care unit admission, respiratory/cardiac failure, or death, in the large cohorts of women who received MgSO$_4$ for neuroprotection when at risk for delivery before 32 weeks' gestation in the published clinical trials. In women with preeclampsia and hypertensive disorders, the authors recommend the lower range of dosing used in the clinical cohorts. Our proposed dosing schedule is based on the current status of the literature within and beyond obstetrics, as well as clinical experience and published research from our laboratory and others.

PHARMACOLOGIC THERAPIES UNDER CLINICAL INVESTIGATION

Emerging medical therapies are being tested to help prevent CP at delivery. In broad categories, these include medications designed to increase oxygen supply to the brain using red blood cells or stem cells, neuromodulators, cell membrane stabilizers, and therapies combining different mechanisms of action.

Erythropoietin and Darbepoetin

These hormones are known to act to increase the number of circulating red blood cells, thereby increasing oxygen carrying capacity and neurogenesis. Moreover, iron

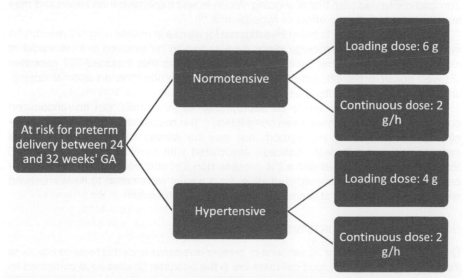

Fig. 2. Algorithm for MgSO4 administration with neuroprotective intent. Loading doses are administered over 30 minutes, with continuous intravenous infusion until delivery or threat of imminent delivery subsides. GA, gestational age.

plays a key role in nerve fiber myelination. Evidence from cord milking and delayed cord clamping studies provides indirect proof of concept as to why these medications may mediate neuroprotection. The ongoing Mild Encephalopathy in the Newborn Treated With Darbepoetin (MEND) trial is currently studying the protective effect of darbepoetin.[10]

Bone Marrow and Mesenchymal Derived Stem Cells

Cellular therapies have been trialed as well and are thought to work by decreasing inflammation and oxidative stress and enhancing regeneration.[10] Experimental animal models have shown that this occurs through various mechanisms using umbilical cord blood cells derived from both bone marrow–derived mesenchymal stem cells (MSCs) and umbilical cord blood–derived MSCs.[46] Both of these MSCs exhibit paracrine effects secreting trophic and immunomodulatory factors that help in brain injury repair. One model of preterm global hypoxic injury showed that intravenous mesenchymal stem cells induced T-cell tolerance.[47] Stem cell therapies are the subject of active clinical trials and have shown much potential with a satisfactory safety profile.[48]

Postnatal Magnesium Sulfate

Magnesium sulfate may also be helpful in neonates postdelivery, although there is inconsistent benefit and little consensus in dose and timing. There is a risk of hypotension and bradycardia with $MgSO_4$, similar to that seen with placental exposure before delivery.[10]

EMERGING PHARMACOLOGIC THERAPIES

Several different neuromodulators are currently being studied in both animal and early human trials. These include vasopressin, endocannabinoids, melatonin, xenon, argon, allopurinol, and topiramate. These medications are hypothesized to decreased glutamate toxicity, NMDA inhibition, enhancement of gamma-aminobutyric acid, and decreased oxidative stress. Melatonin also plays a role in glial development and a randomized controlled pilot trial is ongoing. Argon is less expensive than xenon and may augment the therapeutic effect of hypothermia.[10]

Monosialoganglioside is being investigated for its role in maintaining cell membrane integrity,[39] because ganglioside levels were shown to be reduced in a rat model of neonatal hypoxic ischemic injury.[49] One meta-analysis that included 787 neonates showed possible benefit, although there is limited information on optimal dosing, safety, and long-term outcomes.[50]

Creatine has been shown to be neuroprotective in animals, but no randomized controlled human trials have been completed.[51] The mechanism of action for creatinine is not completely understood, but may be related to the inhibition of the caspase-induced cell death cascade associated with cerebral ischemia. Induced focal ischemia in mice fed with a 2% creatine-rich diet and then exposed to a middle cerebral artery occlusion–mediated injury for 4 weeks were noted to have improved neurologic and behavioral scores 24 hours after reperfusion.[52]

NONPHARMACEUTICAL INTERVENTIONS

Delayed cord clamping of 30 seconds or greater is recommended in preterm infants to increase circulating red blood cell numbers in the neonate. Studies have confirmed its safety, observing decreased delivery room intubation and metabolic acidosis at birth, with less respiratory distress syndrome. Delayed cord clamping was also associated with reduced early blood transfusions and intraventricular hemorrhage.[53,54] It is theorized that delayed cord clamping may act by increasing the oxygen carrying capacity and thereby increasing neonatal brain oxygenation.

Another investigative therapy used for neuroprotection in term and late preterm neonates is therapeutic hypothermia. This therapy should be started within 6 hours of birth and continued for 72 hours. This therapy is only available in some tertiary care centers and is likely not a viable solution in smaller remote community centers. One small study with 31 preterm neonates (34–35 weeks' gestation) showed that therapeutic hypothermia is feasible in this population but is associated with increased rates of complications, including significant differences in hyperglycemia (58.1% vs 31.3%, $P = .03$) and early rewarming (19.4% vs 0%, $P = .009$) compared with 32 term neonates.[55]

Another proposed intervention is remote ischemic preconditioning, which is performed by inducing sublethal ischemia to peripheral tissue remote from the area of damage to induce endogenous repair within the central nervous system. This technique is currently being studied in rat models in which the ischemia is induced in the extremities in order to enhance central endogenous repair. Mediators for this response are thought to include phosphorylation, nitric oxide, transporter regulation, inflammatory response, increased glucose metabolism, and angiogenesis.[56]

EXPERIMENTAL PREDICTORS
Biomarkers

Another field of active research interest is in the identification of biomarkers to predict the likelihood of developing CP. If found to be accurate and reliable, this has the potential to significantly change clinical management. At present, there are no specific marketed biomarkers that are useful in the diagnosis or prediction of CP. Different markers being investigated include S100B (a calcium binding marker that is released by damaged neurons), neuron-specific enolase (released after neuronal death), glial fibrillary acidic protein (released by damaged astroglia), total tau proteins, and ubiquitin carboxyl terminal hydrolase. Inflammatory markers are also being investigated for their ability to predict or diagnose CP, including interleukin (IL)-6, IL-16, IL-8, and vascular endothelial growth factor. Metabolites such as arachidonic acid, butanoic acid, citric acid, lactate, fumaric acid, malate, propanoic acid, and succinic acid are also being considered.[10]

Imaging

Magnetic resonance (MR) spectroscopy is being used to help predict neonatal brain damage but should be performed within 6 hours of delivery in order to be helpful in predicting CP. MR spectroscopy estimates levels of phosphocreatine, inorganic phosphate, or lactate within the brain tissue with levels of phosphocreatine considered protective, whereas high inorganic phosphate and lactate levels are associated with harm.[10] The Magnetic Resonance Biomarkers in Neonatal Encephalopathy (MARBLE) study across 8 neonatal intensive care units in the United States and United Kingdom showed that thalamic proton MR spectroscopy of N-acetyl aspartate concentrations acquired within 14 days of birth in neonates between 36 and 43 weeks' gestation who also received therapeutic hypothermia provided the single best prognostic indicator of CP at 23 months of age.[57]

Discussion

Delivery before 32 weeks' gestation is responsible for approximately one-third of all new cases of CP.[3] The enormous economic and societal costs associated with CP underscores the need for primary and secondary neuroprotection measures. Although this article reviews several promising therapies that are under clinical or preclinical investigation, delayed umbilical cord clamping and antepartum MgSO$_4$ administration are the only interventions shown to be effective at this time. These neuroprotective strategies, in conjunction with antenatal corticosteroid therapy for fetal lung maturity and tocolysis to optimize completion of steroid therapy, are the only effective interventions currently available to decrease the morbidity associated with preterm delivery. The absence of a clear consensus regarding MgSO$_4$ dosing for neuroprotection remains a barrier to widespread implementation. Our recommendation is based on the current status of the literature, clinical experience, and existing research. Further head-to-head comparison trials are needed to determine the best dosing and duration of magnesium therapy in order to provide neuroprotection and prevent CP.

REFERENCES

1. Martin JA, Hamilton BE, Ventura SJ, et al. Births: final data for 2010. Natl Vital Stat Rep 2012;61(1):1–72.
2. Jelin AC, Salmeen K, Gano D, et al. Perinatal neuroprotection update. F1000Res 2016;5.
3. Bax M, Goldstein M, Rosenbaum P, et al. Proposed definition and classification of cerebral palsy, April 2005. Dev Med Child Neurol 2005;47(8):571–6.
4. Winter S, Autry A, Boyle C, et al. Trends in the prevalence of cerebral palsy in a population-based study. Pediatrics 2002;110(6):1220–5.
5. Reddihough DS, Collins KJ. The epidemiology and causes of cerebral palsy. Aust J Physiother 2003;49(1):7–12.
6. Nelson KB, Dambrosia JM, Grether JK, et al. Neonatal cytokines and coagulation factors in children with cerebral palsy. Ann Neurol 1998;44(4):665–75.
7. Leviton A. Preterm birth and cerebral palsy: is tumor necrosis factor the missing link? Dev Med Child Neurol 1993;35:553–8.
8. Girard S, Kadhim H, Roy M, et al. Role of perinatal inflammation in cerebral palsy. Pediatr Neurol 2009;40:168–74.
9. Dammann O, Leviton A. Maternal intrauterine infection, cytokines, and brain damage in the preterm newborn. Pediatr Res 1997;42:1–8.
10. Nair J, Kumar VHS. Current and emerging therapies in the management of hypoxic ischemic encephalopathy in neonates. Children (Basel) 2018;5(7) [pii:E99].
11. Centers for Disease Control and Prevention (CDC). Economic costs associated with mental retardation, cerebral palsy, hearing loss, and vision impairment– United States, 2003. MMWR Morb Mortal Wkly Rep 2004;53(3):57–9.
12. Cahill AG, Odibo AO, Stout MJ, et al. Magnesium sulfate therapy for the prevention of cerebral palsy in preterm infants: a decision-analytic and economic analysis. Am J Obstet Gynecol 2011;205(6):542.e1-7.
13. Shih STF, Tonmukayakul U, Imms C, et al. Economic evaluation and cost of interventions for cerebral palsy: a systematic review. Dev Med Child Neurol 2018; 60(6):543–58.
14. Nelson KB, Grether JK. Can magnesium sulfate reduce the risk of cerebral palsy in very low birthweight infants? Pediatrics 1995;95(2):263–9.
15. Caddell JL, Graziani LJ, Wiswell TE, et al. The possible role of magnesium in protection of premature infants from neurological syndromes and visual impairments and a review of survival of magnesium-exposed premature infants. Magnes Res 1999;12(3):201–16.

16. Duley L, Gülmezoglu AM, Henderson-Smart DJ, et al. Magnesium sulphate and other anticonvulsants for women with pre-eclampsia. Cochrane Database Syst Rev 2010;(11):CD000025.

17. Crowther CA, Brown J, McKinlay CJD, et al. Magnesium sulphate for preventing preterm birth in threatened preterm labour. Cochrane Database of Systematic Reviews 2014;(8). Art. No.: CD001060. 10.1002/14651858.CD001060.pub2.

18. Grimes DA, Nanda K. Magnesium sulfate tocolysis: time to quit. Obstet Gynecol 2006;108:986–9.

19. Mittendorf R, Dambrosia J, Pryde PG, et al. Association between the use of antenatal magnesium sulfate in preterm labor and adverse health outcomes in infants. Am J Obstet Gynecol 2002;186(6):1111–8.

20. Crowther CA, Hiller JE, Doyle LW, et al. Effect of magnesium sulfate given for neuroprotection before preterm birth: a randomized controlled trial. JAMA 2003;290: 2669–76.

21. Marret S, Marpeau L, Zupan-Simunek V, et al. Magnesium sulphate given before very-preterm birth to protect infant brain: the randomised controlled PREMAG trial*. BJOG 2007;114(3):310–8.

22. Rouse DJ, Hirtz DG, Thom E, et al. A randomized, controlled trial of magnesium sulfate for the prevention of cerebral palsy. N Engl J Med 2008;359(9):895–905.

23. Costantine MM, Weiner SJ. Effects of antenatal exposure to magnesium sulfate on neuroprotection and mortality in preterm infants: a meta-analysis. Obstet Gynecol 2009;114:354–64.

24. Doyle LW, Crowther CA, Middleton P, et al. Magnesium sulphate for women at risk of preterm birth for neuroprotection of the fetus. Cochrane Database Syst Rev 2009;(1):CD004661.

25. American College of Obstetricians and Gynecologists Committee on Obstetric Practice, Society for Maternal-Fetal Medicine. Committee opinion no. 455: magnesium sulfate before anticipated preterm birth for neuroprotection. Obstet Gynecol 2010;115(3):669–71.

26. Reeves SA, Gibbs RS, Clark SL. Magnesium for fetal neuroprotection. Am J Obstet Gynecol 2011;204(3):202.e1-4.

27. Bain E, Middleton P, Crowther CA. Different magnesium sulphate regimens for neuroprotection of the fetus for women at risk of preterm birth. Cochrane Database Syst Rev 2012;(2):CD009302.

28. Zeng X, Xue Y, Tian Q, et al. Effects and safety of magnesium sulfate on neuroprotection: a meta-analysis based on PRISMA guidelines. Medicine (Baltimore) 2016;95(1):e2451.

29. Crowther CA, Middleton PF, Voysey M, et al. Assessing the neuroprotective benefits for babies of antenatal magnesium sulphate: an individual participant data meta-analysis. PLoS Med 2017;14(10):e1002398.

30. Shepherd E, Salam RA, Middleton P, et al. Antenatal and intrapartum interventions for preventing cerebral palsy: an overview of Cochrane systematic reviews. Cochrane Database Syst Rev 2017;(8):CD012077.

31. Conde-Agudelo A, Romero R. Antenatal magnesium sulfate for the prevention of cerebral palsy in preterm infants less than 34 weeks' gestation: a systematic review and metaanalysis. Am J Obstet Gynecol 2009;200(6):595–609.

32. Suzuki-Kakisaka H, Sugimoto J, Tetarbe M, et al. Magnesium sulfate increases intracellular magnesium reducing inflammatory cytokine release in neonates. Am J Reprod Immunol 2013;70(3):213–20.

33. Sugimoto J, Romani AM, Valentin-Torres AM, et al. Magnesium decreases inflammatory cytokine production: a novel innate immunomodulatory mechanism. J Immunol 2012;188(12):6338–46.

34. Lecuyer M, Rubio M, Chollat C, et al. Experimental and clinical evidence of differential effects of magnesium sulfate on neuroprotection and angiogenesis in the fetal brain. Pharmacol Res Perspect 2017;5(4).

35. Goñi-de-Cerio F, Alvarez A, Lara-Celador I, et al. Magnesium sulfate treatment decreases the initial brain damage alterations produced after perinatal asphyxia in fetal lambs. J Neurosci Res 2012;90:1932–40.

36. Burd I, Balakrishnan B, Kannan S. Models of fetal brain injury, intrauterine inflammation, and preterm birth. Am J Reprod Immunol 2012;67:287–94.

37. Yuen AW, Sander JW. Can magnesium supplementation reduce seizures in people with epilepsy? A hypothesis. Epilepsy Res 2012;100(1–2):152–6.

38. Maroso M, Balosso S, Ravizza T, et al. Toll-like receptor 4 and high-mobility group box-1 are involved in ictogenesis and can be targeted to reduce seizures. Nat Med 2010;16(4):413–9.

39. Taber EB, Tan L, Chao CR, et al. Pharmacokinetics of ionized versus total magnesium in subjects with preterm labor and preeclampsia. Am J Obstet Gynecol 2002;186(5):1017–21.

40. Brookfield KF, Elkomy M, Su F, et al. Optimization of maternal magnesium sulfate administration for fetal neuroprotection: application of a prospectively constructed pharmacokinetic model to the BEAM cohort. J Clin Pharmacol 2017; 57(11):1419–24.

41. Krauer B, Krauer F. Drug kinetics in pregnancy. Clin Pharmacokinet 1977;2(3):167–81.

42. Chollat C, Sentilhes L, Marret S. Fetal neuroprotection by magnesium sulfate: from translational research to clinical application. Front Neurol 2018;9:247.

43. Nassar AH, Sakhel K, Maarouf H, et al. Adverse maternal and neonatal outcome of prolonged course of magnesium sulfate tocolysis. Acta Obstet Gynecol Scand 2006;85(9):1099–103.

44. Magpie Trial Follow-Up Study Collaborative Group. The Magpie Trial: a randomised trial comparing magnesium sulphate with placebo for pre-eclampsia. Outcome for children at 18 months. BJOG 2007;114(3):289–99.

45. American College of Obstetricians and Gynecologists' Committee on Practice Bulletins—Obstetrics. Practice bulletin no. 171: management of preterm labor. Obstet Gynecol 2016;128(4). e155–164.

46. Mitsialis SA, Kourembanas S. Stem cell-based therapies for the newborn lung and brain: possibilities and challenges. Semin Perinatol 2016;40(3):138–51.

47. Jellema RK, Wolfs TG, Lima Passos V, et al. Mesenchymal stem cells induce T-cell tolerance and protect the preterm brain after global hypoxia-ischemia. PLoS One 2013;8(8):e73031.

48. Nabetani M, Shintaku H, Hamazaki T. Future perspectives of cell therapy for neonatal hypoxic-ischemic encephalopathy. Pediatr Res 2018;83(1–2):356–63.

49. Ramirez MR, Muraro F, Zylbersztejn DS, et al. Neonatal hypoxia–ischemia reduces ganglioside, phospholipid and cholesterol contents in the rat hippocampus. Neurosci Res 2003;46(3):339–47.

50. Sheng L, Li Z. Adjuvant treatment with monosialoganglioside may improve neurological outcomes in neonatal hypoxic-ischemic encephalopathy: a meta-analysis of randomized controlled trials. PLoS One 2017;12(8):e0183490.

51. Dickinson H, Bain E, Wilkinson D, et al. Creatine for women in pregnancy for neuroprotection of the fetus. Cochrane Database Syst Rev 2014;(12):CD010846.

52. Zhu S, Li M, Figueroa BE, et al. Prophylactic creatine administration mediates neuroprotection in cerebral ischemia in mice. J Neurosci 2004;24(26):5909–12.
53. Ruangkit C, Moroney V, Viswanathan S, et al. Safety and efficacy of delayed umbilical cord clamping in multiple and singleton premature infants - a quality improvement study. J Neonatal Perinatal Med 2015;8(4):393–402.
54. Chiruvolu A, Tolia VN, Qin H, et al. Effect of delayed cord clamping on very preterm infants. Am J Obstet Gynecol 2015;213(5):676.e1-7.
55. Rao R, Trivedi S, Vesoulis Z, et al. Safety and short-term outcomes of therapeutic hypothermia in preterm neonates 34-35 weeks gestational age with hypoxic-ischemic encephalopathy. J Pediatr 2017;183:37–42.
56. Adstamongkonkul D, Hess DC. Ischemic conditioning and neonatal hypoxic ischemic encephalopathy: a literature review. Cond Med 2017;1(1):9–16.
57. Lally PJ, Montaldo P, Oliveira V, et al. Magnetic resonance spectroscopy assessment of brain injury after moderate hypothermia in neonatal encephalopathy: a prospective multicentre cohort study. Lancet Neurol 2019;18(1):35–45.

Medications that Cause Fetal Anomalies and Possible Prevention Strategies

Elizabeth Kiernan, MPH, Kenneth L. Jones, MD*

KEYWORDS

- Teratology • Medications • Frequently used drugs during pregnancy

KEY POINTS

- It is commonly, but incorrectly, believed that prenatal exposure to most drugs is a high risk for fetal development.
- It is not possible at the present time to document the safety of drugs in the prenatal period.
- Most of the known human teratogens are associated with a pattern of 3 or more minor anomalies, not a single major malformation.

INTRODUCTION

Before 1960 all birth defects were believed to have a genetic cause. The fetus was thought to occupy a privileged site within an iron-clad uterus, safe from the ravages of the external environment. That all changed in the early 1960s when Lenz in Germany and McBride in Australia suggested that prenatal exposure to a drug, thalidomide, led to serious problems in fetal structural development. Based on increased awareness over the years of the potential danger of a variety of drugs on fetal development, the pendulum has now swung in the opposite direction. Today, most drugs are believed to be harmful to the developing fetus. As a result, during their pregnancy, women with certain chronic diseases that require specific medications often decrease or even discontinue taking a drug that is necessary for their own health, potentially leading to greater harm to the fetus than the drug itself. The purpose of this article is to outline what is known and what is not known about some of the more common pharmacologic agents that pregnant women come into contact with during pregnancy, and to suggest possible prevention strategies.

Disclosure Statement: None.
Department of Pediatrics, University of California, San Diego, 9500 Gilman Drive, Mail Code #0828, La Jolla, CA 92039, USA
* Corresponding author.
E-mail address: klyons@ucsd.edu

Clin Perinatol 46 (2019) 203–213
https://doi.org/10.1016/j.clp.2019.02.003
0095-5108/19/© 2019 Elsevier Inc. All rights reserved.
perinatology.theclinics.com

PHARMACOLOGIC AGENTS COMMONLY TAKEN DURING PREGNANCY

There are many drugs that are used for the treatment of conditions that occur more frequently in women in their childbearing years or for the treatment of diseases that are limited to pregnancy. This article will focus on those medications.

Asthma During Pregnancy

Asthma is the most common chronic condition in pregnant women. Studies show increasing prevalence in the past decade, with estimates of up to 8% of women affected in the United States, and up to 12% affected globally.[1] Asthma control is critically important in helping to maintain a healthy pregnancy, and medications play a key role in treating and preventing exacerbations that can decrease oxygen levels reaching the fetus. Asthma may worsen in the second and third trimesters; consequently, monthly monitoring of asthma and the effectiveness of asthma medications is recommended. Pregnant women may be hesitant to take their asthma medications, but uncontrolled asthma increases risks for complications that affect the mother and child, including preterm delivery, cesarean section, low birth weight, preeclampsia, congenital malformations, gestational diabetes, placenta previa, placental abruption, premature rupture of membranes, neonatal hospitalization, and neonatal death.[1–3] Therefore, adequate treatment of asthma improves pregnancy outcomes.

This section will describe the available data for some of the drugs used most commonly to treat asthma: systemic or oral corticosteroids, inhaled corticosteroids, short-acting beta-agonists (SABAs), such as albuterol, long-acting beta-agonists (LABA), and montelukast. As there are challenges to recruiting pregnant women into clinical trials, data are limited in pregnancy, although this is true for most medications used for any condition during gestation. Although more studies are needed, existing data for these more commonly used asthma medications are generally reassuring for the treatment of pregnant women.

Systemic Corticosteroids

Meta-analysis of studies of systemic corticosteroids such as prednisone have shown mixed results, with one showing no overall increased risk for major malformations, and another concluding there is a 3-fold increased risk for oral clefts.[4] Yet no increased risk for oral clefts was seen in the most recent and largest case-control research from the US National Birth Defects Prevention Study (US NBDPS),[5] leading to the conclusion that there may be a small increased risk for oral clefts with first trimester use of corticosteroids. Increased rates of pregnancy complications such as preterm delivery,[6] low birth weight, preeclampsia, and gestational diabetes have been seen in pregnant women treated with systemic steroids, but these were reduced when studies controlled for maternal disease and disease severity. A recent study concluded that there is little evidence to show that use of systemic corticosteroids independently increases risks for preterm birth, low birth weight, or preeclampsia,[7] although maternal disease is associated with increased risk.

Prednisone is excreted into human milk at very low levels and is thought to be compatible with lactation.[8]

Inhaled Corticosteroids

A meta-analysis did not find an increased risk for major malformations for inhaled corticosteroids in general; nor were risks seen for preterm delivery, low birth weight, or gestational hypertension.[9] Furthermore, studies have not demonstrated an increased risk for gestational diabetes or gestational hypertension.[10] For budesonide in particular, one study of more than 2000 exposed women showed no increased risk for major birth defects overall or for oral clefts, and no increased risk in another study of nearly 3000 women for preterm birth, reduced birth weight or length, or stillbirth.[11] For fluticasone, similar results were seen, no increased risk for major malformations compared with women exposed to other inhaled corticosteroids[12] and stratified by severity.

Because the amounts of inhaled corticosteroids absorbed into the bloodstream and excreted into breastmilk are small, use by a nursing mother is not expected to cause adverse reactions in a breastfed infant.[13]

Albuterol and Other Short-Acting Beta-Agonists

In studies of albuterol-exposed pregnancies, no increased rate of birth defects was seen with first-trimester exposure,[14] although modest increased risks (<2.0 or <3.0) for isolated oral clefts, any cardiac defect, gastroschisis, anorectal or esophageal atresia, or omphalocele[15,16] have been noted in some studies. Additional study is required to discern if these findings are because of SABA exposure, maternal disease, disease severity, or another factor. Research on more than 1800 pregnancies exposed to any SABAs has not revealed increases in rates of preterm delivery, low birth weight, gestational hypertension, or small for gestational age infants.[6]

An expert panel concluded that use of albuterol is compatible with breastfeeding even in the absence of published studies, because of low bioavailability and low maternal serum levels.[17]

Long-Acting Beta-Agonists

First-trimester exposure to LABAs increased the risk for major cardiac defects and "other and unspecified" major malformations[14] in a data linkage study. The authors suggest that this could be because of the medication, to an association with more severe and uncontrolled asthma that is found with LABA users, to chance, or to the fact that some of these malformations are common among preterm infants, and preterm birth occurs more often among LABA users than non-users. Other studies have not found an increased risk for major birth defects with LABA use.[18] Studies conducted on salmeterol exposure in 126 pregnant women compared use with (1) pregnant women who took SABAs and (2) healthy controls, and found no increased risk for major birth defects, preterm birth, or low birth weight.[19]

Similar to albuterol, many experts consider inhaled bronchodilators such as salmeterol and formoterol compatible with breastfeeding because of the low bioavailability and low maternal serum levels after dosing.[20]

Leukotriene Receptor Antagonists

No increased risk for major birth defects was seen in a claims study of 1164 first-trimester-exposed pregnancies,[21] or in a study of 180 exposures reported to 7 teratogen information services.[22] Similar results were seen in a Danish registry study of preconception and first-trimester-exposed pregnancies.[23] This study also showed a higher risk for preeclampsia and gestational diabetes, although these are associated with more severe asthma and likely not specific to montelukast. No increased risk for pregnancy loss, gestational diabetes, preeclampsia, low maternal weight gain, preterm delivery, low Apgar scores, or small size was seen in a study of 96 infants exposed to leukotriene receptor antagonists in pregnancy.[24] Further, no pattern of major anomalies could be identified, and malformation rates were not significantly higher among the infants of asthmatics who took leukotriene receptor antagonists or SABAs. Similarly, no increased risk has been shown for low birth weight, shortened gestational age, preterm delivery, or preeclampsia in studies comparing exposed pregnancies with those of other asthmatic women not exposed to montelukast.[22]

Montelukast is excreted into breastmilk in very low levels[25] and has been used in neonates at levels higher than would be found in milk. No adverse reactions are expected in the infant of a nursing mother taking montelukast.[26]

Drugs Used for Treatment of Nausea and Vomiting of Pregnancy

Ondansetron

Nausea and vomiting of pregnancy (NVP) is the most common medical condition that occurs during pregnancy, with an estimated incidence of 85% of pregnant women.[27] Most of those women take antiemetic drugs to mitigate their symptoms. Based on a study of antiemetic use from an insured population of pregnant women in the United States who delivered live-born babies, Taylor and colleagues[27] observed a marked increase in the use of ondansetron for treatment of NVP from less than 1% of pregnancies in 2001 to 22.25% in 2014.

Ondansetron is a serotonin 5-HT3 receptor antagonist. It was originally marketed for nausea and vomiting associated with chemotherapy, radiation therapy, and surgery. Its use in NVP is off-label. Studies evaluating the effect of ondansetron on fetal development are few and the data are conflicting.

Anderka and colleagues,[28] used data from the US NBDPS to determine if NVP or its treatment was associated with an increased risk for the most common non-cardiac defects including non-syndromic cleft lip with or without cleft palate, cleft palate alone, neural tube defects, and hypospadias. NVP was not associated with any of the 4 non-cardiac defects. However ondansetron was associated with an increased risk for cleft palate alone (adjusted odds ratio = 2.37; 95% CI: 1.18–4.76).

There was one additional study showing an increased risk for structural defects following prenatal exposure to ondansetron. Published by Danielsson and colleagues,[29] data from the Swedish Medical Birth Register combined with the Swedish Register of Prescribed Drugs were used to recruit 1349 infants whose mothers took ondansetron in early pregnancy. Although there was no statistically increased risk for major malformations, the risk for cardiovascular defects, particularly cardiac septal defects, was statistically significantly increased (odds ratio = 1.62, 95% CI: 1.04–2.14 and relative risk = 2.05, 95% CI: 1.19–3.28). No cases of cleft palate were reported in the offspring of exposed women in that study.

Three other studies have shown the opposite result.

Based on a study using data from the Medical Birth Registry and the National Patient Registry in Denmark, Pasternak and colleagues,[30] compared major birth defect outcomes among the offspring of 1233 women exposed to ondansetron in the first trimester compared with the offspring of 4932 unexposed women. Prenatal exposure to ondansetron was not associated with an increased risk when compared with the offspring of unexposed women for any major malformation (2.9% and 2.9%, respectively; prevalence odds ratio, 1.12; 95% CI: 0.69–1.82). Einarson and colleagues[31] published data from a prospective comparison study involving 176 pregnancy outcomes in women taking ondansetron in the first trimester, 176 women taking another antiemetic, and 176 women with non-teratogenic exposures. There were no statistically significant differences in the prevalence of major malformations in the 3 groups.

Fejzo and colleagues[32] reported pregnancy outcome in 1070 women who took ondansetron in pregnancy for the treatment of hyperemesis gravidarum

(HG) compared with pregnancy outcome in 771 pregnant women with a history of HG, but who reported no ondansetron exposure and 1555 pregnant women with no HG and no ondansetron exposure. There was no difference in major malformations in the HG/ondansetron group compared with the HG/No ondansetron group.

Based on the sparsity of studies and the lack of agreement between the studies that are available, it is not possible to state whether ondansetron is associated with a small risk for cleft palate or for cardiac defects. However, given the large number of women who are taking this drug during the first trimester of their pregnancy, more research into its prenatal effects is critical.

Drugs Used for the Treatment of Hyperthyroidism During Pregnancy

The presence of clinical hyperthyroidism in the childbearing years occurs in from 0.1% to 0.4%, and the most common cause is Graves' disease.[33] Graves' disease is an autoimmune disease in which an individual's own immune system makes thyrotropin receptor antibodies that bind to receptors on the surface of thyroid cells and cause them to overproduce and release thyroid hormone.[34] Methimazole (MMI)/carbimazole (CMZ), and propylthiouracil are the drugs of choice for hyperthyroidism in pregnancy.[35]

Primarily case reports and a few epidemiologic studies have shown that MMI/CMZ is a human teratogen when taken during the first trimester of pregnancy, although the occurrences are rare. Milham and Elledge first suggested, in 1972, that MMI was a human teratogen based on the observation that 2 of 11 newborns with midline scalp defects were born to women treated with MMI for the treatment of hyperthyroidism during pregnancy.[36] Thereafter Clementi and colleagues[37] suggested that MMI was associated with a specific pattern of structural defects. Identical features have been associated with CMZ, which is converted to MMI after absorption. It has been suggested that the critical window for exposure is between the third and ninth gestational weeks. The pattern of malformations documented in 72 case reports comprise: ectodermal defects including scalp aplasia cutis congenita, aplasia/hypothelia, and hypoplastic/dystrophic nails; gastrointestinal defects including esophageal atresia, hypoplastic/absent gall bladder, and patent omphalomesenteric duct; *abdominal wall defects* including omphalocele and gastroschisis, as well as other anomalies including choanal atresia, coloboma, heart defects, renal anomalies, and intellectual disability in 60% of cases.[37]

Propylthiouracil

Andersen and colleagues[38] evaluated the presence of birth defects in the offspring of women who redeemed a prescription for propylthiouracil (PTU) from a nationwide registry of all children born in Denmark from 1996 to 2008. Fourteen children with birth defects were identified following PTU exposure early in pregnancy. Of those 14 children, 7 had defects involving the face and neck and 7 had defects involving the urinary tract. Among those children the adjusted hazard ratio (HR) for children having a defect of the face and neck was 4.92 (95% CI: 2.04–11.86) and for the urinary system the adjusted HR was 2.73 (95% CI: 1.22–6.07).

Of the 7 children with a birth defect of the face and neck, most had a preauricular or branchial fistula/cyst, and of the 7 children with urinary tract defects most had a single cyst of the kidney or hydronephrosis.

This study is in contrast to 3 previous studies that showed no increase in the risk of birth defects in offspring of women using PTU in pregnancy.[39–41]

Treatment of Pain and Fever During Pregnancy

Acetaminophen (paracetamol)

Acetaminophen is the most common drug used in pregnancy for the treatment of pain and fever. Various studies have shown that the drug is used by up to 60% of women at some time during their pregnancy.[42] Several studies have recently evaluated neurobehavioral outcome in children prenatally exposed to acetaminophen. Although the results of these studies have varied, there is clearly reason that the effect of prenatal exposure to this drug on neurodevelopment needs to be more fully studied.

A study published in 2013 used data from the Norwegian Mother and Child Cohort Study, which included 2919 same-sex sibling pairs who were used to adjust for familial and genetic factors.[43] A total of 134 (4.6%) were discordant for prenatal exposure to acetaminophen for ≥28 days during the pregnancy and 805 were discordant for prenatal exposure for less than 28 days. Those children prenatally exposed for ≥28 days had poorer gross motor development, poorer communication skills, externalizing and internalizing behavioral problems, and higher activity levels. Those prenatally exposed for less than 28 days had poorer gross motor functioning.

Another study evaluated neurobehavioral development using 64,322 live-born children and their mothers enrolled in the Danish National Birth Cohort.[44] Children prenatally exposed to acetaminophen during pregnancy were at higher risk for receiving a hospital diagnosis of hyperkinetic disorder (HR = 1.37; 95% CI: 1.15–1.59); having attention-deficit/hyperactivity disorder-like behaviors at age 7 years (relative risk = 1.13; 95% CI: 1.01–1.27); and use of attention-deficit/hyperactivity disorder medications (HR = 1.29; CI: 1.15–1.44). There was a stronger association observed with use of the drug in more than one trimester of pregnancy.

Language development at 30 months of age was evaluated in the offspring of 754 women who enrolled in the Swedish Environmental Longitudinal, Mother and Child, Asthma and Allergy study.[45] Language delay in girls but not in boys at 30 months of age was noted to be associated with prenatal exposure to acetaminophen in the first trimester of pregnancy. Similarly, first-trimester exposure to acetaminophen was associated with poorer overall attention scores in childhood and parent-rated subnormal executive function. The risk was increased with longer duration of exposure during pregnancy.

A study of the prenatal use of acetaminophen on child IQ provides further reason to suggest that a study to more appropriately evaluate the effect of this drug on neurodevelopment needs to be done. Data from the Danish National Birth Cohort was used to assess the prenatal effect of maternal fever and acetaminophen on the IQ of the child.[46] Children born to mothers who took acetaminophen without fever had on average a 3.4 lower performance IQ compared with those born to women who neither took acetaminophen nor had fever during their pregnancy. In addition, women who experienced fever, but did use acetaminophen during pregnancy, scored lower on verbal and performance IQ. However, for women with fever who took acetaminophen during pregnancy, there was no effect on IQ score suggesting that by decreasing the fever its effect on child IQ was lessened.

In summary, although the prenatal effect of this drug on fetal neurodevelopment may be small, the large number of women taking this drug during pregnancy raises concern that its impact may be great.

Depression During Pregnancy

Depression is one of the most common conditions occurring in pregnancy, with a prevalence of greater than 10%. The most common drugs used for the treatment of depression during pregnancy are the selective serotonin reuptake inhibitors (SSRIs). A study conducted by the US NBDPS evaluated pregnancy outcome following maternal exposure to 5 SSRIs including fluoxetine, paroxetine, citalopram, escitalopram, and sertraline from 1 month before conception through the third month of pregnancy.[47] A Bayesian analysis was used in that study to interpret new data in the context of previous reports. The authors reviewed the medical literature to find previous reports of specific birth defects noted in association with prenatal exposure to an SSRI that was included in the US NBDPS. They found no association with prenatal exposure to citalopram or escitalopram monotherapy for any or the 5 birth defects seen in previous reports, including anencephaly, cardiac septal defects, anal atresia, any limb reduction defect, or omphalocele. However, for the 7 previously reported birth defects associated with prenatal exposure to paroxetine, significant associations were seen in 5 of them, including anencephaly, atrial septal defect, right ventricular outflow tract obstruction, gastroschisis, and omphalocele. No association was seen for cleft palate or hypospadias. It was concluded from that study that the various SSRIs need to be evaluated separately as opposed to as a group with respect to pregnancy outcome, and that, although the data were reassuring relative to pregnancy outcome for some of the SSRIs, there was concern for others.

In addition, a study by Chambers and colleagues[48] has documented the risk for persistent pulmonary hypertension of the newborn (PPHN) following late third-trimester exposure to fluoxetine. In that study, 377 infants with PPHN and 836 control infants were ascertained through the Slone Epidemiology Center. Fourteen of the infants had been exposed to an SSRI after completion of the 20th week of gestation as opposed to 6 control infants (adjusted odds ratio, 6.1; 95% CI: 2.2–16.8). None of the infants with SSRI exposure before the 20th week of gestation developed PPHN. These observations have some biologic plausibility. It is known that SSRIs accumulate in the lung and have vasoconstrictive capabilities. Secondly SSRIs are known to inhibit the synthesis of nitric oxide, which is a vasodilator that regulates vascular tone.

Finally, it is important to realize that increased risk with regard to pregnancy outcome in women taking antidepressants must always take into consideration the extent of untreated maternal depression on pregnancy outcome. A study documenting relapse of major depression during pregnancy in women who maintained or discontinued antidepressant treatment is particularly relevant.[49] Of the 82 women in that study who continued to take their antidepressant medication during pregnancy, 21 (26%) of them relapsed, as opposed to 44 (68%) of the 65 women who discontinued their medication during pregnancy, a statistically significant difference.

POSSIBLE PREVENTION STRATEGIES

The U.S. Food and Drug Administration has the responsibility for protection of and promotion of public health through the control and supervision of, among other things, medications (prescription and over-the-counter pharmaceutical drugs). The safety of medication use during pregnancy represents a unique situation. Giving a woman a medication during pregnancy to test whether the drug causes birth defects or other adverse pregnancy outcomes is impossible to justify. Therefore, it becomes necessary to resort to post-marketing surveillance studies to determine the safety of medications during pregnancy.

In 1985, a multicenter prospective cohort methodology using the Organization of Teratology Services (OTIS) for the identification of human teratogens was established.[50] Twenty Teratology Information Services were established through the United States and Canada with the purpose of providing information about the risk of adverse pregnancy outcome to women contemplating pregnancy, pregnant and breastfeeding women and their physicians, as well as to gain new information about the effect of medications about which pregnancy outcome data are unknown. The formation of this organization has facilitated communication among individual programs, has allowed for access to common database information, has increased public visibility of the individual services and has provided a forum for utilizing prospective pregnancy outcome data in a scientific manner that can be provided to the public. With respect to the latter, this cohort study design allows for documentation of a wide range of adverse pregnancy outcomes including spontaneous abortion, intrauterine growth retardation, prematurity, intellectual disability, and birth defects. Although the sample size of the studies limits in most cases the identification of an increased risk for single major malformations, the capability to do careful dysmorphology examinations, blind to prenatal exposure of the child, provides the ability to identify a specific pattern of minor anomalies. This is particularly important in that most of the known human teratogens are associated with a pattern of 3 or more minor anomalies, not a single major malformation. Through the use of this methodology OTIS studies have been used to document the risk or lack of risk of a number of agents. Clearly there are many limitations of this methodology including the use of volunteer subjects; the bias that could occur as a result of prenatal diagnosis (this has been dealt with by excluding women who have already had prenatal diagnosis before recruitment); the assessment of spontaneous abortion. (Most women who enroll in the study do so after pregnancy recognition. Therefore the relative risk for spontaneous abortion is confined to late first- or early second-trimester occurrences.)

There are some very important advantages about the OTIS methodology, particularly when it comes to counseling women contemplating pregnancy who have a concern about a particular medication they are taking. An increasing number of women are contacting OTIS services in the preconception period. Communicating with those women gives Teratology Information Specialists the opportunity to provide women information that can have a major impact on their risk of having a child with birth defects and other adverse pregnancy outcomes.

REFERENCES

1. Murphy VE. Managing asthma in pregnancy. Breathe (Sheff) 2015;11:258–67.
2. Murphy V, Wang G, Namazy J, et al. The risk of congenital malformations, perinatal mortality and neonatal hospitalisation among pregnant women with asthma: a systematic review and meta-analysis. BJOG 2013;120:812–22.
3. Wang G, Murphy VE, Namazy J, et al. The risk of maternal and placental complications in pregnant women with asthma: a systematic review and meta-analysis. J Matern Fetal Neonatal Med 2014;27(9):934–42.
4. Park-Wyllie L, Mazzotta P, Pastuszak A, et al. Birth defects after maternal exposure to corticosteroids: prospective cohort study and meta-analysis of epidemiological studies. Teratology 2000;62:385–92.
5. Skuladottir H, Wilcox AJ, Ma C, et al. Corticosteroid use and risk of orofacial clefts. Birth Defects Res A Clin Mol Teratol 2014;100(6):499–506.
6. Schatz M, Dombrowski MP, Wise R, et al, for The National Institute of Child Health and Development Maternal-Fetal Medicine Units Network and The National Heart, Lung, and Blood Institute. The relationship of asthma medication use to perinatal outcomes. J Allergy Clin Immunol 2004;113(6):1040–5.

7. Bandoli G, Palmsten K, Forbess Smith CJ, et al. A review of systemic corticosteroid use in pregnancy and the risk of select pregnancy and birth outcomes. Rheum Dis Clin North Am 2017;43(3):489–502.

8. LactMed. 2018. Available at: Toxnet.nlm.nih.gov; https://toxnet.nlm.nih.gov/cgi-bin/sis/search2/f?./temp/~AywlHw:1. Accessed August 12, 2018.

9. Rahimi R, Nikfar S, Abdollahi M. Meta-analysis finds use of inhaled corticosteroids during pregnancy safe: a systematic meta-analysis review. Hum Exp Toxicol 2006;25(8):447–52.

10. Lee C-H, Kim J, Jang EJ, et al. Inhaled corticosteroids use is not associated with an increased risk of pregnancy-induced hypertension and gestational diabetes mellitus: two nested case-control studies. Medicine 2016;95(22):e3627.

11. Norjavaara E, de Verdier MG. Pregnancy outcomes in a population-based study including 2968 pregnant women exposed to budesonide. J Allergy Clin Immunol 2003;111(4):736–42.

12. Charlton RA, Snowball JM, Nightingale AL, et al. Safety of fluticasone propionate prescribed for asthma during pregnancy: a UK population-based cohort study. J Allergy Clin Immunol 2015;3(5):772–9.e3.

13. LactMed. 2018. Available at: Toxnet.nlm.nih.gov; https://toxnet.nlm.nih.gov/cgi-bin/sis/search2/f?./temp/~Qg2Z2g:2 https://toxnet.nlm.nih.gov/cgi-bin/sis/search2/f?./temp/~Qg2Z2g:4. Accessed August 12, 2018.

14. Eltonsy S, Forget A, Blais L. Beta2-agonists use during pregnancy and the risk of congenital malformations. Birth Defects Res A Clin Mol Teratol 2011;91:937–47.

15. Munsie JW, Lin S, Browne ML, et al. Maternal bronchodilator use and the risk of orofacial clefts. Hum Reprod 2011;26(11):3147–54.

16. Lin S, Munsie JPW, Herdt-Losavio ML, et al. Maternal asthma medication use and the risk of selected birth defects. Pediatrics 2012;129(2):e317–24.

17. LactMed. 2018. Available at: Toxnet.nlm.nih.gov; https://toxnet.nlm.nih.gov/cgi-bin/sis/search2/f?./temp/~IfiZKV:1. Accessed August 12, 2018.

18. Wilton LV, Pearce GL, Martin RM, et al. The outcomes of pregnancy in women exposed to newly marketed drugs in general practice in England. Br J Obstet Gynaecol 1998;105:882–9.

19. Jones KL, Johnson DL, D Van Maarseveen N, et al. Salmeterol use and pregnancy outcome: a prospective multi-center study. J Allergy Clin Immunol 2002; 109(1):S156.

20. LactMed. 2018. Available at: Toxnet.nlm.nih.gov; https://toxnet.nlm.nih.gov/cgi-bin/sis/search2/f?./temp/~LKPv2F:5. Accessed August 12, 2018.

21. Nelsen LM, Shields KE, Cunningham ML, et al. Congenital malformations among infants born to women receiving montelukast, inhaled corticosteroids, and other asthma medications. J Allergy Clin Immunol 2012;129(1):251–4.e1-6.

22. Sarkar M, Koren G, Kalra S, et al. Montelukast use during pregnancy: a multi-centre, prospective, comparative study of infant outcomes. Eur J Clin Pharmacol 2009;65:1259–64.

23. Cavero-Carbonell C, Vinkel-Hansen A, Rabanque-Hernández MJ, et al. Fetal exposure to montelukast and congenital anomalies: a population based study in Denmark. Birth Defects Res 2017;109:452–9.

24. Bakhireva LN, Jones KL, Schatz M, et al, Organization of Teratology Information Specialists Collaborative Research Group. Safety of leukotriene receptor antagonists in pregnancy. J Allergy Clin Immunol 2007;119:618–25.

25. Datta P, Rewers-Felkins K, Baker T, et al. Transfer of montelukast into human milk during lactation. Breastfeed Med 2017;12(1):54–7.

26. LactMed. 2018. Available at: Toxnet.nlm.nih.gov; https://toxnet.nlm.nih.gov/cgi-bin/sis/search2. Accessed August 13, 2018.

27. Taylor LG, Bird ST, Sahin L, et al. Antiemetic use among pregnant in the United States; the escalating use of ondansetron. Pharmacoepidemiol Drug Saf 2017; 26:592–6.

28. Anderka M, Mitchell AA, Louik C, et al. Medications used to treat nausea and vomiting of pregnancy and the risk of selected birth defects. Birth Defects Res A Clin Mol Teratol 2012;94:22–30.

29. Danielsson B, Wikner BN, Kallen K. Use of Ondansetron during pregnancy and congenital malformations in the infant. Reprod Toxicol 2014;50:134–7.

30. Pasternak B, Svanstrom H, Hviid A. Ondansetron in pregnancy and risk of adverse fetal outcomes. N Engl J Med 2013;368:814–23.

31. Einarson A, Maltepe C, Nsavioz Y, et al. The safety of Ondansetron for nausea and vomiting pf pregnancy: a prospective comparison study. BJOG 2004;111: 940–3.

32. Fejzo MS, MacGibbon KW, Mullen PM. Ondansetron in pregnancy and risk of adverse fetal outcomes in the United States. Reprod Toxicol 2002;62:87–91.

33. Mestman JH. Hyperthyroidism in pregnancy. Best Pract Res Clin Endocrinol Metab 2004;18:267–88.

34. Menconi F, Marcocci C, Marino M. Diagnosis and classification of Graves' disease. Autoimmun Rev 2014;13:398–402.

35. Clementi M, Di Gianantonio E, Cassina M, et al. Treatment of hyperthyroidism in pregnancy and birth defects. J Clin Endocrinol Metab 2010;95:E337–41.

36. Melham S, Elledge W. Maternal methimazole and congenital defects in children. Teratology 1972;5:125–6.

37. Jones KL, Jones MC, del Campo M. Smith's recognizable patterns of human malformation. 7th edition. Philadelphia: Elsevier; 2013. p. 744–5.

38. Andersen SL, Olsen J, Wu CS, et al. Severity of birth defects after propylthiouracil exposure in early pregnancy. Thyroid 2014;24:1533–40.

39. Yoshihara A, Noh J, Yamaguchi T, et al. Treatment of Graves' disease with antithyroid drugs in the first trimester of pregnancy and the prevalence of congenital malformations. J Clin Endocrinol Metab 2012;97:2396–403.

40. Rosenfeld H, Ornoy A, Shechtman S, et al. Pregnancy outcome, thyroid dysfunction, and fetal goiter after in utero exposure to propylthiouracil: a controlled cohort study. Br J Clin Pharmacol 2009;68:609–17.

41. Chen CH, Xirasagar S, Lin CC, et al. Risk of adverse perinatal outcomes with antithyroid treatment during pregnancy: a nationwide population-bases. BJOG 2011; 118:1365–73.

42. Werler MM, Mitchell AA, Hernandez-Diaz S, et al. Use of over-the-counter medications during pregnancy. Am J Obstet Gynecol 2005;193:771–7.

43. Brandlistuen RE, Ystrom E, Nulman I, et al. Prenatal paracetamol exposure and child neurodevelopment: a sibling-controlled cohort study. Int J Epidemiol 2013;42:1702–13.

44. Liew Z, Ritz B, Rebordosa C, et al. Acetaminophen use during pregnancy, behavioral problems and hyperkinetic disorders. JAMA Pediatr 2014;168:313–20.

45. Bornehag C-G, Reichenberg A, Hallerback MU, et al. Prenatal exposure to acetaminophen and children's language development at 30 months. Eur Psychiatry 2018;51:98–103.

46. Liew Z, Ritz B, Virk J, et al. Prenatal use of acetaminophen and child IQ: a Danish cohort study. Epidemiology 2016;27:912–8.

47. Reefhuis J, Devine O, Friedman JM, et al. Specific SSRIs and birth defects: Bayesian analysis to interpret new data in the context of previous reports. BMJ 2015;350:h3190.
48. Chambers CD, Hernandez S, Van Marter LJ, et al. Selective serotonin-reuptake inhibitors and risk of persistent pulmonary hypertension of the newborn. N Engl J Med 2006;354:579–87.
49. Cohen LS, Altshuler LL, Harlow BL, et al. Relapse of major depression during pregnancy in women who maintain of discontinue antidepressant treatment. JAMA 2006;295:295–507.
50. Chambers CH, Braddock SR, Briggs GG, et al. Post marketing surveillance for human teratogenicity: a model approach. Teratology 2001;64:252–61.

Safety of Psychotropic Medications During Pregnancy

Edwin R. Raffi, MD, MPH*, Ruta Nonacs, MD, PhD, Lee S. Cohen, MD

KEYWORDS

- Perinatal reproductive psychiatry • Women's mental health • Pregnancy
- Psychopharmacology • Perinatal addiction

KEY POINTS

- Common psychiatric disorders during pregnancy and risks of no treatment in patients with moderate and severe disorder, including substance use disorders are reviewed.
- Selecting the best medications during pregnancy and the reproductive safety of psychotropic medications is discussed.
- Management of substance use disorders in pregnancy using medication-assisted treatments is explored.

INTRODUCTION

The objective of this article is to discuss the safety and efficacy of psychotropic medications during pregnancy. The common disorders and the risks of not receiving treatment of certain psychiatric conditions, including substance use disorders (SUDs), also are discussed.

Pregnancy is a time of stress. Stressing the nervous system—whether positive stress (eg, weddings and graduations) or negative stress, also referred to as distress

Disclosure Statement: Dr E.R. Raffi has no disclosure for any relationship with a commercial company that has a direct financial interest in subject matter or materials discussed in article or with a company making a competing product. Dr R. Nonacs: Simon & Schuster. Dr L.S. Cohen: Research support for the National Pregnancy Registry for Atypical Antipsychotics (tAlkermes Biopharmaceuticals; Forest/Actavis Pharmaceuticals; Otsuka Pharmaceuticals; Sunovion Pharmaceuticals, Inc.; and Teva Pharmaceutical Industries). Other research support: Brain & Behavior Research Foundation; JayMac Pharmaceuticals; National Institute on Aging; National Institutes of Health; and SAGE Therapeutics. Advisory/Consulting: Alkermes Biopharmaceuticals (through MGH Clinical Trials Network Initiative).
Perinatal and Reproductive Psychiatry Program, Massachusetts General Hospital Center for Women's Mental Health, Harvard Medical School, Simches Research Building, 185 Cambridge Street, Suite 2200, Boston, MA 02114, USA
* Corresponding author.
E-mail address: eraffi@mgh.harvard.edu

Clin Perinatol 46 (2019) 215–234
https://doi.org/10.1016/j.clp.2019.02.004
0095-5108/19/© 2019 Elsevier Inc. All rights reserved.

(eg, loss of a loved one)—can precipitate psychiatric symptoms, especially in a mental health–vulnerable individual. Data show that pregnancy does not protect against relapse of symptoms in disorders, such as depression.[1]

Treatment recommendations for patients often are individualized. When developing a management plan, the provider should consider the patient's detailed psychiatric history: diagnostic work-up, previous treatment regimens that have failed, treatment modalities that have resulted in achieving euthymia (including past and current medication responses), current presentation, history of mental health during previous pregnancies, family history, social history, substance use history, and the timeline during which the course of treatment is proposed (whether or not the patient currently is pregnant or planning a pregnancy and so forth).

We will first start by reviewing common psychiatric disorders during pregnancy and risk of no treatment followed by a discussion of psychotropic medications in 6 drug categories as follows:

1. Considering psychopharmacology during pregnancy: common psychiatric disorders and risk of no treatment
2. Antidepressant medications, including selective serotonin reuptake inhibitors (SSRIs), serotonin-norepinephrine uptake inhibitors (SNRIs), bupropion, and other antidepressants
3. Mood-stabilizing medications, including lithium, lamotrigine, valproic acid, other antiepileptic mood stabilizers, and antipsychotics as mood stabilizers
4. Antipsychotic medications, both typical antipsychotics and atypical antipsychotics
5. Anxiolytic/sedative hypnotic medications, including benzodiazepines, gabapentin, and other anxiolytics
6. Stimulants in pregnancy
7. Medication-assisted treatment (MAT) of SUDs, including opioid use disorders (OUDs), alcohol use disorder, smoking cessation, and cocaine/stimulant use disorder

If patient and provider decide to use pharmacologic treatment during pregnancy, efforts should be made to

- Select medications that have a well-studied reproductive safety profile. Ideally, all women of reproductive age should be continued on medication regimens that are safe in case of an unplanned pregnancy.
- Make modifications to medication regimens prior to pregnancy when possible, to confirm a stable and euthymic state on the new regimen prior to conception
- Limit the number of medication exposures to the fetus during pregnancy by maximizing 1 medication at effective doses instead of using multiple medications at lower doses.

In December 2014, the Food and Drug Administration (FDA) published the Content and Format of Labeling for Human Prescription Drug and Biological Products; Requirements for Pregnancy and Lactation Labeling, referred to as the Pregnancy and Lactation Labeling Rule.[2] This new system removes the previous letter categories—A, B, C, D, and X—as a means of determining medication safety for treatment of pregnant and lactating mothers. It requires a change to the content of the prescription drug labeling, which would now have to include up-to-date data to allow providers and mothers to make educated decisions.[2] As such, the following information aims to help providers guide patients in their decision-making process within the new and improved FDA guidelines.

Considering Psychopharmacology During Pregnancy: Common Psychiatric Disorders and Risk of No Treatment

When making considerations for treatment, variables to consider are severity of underlying disorder (during current episode and in the past), history of response to treatment, and patient preference and attitude toward treatment. The effect of maternal psychiatric illness (eg, depression) on fetal and neonatal well-being must be taken into account in the risk-benefit decision-making process with respect to use or choice to defer use of medication (ie, no treatment).[3–7]

Discontinuation of medication can be considered for people with a history of mild psychiatric illness. This change ideally should be done in conjunction with continuation or addition of nonpharmacologic treatments modalities.[8] In treatment of depression, for example, such modalities can include supportive therapy, cognitive-behavior therapy, or interpersonal therapy.[9–12]

Many women with history of depression who discontinue antidepressant medications during pregnancy may experience recurrent symptoms.[13] In a prospective study of 201 women, Cohen and colleagues[1] showed that patients who discontinued their antidepressants were 5 times more likely to relapse (rate of relapse of 68%) compared with women who maintained their antidepressants across pregnancy. This study also showed that 26% of women who continue antidepressants had a relapse of major depressive disorder during pregnancy.

Bipolar illness in pregnant patients carries a high risk of poor prenatal outcomes,[14,15] including but not limited to risk of self-harm, substance use, and poor compliance with prenatal care. Relapse rates in women with bipolar disorder are high in women who discontinue mood stabilizers proximate to conception (71% according to 1 study[15]).

Emergence of psychosis during pregnancy is an obstetric and psychiatric emergency. Psychosis could pose a risk to the mother and her infant. It can also hinder a patient's capability to participate in prenatal care or cooperate with care during delivery.[16,17]

More than 10% of women experience clinically significant symptoms of anxiety during pregnancy,[18] particularly during the first trimester. Pathologic anxiety has been correlated with a variety of poor obstetric outcomes, including increased rates of premature labor, low Apgar scores, and placental abruption.[19]

Many women with polysubstance use disorder are likely to attempt to abstain from using during pregnancy.[20] Continued use or relapse of SUD during pregnancy, however, can have devastating results.

Illicit opioid use is most prominent in the under-25 age group, which includes women of reproductive age. Withdrawal from opioids is known to cause premature labor, miscarriages, and fetal distress. There also is an increased risk for relapse, overdose, and death by patients who go through withdrawals.[21] In addition to OUD, alcohol use disorder (leading to fetal alcohol syndrome), cocaine/stimulant use disorder, nicotine use disorder, and other substances pose a danger to the health of young women of reproductive age and their fetuses during pregnancy.

Early screening, diagnosis, and intervention prior to and/or during pregnancy often reduce morbidity and mortality of mental health disorders for mothers and infants.

Pharmacologic treatment is usually recommended when nonpharmacologic strategies have not been efficacious and/or the risks of being psychiatrically ill during pregnancy might outweigh the benefits of nontreatment or the risks of fetal exposure to the medication.

Clinicians should attempt to make modifications to medication regimens prior to pregnancy to confirm a stable and euthymic state on the new regimen prior to conception. The goal also should be to limit the number of medications exposures to infant during pregnancy. Maximizing 1 medication at affective doses is preferred to using more medications at lower doses.

Regardless of whether or not medication is used, vulnerable patients should be monitored closely because they are at a high risk for relapse during pregnancy and in the postpartum period.

ANTIDEPRESSANT MEDICATIONS
Risks Associated with Fetal Exposure to Antidepressant Medications

Most studies related to fetal risks associated with antidepressant use during pregnancy have been on SSRIs and tricyclic antidepressants (TCAs.) These studies have provided reassurance that SSRI medications, as a group, are not considered teratogenic[5,22,23]; however, research on the complete safety profile of these medications remains ongoing.

Although the relative safety of this class of medication with respect to fetal exposure has been reported,[24–26] other reports have described adverse perinatal outcomes, such as decreased gestational age, poor neonatal adaptation, and low birthweight. These studies are controversial, however, because other investigators have not observed the same associations.[27–29] Side effects, such as neurocognitive sequelae, are controversial at best, and further investigations are needed to determine if these are a direct result of antidepressants or of other confounders, such as parental ailment.[30–32]

A majority of reports studying the potential adverse outcomes of peripartum exposure to SSRI medications have been limited by nonsystematic assessment of infant outcomes, nonblinded raters, and small sample sizes. Most of such studies fail to assess the impact of other confounders, especially maternal depression or other psychiatric comorbidities, which by themselves can be associated with compromised perinatal outcomes.[33]

Neonatal adaptation is of some concern with antidepressant medications.[34] Symptoms include jitteriness, tachypnea, tremulousness, which usually are mild, are transient, and resolve without much medical intervention within the first few days of birth. It is important for pediatricians to be aware of infants' exposure and monitor them for supportive therapy.

Some studies have associated SSRI use in late pregnancy with persistent pulmonary hypertension of the newborn (PPHN), a serious and rare developmental lung condition. Chambers and colleagues[35] reported the risk of PPHN with exposure to SSRIs after 20 weeks at approximately 1%. Multiple large studies, however, have shown there is much lower risk of PPHN or no association at all between SSRI use and PPHN.[36,37] A large Medicaid database studied 3.8 million pregnancy outcomes and demonstrated that the risk of PPHN was 0.3% for women who were treated with SSRIs versus 0.2% among the nonexposed.[38] PPHN is correlated with multiple other risk factors that are not associated with SSRI use, such as cesarean delivery, race, and body mass index.[38]

There are fewer reports and sparse research conducted on the long-term sequelae of prenatal antidepressant exposure. In children (followed through early childhood), exposure to fluoxetine, venlafaxine, TCAs, or no medication has shown no differences in behavioral or cognitive development. These measures include IQ, language, temperament, behavior, reactivity, mood, distractibility, and activity level.[39,40] At least 1 study has shown no difference between children exposed to fluoxetine or TCAs during pregnancy and those not exposed in relation to the neurocognitive measures discussed preivously.[28,39]

Although some studies have reported that autism spectrum disorders, anxiety, and attention-deficit disorder (ADD) are more common in antidepressant-exposed children,[41] these studies do not account for many confounders, perhaps the most important of which is maternal psychiatric illness as a major contributing confounder.[42,43] The intuitive notion that the higher prevalence of these disorders is likely due to genetics or maternal illness is supported by studies that have controlled for variables, such as maternal psychiatric diagnosis and exposure to other medications.[44–47]

The data suggest that the risk of postpartum hemorrhage seems slightly increased in women taking serotonin reuptake inhibitors near the time of delivery.[48–50] Given the inconsistencies across findings on this topic and the small increase in risk observed in studies on this issue, there is no compelling evidence to change prescribing practices during pregnancy. Obstetricians, however, should be alert to the possibility of an increased risk of postpartum hemorrhage in this population, so that hemorrhage, should it occur, may be managed aggressively, with the goal of minimizing maternal morbidity.

Selective Serotonin Reuptake Inhibitor Medications: Sertraline, Fluoxetine, Citalopram, Escitalopram, Paroxetine, and Fluvoxamine

A large Medicaid data study (n = 949,504) by Huybrechts and colleagues[51] and another by Furu and colleagues[52] have concluded that SSRI (fluoxetine, citalopram, paroxetine, sertraline, fluvoxamine, or escitalopram) exposure was not associated with an increased risk of any specific congenital malformations. This has also been shown in various other meta-analyses, which has been reassuring.[16]

Paroxetine is the 1 antidepressant, however, with previously concerning yet still controversial risks for fetal malformations. Reports have suggested that first-trimester exposure to paroxetine is correlated with an increased risk of cardiac malformations, such as atrial and ventricular septal defects.[53,54] Again, other peer-reviewed studies, including 2 independent, comprehensive meta-analysis studies, have not demonstrated the same increased risks of teratogenicity with first-trimester exposure to paroxetine.[55–58] Thus, although some still avoid paroxetine as first-line medication for an antidepressant-naive woman of reproductive age, this medication should surely be considered as a treatment option during pregnancy, given the previously noted reassuring data.

It has generally been assumed that the reproductive safety of escitalopram would be similar to that of the parent drug citalopram, because "S"-citalopram is 1 component of this racemic mixture. An observational multicenter prospective cohort study showed escitalopram does not seem associated with an increased risk for major malformations.[59] As seen in other studies of antidepressants, escitalopram was associated with higher rates of low birthweight (<2500 g). As is often seen in such studies, without a comparison group of women diagnosed with depression who are not taking an antidepressant, it is difficult to determine whether this adverse effect is due to the depression itself or exposure to the drug. This is particularly relevant given the multiple studies that have associated low birthweight with untreated depression and anxiety.

Fluvoxamine, a newer SSRI antidepressant, is FDA approved specifically for treatment of obsessive-compulsive disorder (OCD). Some patients who might not have responded to first-line antidepressant for the obsessive qualities of their anxiety may respond to this medication. Two large studies have shown no major congenital malformations in infants exposed to fluvoxamine compared with the unexposed infants.[52,60] The current data on fluvoxamine, however, is not as expansive of that of other antidepressants, simply due to the fact that it is not as widely prescribed.

Serotonin-Norepinephrine Uptake Inhibitor Medications: Duloxetine and Venlafaxine

Although there are fewer data on SNRI medications than on SSRI medications, so far these medications seem comparable in safety profile. A 2015 article, pooling data from 8 large cohort studies (3186 exposed to venlafaxine and 668 exposed to duloxetine), provides reassuring information regarding the reproductive safety of both venlafaxine and duloxetine after first-trimester exposure, concluding no association between exposure and increased risk of major congenital malformations.[61]

Currently, there are more data about the general safety of venlafaxine[52,62] compared with duloxetine. There is mounting evidence, however, for general safety of the latter during pregnancy. Despite some studies discussing possible association between duloxetine and increased risk of spontaneous abortion and poor neonatal adaptation syndrome,[63,64] causation is difficult and complicated to determine because it seems that having depression itself may have an impact on the risk of miscarriage.[65] Two prospective observational studies of safety of duloxetine can be combined to show that in 439 pregnancies, there were a total of 9 malformations (approximately 2.1%), which is comparable to the rate seen in the general population.

Gestational hypertension has been found significantly associated with the use of SNRI medications; thus, women on these medications should be monitored for hypertension. In a study of 686 women, gestational hypertension was significantly associated with the use of psychostimulants (odds ratio [OR] 6.11; 95% CI, 1.79–20.9) and SNRIs (OR 2.57; 95% CI, 1.34–4.93) after 20 weeks of gestation. Use of serotonin reuptake inhibitors was not associated with increased risk for hypertension. In women taking the SNRI venlafaxine or amphetamine stimulants, risk for gestational hypertension was seen more commonly at higher medication doses.[66]

Bupropion

There are data supporting the use of bupropion during pregnancy.[67–69] The Bupropion Pregnancy Registry concludes no major congenital malformation in association with this exposure in early pregnancy (n = 806).[67]

Although this information regarding the overall risk of malformation is reassuring, earlier reports had concerns of cardiac malformations in bupropion-exposed infants. To more carefully quantify this, a large insurance claims–based study was conducted. This retrospective cohort study, including more than 1200 infants exposed to bupropion during the first trimester, did not demonstrate an increased risk for cardiovascular malformations.[69]

Bupropion can be especially useful for patients with comorbid nicotine use disorder who are motivated to quit smoking and/or those with ADD (discussed later). Further studies are required to assess the risk of neonatal symptoms in bupropion-exposed infants and to better evaluate the long-term neurobehavioral effects of bupropion exposure.

Other Antidepressant Medications: Tricyclic Antidepressants, Mirtazapine, and Trazodone

TCAs, as a class, are not contraindicated for use during pregnancy. This class of medication, however, is not considered first line for treatment of mood and anxiety disorders due to generally increased and unwanted side effects (sedation, anticholinergic side effects, and so forth).[5,70,71] Desipramine and nortriptyline are preferred TCAs due to their less anticholinergic profile and less likely to exacerbate orthostatic hypotension during pregnancy.[72,73]

Data on the safety profile of mirtazapine for infants exposed in utero are considered limited (although reassuring)[6,74,75] and thus this medication should not be used as first-line treatment of mood or anxiety. Unlike typical SSRI medications, mirtazapine seems to have antiemetic properties[74] and has been used in case reports for treatment of hyperemesis gravidarum.[76] Given that hyperemesis gravidarum often is associated with significant anxiety, this medication may be a promising intervention for women with these comorbidities in the future.

The same is true for trazodone (often used as a sleep aid). Despite minimal reassuring data,[77] this medication should not use as first line for treatment of insomnia during pregnancy.

MOOD-STABILIZING MEDICATIONS

The 2 mood stabilizers most commonly considered during pregnancy are lithium and lamotrigine. Antipsychotic medications also play a major role in treatment of patients with manic-depressive disorder.

Lithium

The risk of prenatal exposure to lithium is notoriously coupled with fears of cardiovascular malformations (eg, Ebstein anomaly).[78] Previous reports have indicated that, although a signal for an increased risk of this cardiovascular malformation might be present, this risk is rare. In comparison to the general population, in which Ebstein anomaly occurs in 1/20,000 live births, lithium exposure in the first trimester was estimated to change this risk to at most 1/1000.[79] Despite approximately 50 years of data on this medication, new studies on the reproductive safety of this medication still continue.

A large retrospective cohort study of 1,325,563 pregnant women studied in utero exposure to lithium and risks of cardiovascular malformations.[80] This study, which included 663 women who used lithium during the first trimester of pregnancy, is the largest study of prenatal lithium exposure to date. Two comparison groups were women with no lithium exposure and women with bipolar disorder who used lamotrigine as a mood stabilizer. The findings of this study indicate a modest increase in the risk of cardiac malformations in infants with prenatal exposure to lithium. Compared with women with no known exposures, the relative risk of cardiac malformations calculated here was 1.65. Translating this into absolute risk, this means that if the risk of cardiovascular malformations is 1.15% in women with no exposure, the risk rises to approximately 1.90% in infants exposed to lithium. In this study, the risk of right ventricular outflow tract obstruction defects was 0.60 per 100 live births among infants exposed to lithium and 0.18 per 100 among unexposed infants.[80] The researchers also observed the increase in relative risk to be dose related. Such analysis, however, should be considered premature, considering lack of causation and possibility of other confounders.

Although the absolute risk discussed is not dramatic, this study confirms that lithium carries some teratogenic risk. Although the authors try to avoid prescribing teratogens during pregnancy, with lithium, at times, the benefits outweigh the risks.

Prenatal screening with fetal echocardiography and high-resolution ultrasound is recommended in patients who take lithium during pregnancy (approximately 16–18 weeks of gestation).[16]

Lamotrigine

Lamotrigine is another mood stabilizer used for treatment of bipolar disorder in pregnancy. This medication might not be as effective, however, as lithium in protecting against manic symptoms and is usually used for patients with a history of bipolar traits or hypomania (ie, bipolar II disorder).

Earlier reports warned of possible increased risk of increased risk of cleft palate or cleft lip deformity in infants exposed to lamotrigine during the first trimester.[81] Multiple large studies have indicated that this risk is either nonexistent or very low.[82–84] In 1 study, researchers analyzed a total of 21 studies describing pregnancy outcomes and rates of congenital malformations. Compared with disease-matched controls (n = 1412) and healthy controls (n = 774,571), in utero exposure to lamotrigine monotherapy was not associated with an increased risk of major malformations. Rates of miscarriages, stillbirths, preterm deliveries, and small-for-gestational age neonates were similar in lamotrigine-exposed pregnancies compared with the general population.[85]

In short, lamotrigine is believed to be a relatively safe mood stabilizer for use during pregnancy.

Valproic Acid

Prenatal exposure to valproic acid is strongly associated with neural tube defects, such as spina bifida, and many other anomalies, including midface hypoplasia, congenital heart disease, cleft lip and/or cleft palate, growth retardation, and microcephaly, have been observed.[16,86]

In utero valproic acid has also exposure been associated other developmental neurocognitive deficiencies, including lower IQ and impaired cognition across several domains,[87] and increased risks of autism and ADDs later in childhood.[88,89]

As a general rule, women of reproductive age should not be prescribed valproic acid. If this agent is prescribed, patients should be fully educated on the risks profile of this medication, and robust contraceptive measures should be put in place. This medication ideally should be discontinued at least 6 months prior to planning for conception of any new pregnancy. This would allow for ample time to taper off the valproate, start a new medication, and ensure euthymia and mood stabilization on the new regimen.

Other Antiepileptic Mood-Stabilizing Medications

Information about the reproductive safety of other anticonvulsants, such as oxcarbazepine and topiramate is limited. These medications generally are not first line for the treatment of bipolar disorder, and therefore, ideally should be avoided during pregnancy. The same is true for carbamazepine, especially because prenatal exposure to this substance also has been associated with neural tube defects.[90] Teratogenicity is believed to increase with high maternal serum levels of anticonvulsant and exposure to more than 1 anticonvulsant.[16]

For patients exposed to anticonvulsants during pregnancy, neural tube defects should be evaluated with ultrasonography and maternal serum α-fetoprotein. Increase of folic acid supplementation (4 mg a day) prior to conception and during the first trimester is often recommended,[16] although the general efficacy of this intervention is not clear.

Antipsychotic Medications as Mood Stabilizers

Atypical antipsychotic drugs are commonly used in treatment of bipolar affective disorder (discussed later). Judicial use of adjunctive antipsychotic medication, or at times monotherapy, is common in patients with bipolar disorder. As-needed dosing of these medications (such as olanzapine or quetiapine) can be helpful in managing issues related to insomnia, anxiety, agitation, or irritability related to bipolar disorder.

ANTIPSYCHOTIC MEDICATIONS
Typical (First-Generation) Antipsychotics

Due to the long history of use of typical antipsychotics, there are considerable data available on the reproductive safety of these medications. There is no definitive association between typical antipsychotic exposure during pregnancy and risk of congenital malformations.[91,92] When using a typical antipsychotic, a high-potency neuroleptic (eg, haloperidol) should be used. Although lower-potency typical antipsychotics are not contraindicated, some historical data do exist for their increased risk of congenital malformations associated with prenatal exposure.[93]

Haloperidol, which has much historical data, is a good medication for use in medical settings, such as in florid psychosis during labor and delivery. This is especially true because this medication can be used intravenously, intramuscularly, and orally. The wide range of dosing of this drug also can facilitate improvement of symptoms and cooperation with care, improving safety of patient, safety of care providers, and delivery outcomes.[94]

Atypical (Second-Generation) Antipsychotics

The atypical (second-generation) antipsychotics medications currently serve multiple purposes in the treatment of mental health conditions. They also are used more frequently because they are associated with fewer side effects. In addition to treating psychotic disorders, such as schizophrenia, many are approved for treatment of bipolar disorder, and anxiety disorders. For this reason, this class of medication is perhaps the most multifunctional class of medication at the disposal of care providers.

The versatile use of these medications is important in pregnancy, because prescribers should try to minimize a fetus's exposure to multiple medications. Thus, a medication that could serve multiple purposes is of great value (eg, Seroquel for treatment of anxiety, insomnia, and psychosis.)

Although there are fewer data available on the reproductive safety of this class of medication, multiple large studies have shown that, as a class, they do not seem to have an association with any congenital malformations.[91,95–98]

One study concludes that prenatal exposure to quetiapine, aripiprazole, olanzapine, and ziprasidone does not increase the risk for congenital malformation or cardiac malformations. The possible exception noted is risperidone.[92] The data regarding the safety profile of risperidone are not easy to interpret. Another similar study on risperidone notes that data "should be interpreted with caution because no apparent biological mechanism can readily explain this outcome, and the possibility of a chance finding cannot be ruled out."[99] That said, even if we assume an increased risk is associated with the use of risperidone exists, the risk appears to be small.

Newer antipsychotics, such as lurasidone, iloperidone, and brexpiprazole, are under-represented in most large-scale studies, and more studies need to be done on their perinatal safety profile.

Pregnant patients on second-generation antipsychotics should be closely monitored and screened for gestational diabetes mellitus. Polypharmacy should be avoided to the extent possible to minimize the exposure to the fetus.

ANXIOLYTIC/SEDATIVE HYPNOTIC MEDICATIONS
Benzodiazepines

According to 1 study, 3.9% of American women with private insurance use a benzodiazepine during pregnancy.[100] First-trimester exposure to benzodiazepines has been reported to increase the risk for oral cleft formation for infants (estimated increase of

0.6%).[101] Other studies (including studies with pooled data analysis),[102–104] however, have not supported this association. Although some patients might avoid first-trimester exposure to benzodiazepines, this class of medication can be useful during the second and third trimesters, especially on an as-needed basis.

A 2018 prospective study compared 144 pregnancies exposed to benzodiazepines to a group of 650 unexposed. Infants exposed to benzodiazepines in utero were more likely to be admitted to a neonatal ICU (OR 2.02; 95% CI, 1.11–3.66) and to have a small head circumference (OR 3.89; 95% CI, 1.25–12.03) compared with unexposed infants. Other adverse effects, such as low birthweight, preterm birth, respiratory distress, and muscular symptoms, including hypotonia, were not observed.[105] This study did not find a significant increase in respiratory difficulties, as observed by Yonkers and colleagues.[106] There are reports of peripartum sedation, decreased muscle tone (floppiness), and breathing problems in some infants exposed to benzodiazepines.[107,108] In general, these symptoms appear infrequently and likely are more common in women who take high dosages of these medications.

The results of most benzodiazepine studies are challenging to analyze because in most cases of benzodiazepine exposure, women were also treated with other psychotropic medications. Some providers recommend tapering and discontinuing benzodiazepines around the time of parturition. This rationale is not fully supported, however, given the risk of puerperal worsening of anxiety disorders in women with a history of panic disorder and OCD.[109,110] In a case series, clonazepam-only use during pregnancy and labor did not cause any maternal or fetal compromise.[111]

For patients who conceive on benzodiazepines and do not wish to continue to take these medications over the course of their pregnancy, a gradual taper of these medications is required to prevent rebound anxiety, panic, insomnia, and serious withdrawal side effects, such as seizures. The slower the taper, the better it is tolerated.

Gabapentin

Gabapentin is used in a wide variety of clinical settings (epilepsy, pain management, restless leg syndrome, anxiety, and sleep disturbance); however, there is small amount of information available in regard to the reproductive safety of this medication,[112] and a greater number of exposed infants are required to definitively quantify the reproductive risk profile of this medication. One report reviews the accumulated data regarding the reproductive safety of gabapentin. Pooling all of the available data estimated the risk of malformation in gabapentin only–exposed infants to be less than that of the congenital malformations observed in the general population.[113]

Other Anxiolytics: Antipsychotics, Hydroxyzine, and Buspirone

Antipsychotic medications, such as Seroquel and olanzapine, can be used for as-needed treatment of anxiety (discussed previously). Hydroxyzine has limited but reassuring reproductive safety data.[114] Currently, no systematic data are available on the reproductive safety of buspirone.

STIMULANT MEDICATIONS AND PREGNANCY

Psychostimulants may be used for treatment of variety of reasons, including ADD, management of side effects (such as fatigue and cognitive deficits), enhancement of antidepressant medications, and treatment of narcolepsy.

A 2017 study has shown that infants exposed during pregnancy had increased risk for neonatal ICU admission, were more likely to have central nervous system–related disorders and were more often moderately preterm than nonexposed infants. There was no increased risk for congenital malformations or perinatal death.[115] These findings are consistent with previous studies. What makes this study more useful and clinically relevant, however, is that it focuses on exposure to stimulants prescribed in standard doses as opposed to previous studies, which studied outcomes primarily in women who were abusing or misusing stimulants in combination with other substances.

Most of the studies that have focused on risk for major malformations have not demonstrated any increase in risk of major malformations with first-trimester exposure to methylphenidate. There are fewer available data on dextroamphetamine and amphetamine but still no evidence of teratogenesis.

Gestational hypertension also has been found significantly associated with the use of psychostimulants and seems dose-dependent.[66] Some studies of stimulants, including in women who abuse stimulants, have suggested higher rates of preterm birth, lower birthweight, and other adverse outcomes in infants exposed to stimulants during pregnancy.

The recommendations for use of these medications during pregnancy should be to try to taper off the medications, if feasible, or alternatively decrease the medication to the lowest possible dose and take it at the least number of times possible, on an as-needed basis. There are exceptions to this approach for patients who have challenged functionality if these medications are discontinued. Some examples include severe cases of attention-deficit/hyperactivity disorder (ADHD), leading to accidental injuries, such as car accidents, or cases of treating narcolepsy.

In some cases, bupropion, can be a consideration for replacement of stimulants during pregnancy. This can especially be useful for patients with comorbid depression and/or nicotine use disorder (discussed previously). Bupropion is also used by some providers (off table) for treatment of Attention Deficit Disorder.

MEDICATION-ASSISTED TREATMENT FOR SUBSTANCE USE DISORDERS
Opioid Maintenance Therapy: Methadone Versus Buprenorphine

Treatment with methadone had been considered the gold standard of care for patients requiring opioid maintenance therapy during pregnancy.[116,117] There is a growing body of evidence, however, that indicates buprenorphine should be considered equally efficacious or even as first-line therapy, especially due to its potential advantages for neonatal outcomes.[118,119] Often the decision to choose between these 2 agents is guided by patient history of use and treatment, preference, history of relapse, and need for closer monitoring.

The Maternal Opioid Treatment: Human Experimental Research (MOTHER) project, an 8-site randomized, double blind, double-dummy, flexible-dosing, parallel-group clinical trial compared treatment with methadone to that of buprenorphine. The study showed that neonates exposed to buprenorphine required shorter hospital stays, lower morphine requirements, and an average of 4.1 days of treatment of neonatal adaptation syndrome compared with 9.9 days for the methadone group ($P<.01$).[119]

SUD is a disorder plagued by risk of relapse, which is a main concern of treatment with buprenorphine (a partial agonist) versus methadone (a full opioid agonist). Full agonists might leave patients with less cravings and lower risk of concomitant opioid use.[120] In the MOTHER study, 33% of women on buprenorphine therapy stopped treatment compared with 18% of the methadone group ($P = .02$).[119] In this study, however, women in both groups had to present to a clinic daily. Buprenorphine in the outpatient setting can be prescribed on a monthly basis for patients in long-standing sustained remission, whereas most patients on methadone maintenance need to present to a specialized methadone clinic daily. As such, retention and compliance between the 2 can differ in the outpatient setting.

Special attention should be paid to the risk of polypharmacy with MAT for OUD for patients and their infants. When opiates were coadministered with psychotropic medications, the risk for neonatal drug withdrawal increased.[121] There also are increased risks for accidents, injuries, and respiratory depression for patients who use both opioids and benzodiazepines.[122,123]

Other Medication-Assisted Treatments for Opioid Use Disorder and Alcohol Use Disorder

Naltrexone is not a first-line treatment during pregnancy, especially for patients who are not on this medication prior to their pregnancy. For women who become pregnant while on treatment with naltrexone, this medication should be discontinued if the risk of relapse is low. In cases of high concern about relapse, risks, benefits, and alternatives should be discussed, including treatment with methadone or buprenorphine. Unfortunately, data on the safety profile of this medication are limited.[124]

Naltrexone is also used for treatment of alcohol use disorder. Other medications used for MAT for alcohol use disorder, including disulfiram and acamprosate, likely should be discontinued during pregnancy. The use of naloxone during pregnancy should be limited to cases of maternal overdose only to save a mother's life.

Medication-Assisted Treatments for Smoking Cessation in Pregnancy

The 3 MATs for nicotine use disorder for the general public are nicotine replacement therapy, bupropion, and varenicline. Data regarding the reproductive safety of nicotine replacement therapy are limited and controversial.[125] According to the American College of Obstetricians and Gynecologists recommendations, nicotine replacement therapy should be undertaken "only with close supervision and after careful consideration of the known risks of continued smoking versus the possible risks of nicotine replacement therapy."[126]

At this point, there is no information regarding the reproductive safety of varenicline; thus, it is generally not used in pregnancy.

In contrast, there are data to support the use of bupropion in pregnancy (discussed previously). This medication would be especially efficacious for patients with comorbid depression or ADHD requiring treatment with medications during pregnancy.

Cocaine/Stimulant Use Disorder In Pregnancy

Patients with a history of cocaine or stimulant dependence are at an increased risk for relapse of primary mood and anxiety disorders in addition to substance-induced mood disorder. Medications aimed at curbing cravings (such as topiramate and naltrexone) have been discussed. Patients with a history of cocaine dependence (with no current use) have an increased risk of hypertension. Thus, caution should be taken when prescribing SNRI medications to patients with current or remote history of cocaine use disorder with close observation for possible gestational hypertension.[66]

Best practices

What is the current best practice?

Psychopharmacology and pregnancy

- Screen, diagnose, and treat common mental health conditions prior to pregnancy when possible and/or otherwise during pregnancy

- Understand risks, benefits, alternatives, and appropriateness of psychopharmacologic treatment, including risk of no treatment

- Select medications that have a well-studied reproductive safety profile

- When possible, make modifications to medication regimens prior to pregnancy to confirm a stable and euthymic state on the new regimen prior to conception.

- Limit the number of medication exposures to infant during pregnancy.

What changes in current practice are likely to improve outcomes?

- Appropriate planning prior to pregnancy

- Early intervention prior to or during pregnancy or postpartum

- Continuous and close monitoring of symptoms

- Further research on safety and efficacy of medications during pregnancy

Major recommendations

- Screen all women of reproductive age for common mental health conditions, including, but not limited to, mood and anxiety disorders, OCD posttraumatic stress disorder (history of trauma past and present), ADHD, psychotic disorders (a medical emergency during pregnancy or postpartum), and SUDs.

- Treat women of reproductive age in need of psychiatric medications with medication that have a known favorable perinatal safety profile.

- Engage patients in conversations about family planning, including contraception, and adjust psychiatric medications before conception.

- Monitor patients during pregnancy and in the postpartum period for recurrence of symptoms, regardless of use of psychotropic medications.

Summary statement

Risks, benefits, alternatives, and appropriateness of psychotropic medications, including risks of no treatment, are discussed. Early screening, diagnosis, and intervention prior to and/or during pregnancy often reduce morbidity and mortality of mental health disorders.

REFERENCES

1. Cohen LS, Altshuler LL, Harlow BL, et al. Relapse of major depression during pregnancy in women who maintain or discontinue antidepressant treatment. JAMA 2006;295:499–507.

2. Research C for DE and. Labeling - pregnancy and lactation labeling (Drugs) final rule. Available at: https://www.fda.gov/drugs/developmentapprovalprocess/developmentresources/labeling/ucm093307.htm. Accessed August 6, 2018.

3. Altshuler LL, Cohen LS, Moline ML, et al. The expert consensus guideline series. Treatment of depression in women. Postgrad Med 2001;(Spec No):1–107.

4. Margulis AV, Abou-Ali A, Strazzeri MM, et al. Use of selective serotonin reuptake inhibitors in pregnancy and cardiac malformations: a propensity-score matched cohort in CPRD. Pharmacoepidemiol Drug Saf 2013;22:942–51.

5. Altshuler LL, Cohen L, Szuba MP, et al. Pharmacologic management of psychiatric illness during pregnancy: dilemmas and guidelines. Am J Psychiatry 1996; 153:592–606.

6. Djulus J, Koren G, Einarson T, et al. Exposure to mirtazapine during pregnancy: a prospective comparative study of birth outcomes. J Clin Psychiatry 2006;67: 1280–4.

7. Bonari L, Pinto N, Ahn E, et al. Perinatal risks of untreated depression during pregnancy. Can J Psychiatry 2004;49:726–35.

8. Yonkers KA, Wisner KL, Stewart DE, et al. The management of depression during pregnancy: a report from the American Psychiatric Association and the American College of Obstetricians and Gynecologists. Obstet Gynecol 2009; 114:703–13.

9. Freeman MP, Davis M, Sinha P, et al. Omega-3 fatty acids and supportive psychotherapy for perinatal depression: a randomized placebo-controlled study. J Affect Disord 2008;110:1420148.

10. King R. Cognitive therapy of depression. Aaon Beck, John Rush, Brian Shaw, Gary Emery. New York: Guilford, 1979. Aust N Z J Psychiatry 2002;36:272–5.

11. Spinelli MG. Interpersonal psychotherapy for depressed antepartum women: a pilot study. Am J Psychiatry 1997;154:1028–30.

12. Weissman MM, Kleramna GL. Interpersonal psychotherapy for depression. Chase (MD): International Psychotherapy Institute; 2015. Available at: https://www.israpsych.org/books/wp-content/uploads/2015/06/interpersonal_ psychotherapy_for_depression_-_myrna_m__weissman_phd.pdf. Accessed August 11, 2018.

13. Cohen LS, Altshuler LL, Stowe ZN, et al. Reintroduction of antidepressant therapy across pregnancy in women who previously discontinued treatment. Psychother Psychosom 2004;73:255–8.

14. Bodén R, Lundgren M, Brandt L, et al. Risks of adverse pregnancy and birth outcomes in women treated or not treated with mood stabilisers for bipolar disorder: population based cohort study. BMJ 2012;345:e7085.

15. Viguera AC, Whitfield T, Baldessarini RJ, et al. Risk of recurrence in women with bipolar disorder during pregnancy: prospective study of mood stabilizer discontinuation. Am J Psychiatry 2007;164:1817–24.

16. Hogan C, Wang B, Freeman M, et al. Psychiatric illness during pregnancy and the postpartum period. In: Stern T, Freudenreich O, Smith F, et al, editors. Massachusetts general hospital handbook of general hospital psychiatry. 7th edition. Philadelphia: Elsevier Inc.; 2018. Available at: https://phstwlp2.partners. org:2093/#!/content/book/3-s2.0-B9780323484114000497. Accessed August 11, 2018.

17. Spielvogel A, Wile J. Treatment and outcomes of psychotic patients during pregnancy and childbirth. Birth 1992;19:131–7.

18. Buist A, Gotman N, Yonkers KA. Generalized anxiety disorder: course and risk factors in pregnancy. J Affect Disord 2011;131:277–83.

19. Cohen LS, Rosenbaum JF, Heller VL. Panic attack-associated placental abruption: a case report. J Clin Psychiatry 1989;50:266–7.

20. Ebrahim SH, Gfroerer J. Pregnancy-related substance use in the United States during 1996-1998. Obstet Gynecol 2003;101:374–9.

21. Tran TH, Griffin BL, Stone RH, et al. Methadone, buprenorphine, and naltrexone for the treatment of opioid use disorder in pregnant women. Pharmacotherapy 2017;37:824–39.

22. Wisner KL, Gelenberg AJ, Leonard H, et al. Pharmacologic treatment of depression during pregnancy. JAMA 1999;282:1264–9.

23. Ornoy A, Koren G. Selective serotonin reuptake inhibitors in human pregnancy: on the way to resolving the controversy. Semin Fetal Neonatal Med 2014;19: 188–94.

24. Chambers CD, Johnson KA, Dick LM, et al. Birth outcomes in pregnant women taking fluoxetine. N Engl J Med 1996;335:1010–5.

25. Zeskind PS, Stephens LE. Maternal selective serotonin reuptake inhibitor use during pregnancy and newborn neurobehavior. Pediatrics 2004;113:368–75.

26. Simon GE, Cunningham ML, Davis RL. Outcomes of prenatal antidepressant exposure. Am J Psychiatry 2002;159:2055–61.

27. Pastuszak A, Schick-Boschetto B, Zuber C, et al. Pregnancy outcome following first-trimester exposure to fluoxetine (Prozac). JAMA 1993;269:2246–8.

28. Nulman I, Rovet J, Stewart DE, et al. Child development following exposure to tricyclic antidepressants or fluoxetine throughout fetal life: a prospective, controlled study. Am J Psychiatry 2002;159:1889–95.

29. Suri R, Altshuler L, Hendrick V, et al. The impact of depression and fluoxetine treatment on obstetrical outcome. Arch Womens Ment Health 2004;7:193–200.

30. Lupattelli A, Wood M, Ystrom E, et al. New research: effect of time-dependent selective serotonin reuptake inhibitor antidepressants during pregnancy on behavioral, emotional, and social development in preschool-aged children. J Am Acad Child Adolesc Psychiatry 2018;57:200–8.

31. Lattimore KA, Donn SM, Kaciroti N, et al. Selective serotonin reuptake inhibitor (SSRI) use during pregnancy and effects on the fetus and newborn: a meta-analysis. J Perinatol 2005;25:595–604.

32. Cohen LS, Nonacs R. Neurodevelopmental implications of fetal exposure to selective serotonin reuptake inhibitors and untreated maternal depression: weighing relative risks. JAMA Psychiatry 2016;73:1170–2.

33. Steer RA, Scholl TO, Hediger ML, et al. Self-reported depression and negative pregnancy outcomes. J Clin Epidemiol 1992;45:1093–9.

34. Levinson-Castiel R, Merlob P, Linder N, et al. Neonatal abstinence syndrome after in utero exposure to selective serotonin reuptake inhibitors in term infants. Arch Pediatr Adolesc Med 2006;160:173–6.

35. Chambers CD, Hernandez-Diaz S, Van Marter LJ, et al. Selective serotonin-reuptake inhibitors and risk of persistent pulmonary hypertension of the newborn. N Engl J Med 2006;354:579–87.

36. Andrade SE, McPhillips H, Loren D, et al. Antidepressant medication use and risk of persistent pulmonary hypertension of the newborn. Pharmacoepidemiol Drug Saf 2009;18:246–52.

37. Huybrechts KF, Bateman BT, Palmsten K, et al. Antidepressant use late in pregnancy and risk of persistent pulmonary hypertension of the newborn. JAMA 2015;313:2142–51.

38. Hernández-Díaz S, Marter LJV, Werler MM, et al. Risk factors for persistent pulmonary hypertension of the newborn. Pediatrics 2007;120:e272–82.

39. Nulman I, Rovet J, Stewart DE, et al. Neurodevelopment of children exposed in utero to antidepressant drugs. N Engl J Med 1997;336:258–62.

40. Nulman I, Koren G, Rovet J, et al. Neurodevelopment of children following prenatal exposure to venlafaxine, selective serotonin reuptake inhibitors, or untreated maternal depression. Am J Psychiatry 2012;169:1165–74.

41. Boukhris T, Sheehy O, Mottron L, et al. Antidepressant use during pregnancy and the risk of autism spectrum disorder in children. JAMA Pediatr 2016;170: 117–24.
42. Malm H, Brown AS, Gissler M, et al. Gestational exposure to selective serotonin reuptake inhibitors and offspring psychiatric disorders: a national register-based study. J Am Acad Child Adolesc Psychiatry 2016;55:359–66.
43. Figueroa R. Use of antidepressants during pregnancy and risk of attention-deficit/hyperactivity disorder in the offspring. J Dev Behav Pediatr 2010;31: 641–8.
44. Hviid A, Melbye M, Pasternak B. Use of selective serotonin reuptake inhibitors during pregnancy and risk of autism. N Engl J Med 2013;369:2406–15.
45. Sørensen MJ, Grønborg TK, Christensen J, et al. Antidepressant exposure in pregnancy and risk of autism spectrum disorders. Clin Epidemiol 2013;5: 449–59.
46. Andrade C. Antidepressant exposure during pregnancy and risk of autism in the offspring: do the new studies add anything new? J Clin Psychiatry 2017;78: e1052–6.
47. Mezzacappa A, Lasica P-A, Gianfagna F, et al. Risk for autism spectrum disorders according to period of prenatal antidepressant exposure: a systematic review and meta-analysis. JAMA Pediatr 2017;171:555–63.
48. Heller HM, Ravelli ACJ, Bruning AHL, et al. Increased postpartum haemorrhage, the possible relation with serotonergic and other psychopharmacological drugs: a matched cohort study. BMC Pregnancy Childbirth 2017;17:166.
49. Hanley GE, Smolina K, Mintzes B, et al. Postpartum hemorrhage and use of serotonin reuptake inhibitor antidepressants in pregnancy. Obstet Gynecol 2016; 127:553–61.
50. Palmsten K, Hernández-Díaz S, Huybrechts KF, et al. Use of antidepressants near delivery and risk of postpartum hemorrhage: cohort study of low income women in the United States. BMJ 2013;347:f4877.
51. Huybrechts KF, Palmsten K, Avorn J, et al. Antidepressant use in pregnancy and the risk of cardiac defects. N Engl J Med 2014;370:2397–407.
52. Furu K, Kieler H, Haglund B, et al. Selective serotonin reuptake inhibitors and venlafaxine in early pregnancy and risk of birth defects: population based cohort study and sibling design. BMJ 2015;350:h1798.
53. Wogelius P, Nørgaard M, Gislum M, et al. Maternal use of selective serotonin reuptake inhibitors and risk of congenital malformations. Epidemiology 2006;17: 701–4.
54. Paroxetine and pregnancy | GSK. Available at: https://www.gsk.com/en-gb/media/resource-centre/paroxetine-information/paroxetine-and-pregnancy/. Accessed August 22, 2018.
55. Alwan S, Reefhuis J, Rasmussen SA, et al, National Birth Defects Prevention Study. Use of selective serotonin-reuptake inhibitors in pregnancy and the risk of birth defects. N Engl J Med 2007;356:2684–92.
56. Louik C, Lin AE, Werler MM, et al. First-trimester use of selective serotonin-reuptake inhibitors and the risk of birth defects. N Engl J Med 2007;356: 2675–83.
57. Gentile S. Pregnancy Exposure to serotonin reuptake inhibitors and the risk of spontaneous abortions. CNS Spectr 2008;13:960–6.
58. Einarson A, Pistelli A, DeSantis M, et al. Evaluation of the risk of congenital cardiovascular defects associated with use of paroxetine during pregnancy. Am J Psychiatry 2008;165:749–52.

59. Klieger-Grossmann C, Weitzner B, Panchaud A, et al. Pregnancy outcomes following use of escitalopram: a prospective comparative cohort study. J Clin Pharmacol 2012;52:766–70.

60. Malm H, Artama M, Gissler M, et al. Selective serotonin reuptake inhibitors and risk for major congenital anomalies. Obstet Gynecol 2011;118:111–20.

61. Lassen D, Ennis ZN, Damkier P. First-trimester pregnancy exposure to venlafaxine or duloxetine and risk of major congenital malformations: a systematic review. Basic Clin Pharmacol Toxicol 2016;118:32–6.

62. Einarson A, Fatoye B, Sarkar M, et al. Pregnancy outcome following gestational exposure to venlafaxine: a multicenter prospective controlled study. Am J Psychiatry 2001;158:1728–30.

63. Andrade C. The safety of duloxetine during pregnancy and lactation. J Clin Psychiatry 2014;75:e1423–7.

64. Hoog SL, Cheng Y, Elpers J, et al. Duloxetine and pregnancy outcomes: safety surveillance findings. Int J Med Sci 2013;10:413–9.

65. Kjaersgaard MIS, Parner ET, Vestergaard M, et al. Prenatal antidepressant exposure and risk of spontaneous abortion - a population-based study. PLoS One 2013;8:e72095.

66. Newport DJ, Hostetter AL, Juul SH, et al. Prenatal psychostimulant and antidepressant exposure and risk of hypertensive disorders of pregnancy. J Clin Psychiatry 2016;77:1538–45.

67. GalxoSmithKline. GSK pregnancy registry for Bupropioin. Available at: http://pregnancyregistry.gsk.com/documents/bup_report_final 2008.pdf. Accessed August 11, 2018.

68. Chun-Fai-Chan B, Koren G, Fayez I, et al. Pregnancy outcome of women exposed to bupropion during pregnancy: a prospective comparative study. Am J Obstet Gynecol 2005;192:932-6.

69. Cole JA, Modell JG, Haight BR, et al. Bupropion in pregnancy and the prevalence of congenital malformations. Pharmacoepidemiol Drug Saf 2007;16:474–84.

70. Emslie G, Judge R. Tricyclic antidepressants and selective serotonin reuptake inhibitors: use during pregnancy, in children/adolescents and in the elderly. Acta Psychiatr Scand 2000;101:26–34.

71. Pariante CM, Seneviratne G, Howard L. Should we stop using tricyclic antidepressants in pregnancy? Psychol Med 2011;41:15–7.

72. Suri R, Altshuler LL. No decision is without risk. J Clin Psychiatry 2009;70:1319–20.

73. Cohen LS, Wang B, Nonacs R, et al. Treatment of mood disorders during pregnancy and postpartum. Psychiatr Clin North Am 2010;33:273–93.

74. Alam A, Voronovich Z, Carley JA. A review of therapeutic uses of mirtazapine in psychiatric and medical conditions. Prim Care Companion CNS Disord 2013;15 [pii:PCC.13r01525].

75. Smit M, Dolman KM, Honig A. Mirtazapine in pregnancy and lactation - a systematic review. Eur Neuropsychopharmacol 2016;26:126–35.

76. Uguz F, Turgut K, Aydin A, et al. Low-dose mirtazapine in major depression developed after hyperemesis gravidarum: a case series. Am J Ther 2018. https://doi.org/10.1097/MJT.0000000000000698.

77. Einarson A, Bonari L, Voyer-Lavigne S, et al. A multicentre prospective controlled study to determine the safety of trazodone and nefazodone use during pregnancy. Can J Psychiatry 2003;48:106–10.

78. Weinstein MR, Goldfield M. Cardiovascular malformations with lithium use during pregnancy. Am J Psychiatry 1975;132:529–31.
79. Newport DJ, Viguera AC, Beach AJ, et al. Lithium placental passage and obstetrical outcome: implications for clinical management during late pregnancy. Am J Psychiatry 2005;162:2162–70.
80. Patorno E, Huybrechts KF, Bateman BT, et al. Lithium use in pregnancy and the risk of cardiac malformations. N Engl J Med 2017;376:2245–54.
81. Holmes LB, Baldwin EJ, Smith CR, et al. Increased frequency of isolated cleft palate in infants exposed to lamotrigine during pregnancy. Neurology 2008; 70:2152–8.
82. Cunnington MC, Weil JG, Messenheimer JA, et al. Final results from 18 years of the International lamotrigine pregnancy registry. Neurology 2011;76:1817–23.
83. Dolk H, Wang H, Loane M, et al. Lamotrigine use in pregnancy and risk of orofacial cleft and other congenital anomalies. Neurology 2016;86:1716–25.
84. Hernández-Díaz S, Smith CR, Shen A, et al. Comparative safety of antiepileptic drugs during pregnancy. Neurology 2012;78:1692–9.
85. Pariente G, Leibson T, Shulman T, et al. Pregnancy outcomes following in utero exposure to lamotrigine: a systematic review and meta-Analysis. CNS Drugs 2017;31:439–50.
86. Wyszynski DF, Nambisan M, Surve T, et al. Increased rate of major malformations in offspring exposed to valproate during pregnancy. Neurology 2005;64: 961–5.
87. Meador KJ, Baker GA, Browning N, et al. Fetal antiepileptic drug exposure and cognitive outcomes at age 6 years (NEAD study): a prospective observational study. Lancet Neurol 2013;12:244–52.
88. Cohen MJ, Meador KJ, Browning N, et al. Fetal antiepileptic drug exposure: adaptive and emotional/behavioral functioning at age 6 years. Epilepsy Behav 2013;29:308–15.
89. Christensen J, Grønborg TK, Sørensen MJ, et al. Prenatal valproate exposure and risk of autism spectrum disorders and childhood autism. JAMA 2013;309: 1696–703.
90. Rosa FW. Spina bifida in infants of women treated with carbamazepine during pregnancy. N Engl J Med 1991;324:674–7.
91. Einarson A, Boskovic R. Use and safety of antipsychotic drugs during pregnancy. J Psychiatr Pract 2009;15:183–92.
92. Huybrechts KF, Hernández-Díaz S, Patorno E, et al. Antipsychotic use in pregnancy and the risk for congenital malformations. JAMA Psychiatry 2016;73: 938–46.
93. Rumeau-Rouquette C, Goujard J, Huel G. Possible teratogenic effect of phenothiazines in human beings. Teratology 1977;15:57–64.
94. Tesar GE, Stern TA. Evaluation and treatment of agitation in the intensive care unit. J Intensive Care Med 1986;1:137–48.
95. McKenna K, Koren G, Tetelbaum M, et al. Pregnancy outcome of women using atypical antipsychotic drugs: a prospective comparative study. J Clin Psychiatry 2005;66:444–9.
96. Habermann F, Fritzsche J, Fuhlbrück F, et al. Atypical antipsychotic drugs and pregnancy outcome: a prospective, cohort study. J Clin Psychopharmacol 2013;33:453–62.
97. Cohen LS, Viguera AC, McInerney KA, et al. Reproductive safety of second-generation antipsychotics: current data from the Massachusetts general

hospital national pregnancy registry for atypical antipsychotics. Am J Psychiatr 2015;173:263–70.

98. Petersen I, Sammon CJ, McCrea RL, et al. Risks associated with antipsychotic treatment in pregnancy: comparative cohort studies based on electronic health records. Schizophr Res 2016;176:349–56.

99. Ennis ZN, Damkier P. Pregnancy exposure to olanzapine, quetiapine, risperidone, aripiprazole and risk of congenital malformations. A systematic review. Basic Clin Pharmacol Toxicol 2015;116:315–20.

100. Hanley GE, Mintzes B. Patterns of psychotropic medicine use in pregnancy in the United States from 2006 to 2011 among women with private insurance. BMC Pregnancy Childbirth 2014;14:242.

101. Safra MJ, Oakley GP. Association between cleft lip with or without cleft palate and prenatal exposure to diazepam. Lancet 1975;2:478–80.

102. Ban L, West J, Gibson JE, et al. First trimester exposure to anxiolytic and hypnotic drugs and the risks of major congenital anomalies: a United Kingdom population-based cohort study. PLoS One 2014;9:e100996.

103. Bellantuono C, Tofani S, Di Sciascio G, et al. Benzodiazepine exposure in pregnancy and risk of major malformations: a critical overview. Gen Hosp Psychiatry 2013;35:3–8.

104. Enato E, Moretti M, Koren G. The fetal safety of benzodiazepines: an updated meta-analysis. J Obstet Gynaecol Can 2011;33:46–8.

105. Freeman MP, Góez-Mogollón L, McInerney KA, et al. Obstetrical and neonatal outcomes after benzodiazepine exposure during pregnancy: results from a prospective registry of women with psychiatric disorders. Gen Hosp Psychiatry 2018;53:73–9.

106. Yonkers KA, Gilstad-Hayden K, Forray A, et al. Association of panic disorder, generalized anxiety disorder, and benzodiazepine treatment during pregnancy with risk of adverse birth outcomes. JAMA Psychiatry 2017;74:1145–52.

107. Fisher JB, Edgren BE, Mammel MC, et al. Neonatal apnea associated with maternal clonazepam therapy: a case report. Obstet Gynecol 1985;66:34S–5S.

108. Whitelaw AG, Cummings AJ, McFadyen IR. Effect of maternal lorazepam on the neonate. Br Med J 1981;282:1106–8.

109. Cohen LS, Sichel DA, Dimmock JA, et al. Postpartum course in women with pre-existing panic disorder. J Clin Psychiatry 1994;55:289–92.

110. Sichel DA, Cohen LS, Dimmock JA, et al. Postpartum obsessive compulsive disorder: a case series. J Clin Psychiatry 1993;54:156–9.

111. Weinstock L, Cohen LS, Bailey JW, et al. Obstetrical and neonatal outcome following clonazepam use during pregnancy: a case series. Psychother Psychosom 2001;70:158–62.

112. Fujii H, Goel A, Bernard N, et al. Pregnancy outcomes following gabapentin use: results of a prospective comparative cohort study. Neurology 2013;80:1565–70.

113. Guttuso T, Shaman M, Thornburg LL. Potential maternal symptomatic benefit of gabapentin and review of its safety in pregnancy. Eur J Obstet Gynecol Reprod Biol 2014;181:280–3.

114. Einarson A, Bailey B, Jung G, et al. Prospective controlled study of hydroxyzine and cetirizine in pregnancy. Ann Allergy Asthma Immunol 1997;78:183–6.

115. Nörby U, Winbladh B, Källén K. Perinatal outcomes after treatment with ADHD medication during pregnancy. Pediatrics 2017;140 [pii:20170747].

116. Krans EE, Cochran G, Bogen DL. Caring for opioid-dependent pregnant women: prenatal and postpartum care considerations. Clin Obstet Gynecol 2015;58:370–9.

117. Winhusen T, Wilder C, Wexelblatt SL, et al. Design considerations for point-of-care clinical trials comparing methadone and buprenorphine treatment for opioid dependence in pregnancy and for neonatal abstinence syndrome. Contemp Clin Trials 2014;39:158–65.
118. American College of Obsetrics and Gynecology. ACOG committee opinion no. 524: opioid abuse, dependence, and addiction in pregnancy. Obstet Gynecol 2012;119:1070–6.
119. Jones HE, Kaltenbach K, Heil SH, et al. Neonatal abstinence syndrome after methadone or buprenorphine exposure. N Engl J Med 2010;363:2320–31.
120. Fischer G, Ortner R, Rohrmeister K, et al. Methadone versus buprenorphine in pregnant addicts: a double-blind, double-dummy comparison study. Addiction 2006;101:275–81.
121. Huybrechts KF, Bateman BT, Desai RJ, et al. Risk of neonatal drug withdrawal after intrauterine co-exposure to opioids and psychotropic medications: cohort study. BMJ 2017;358:j3326.
122. Hirschtritt ME, Delucchi KL, Olfson M. Outpatient, combined use of opioid and benzodiazepine medications in the United States, 1993-2014. Prev Med Rep 2018;9:49–54.
123. Schuman-Olivier Z, Hoeppner BB, Weiss RD, et al. Benzodiazepine use during buprenorphine treatment for opioid dependence: clinical and safety outcomes. Drug Alcohol Depend 2013;132:580–6.
124. National practice guideline. Available at: https://www.asam.org/resources/guidelines-and-consensus-documents/npg. Accessed August 22, 2018.
125. Forinash AB, Pitlick JM, Clark K, et al. Nicotine replacement therapy effect on pregnancy outcomes. Ann Pharmacother 2010;44:1817–21.
126. American College of Obsetrics and Gynecology. ACOG committee opinion no. 721. Smoking cessation during pregnancy. Obstet Gynecol 2017;130:e200–4.

Treatment of Viral Infections During Pregnancy

Sarah C. Rogan, MD, PhD[a], Richard H. Beigi, MD, MSc[b],*

KEYWORDS

- Viral infections • Pregnancy • Herpes simplex virus • Cytomegalovirus
- Viral hepatitis • Human immunodeficiency virus • Maternal-to-child transmission
- Antiviral therapy

KEY POINTS

- Viral infections are common complications of pregnancy. Although some infections have maternal sequelae, many viral infections can be perinatally transmitted to fetuses or infants.
- Safe and effective treatments are available to treat many viral infections during pregnancy.
- Antiviral therapy is indicated to reduce maternal-to-child transmission of diseases such as herpes simplex virus, chronic hepatitis B virus, and human immunodeficiency virus.
- Research is ongoing to further clarify the role of treatments for cytomegalovirus and chronic hepatitis C virus during pregnancy.

INTRODUCTION

Viral infections are common complications of pregnancy, with a wide range of obstetric and neonatal sequelae. Some viruses, such as the common cold, cause a mild maternal illness and generally have no impact on the pregnancy. Other viruses, such as cytomegalovirus (CMV), are typically asymptomatic or mild in the pregnant patient but can cause congenital infection with devastating fetal and neonatal consequences. Yet other viruses, such as hepatitis B (HBV), hepatitis C (HCV), and human immunodeficiency virus (HIV), pose risks to the patient and can be transmitted perinatally to neonates with resulting chronic infection and associated complications.

Treatments of such infections in pregnancy are currently directed at decreasing maternal symptomatology, ameliorating maternal disease, and minimizing and

Disclosure Statement: Drs S.C. Rogan and R.H. Beigi have no conflicts of interest to disclose.
[a] Maternal and Fetal Medicine Division, Department of Obstetrics, Gynecology, and Reproductive Sciences, University of Pittsburgh School of Medicine, 300 Halket Street, Pittsburgh, PA 15213, USA; [b] Department of Obstetrics, Gynecology, and Reproductive Sciences, University of Pittsburgh School of Medicine, University of Pittsburgh Medical Center Magee-Womens Hospital, 300 Halket Street, Pittsburgh, PA 15213, USA
* Corresponding author.
E-mail address: beigrh@upmc.edu

preventing congenital infection or maternal-to-child transmission (MTCT). Pregnancy is a time during which women without routine health care maintenance and surveillance enter the health care system; thus, pregnancy also represents a window of opportunity to identify chronic infections that will require treatment either during or after pregnancy. In this review, the authors address the treatment of several key viral infections including herpes simplex virus (HSV), CMV, HCV, HBV, and HIV.

HERPES SIMPLEX VIRUS

Herpes simplex virus is one of the most commonly encountered viral infections in pregnancy. The herpes virus is a double-stranded DNA virus in the *Herpesviridae* family and has 2 strains, HSV-1 and HSV-2, which both cause human infection of the oropharyngeal and genital tracts. According to World Health Organization (WHO) estimates from 2012, 1387 million and 267 million reproductive-aged (15- to 49-year-old) women worldwide were infected with HSV-1 and HSV-2, respectively, and approximately 322 to 360 million of those women had genital HSV infections.[1,2] In the United States, the prevalence of HSV-1 and HSV-2 among reproductive-aged adults is 47.8% and 11.9%, respectively.[3] Approximately 2% of seronegative pregnant women acquire HSV during pregnancy.[4] Historically, HSV-1 has been associated with oropharyngeal disease, whereas HSV-2 has been associated with genital disease, but both viral strains can cause genital lesions. The proportion of genital HSV caused by HSV-1 has increased among young women in recent years.[5]

In the context of pregnancy, HSV can cause maternal, fetal, and neonatal infection. Maternal outbreaks are often self-limited, but treatment can shorten the duration and severity of symptoms and limit the duration of viral shedding. Fetal infection via transplacental or transcervical passage of the virus is thought to be rare. Neonatal infection is generally acquired peripartum and can result in disseminated, lethal disease. Neonatal infection is more common in cases of primary maternal infection during pregnancy, particularly if genital HSV is acquired shortly before labor.[4,6] Treatment of HSV infection during pregnancy has 2 primary goals: symptomatic treatment of the patient and prevention of neonatal transmission.

Maternal HSV Infection and Treatment

Maternal genital HSV infection presents in several ways. First-episode primary genital herpes refers to a genital outbreak in a patient who was previously seronegative for both HSV-1 and HSV-2. These episodes can be severe. In addition to the typical painful or pruritic genital vesicular lesions and ulcerations, patients can have dysuria and systemic symptoms including fever, malaise, headache, and lymphadenopathy. Conversely, more than 60% of primary infection during pregnancy is asymptomatic.[4] Patients can also present with first-episode nonprimary genital herpes; this presentation consists of the first genital clinical outbreak in a patient with antibodies to a different HSV strain. Such nonprimary diseases are typically less severe than primary diseases. After initial infection, the virus remains latent in sensory neural ganglia but can reactivate to cause recurrent disease with the same HSV subtype as their serum antibodies. Patients can also experience asymptomatic viral shedding during times in which they have no clinical signs or symptoms of disease. Generally, treatment consists of an antiviral medication such as acyclovir or valacyclovir, and symptomatic therapy, which includes acetaminophen, topical anesthetics, sitz baths, and hygienic measures. Oral antiviral treatment regimens endorsed by the Centers for Disease Control and Prevention (CDC)[7] and the American College of Obstetricians and

Table 1
Oral treatment regimens for HSV infection during pregnancy

Clinical Indication	Acyclovir	Valacyclovir	Treatment Duration
Primary first-episode genital HSV	200 mg five times daily or 400 mg three times daily	1000 mg twice daily	7–10 d
Primary non–first-episode or recurrent genital HSV	400 mg three times daily or 800 mg twice daily	500 mg twice daily or 1000 mg daily	5 d
HSV suppression	400 mg three times daily	500 mg twice daily	From 36 wk' gestation until delivery

Data from Workowski KA, Bolan GA. Sexually transmitted diseases treatment guidelines, 2015. MMWR Recomm Rep 2015;64(RR-03):1–137; and ACOG practice bulletin no. 82: management of herpes in pregnancy. Obstet Gynecol 2007;109(6):1489–98.

Gynecologists (ACOG)[8] for maternal symptomatic infection are listed in **Table 1**. For severe primary infections, intravenous acyclovir can also be used.

Suppressive Therapy

In addition to providing maternal symptomatic relief, antiviral treatment of HSV is also used prophylactically in the late third trimester until the onset of labor to decrease complications from HSV at the time of delivery; see **Table 1** for suppressive therapy regimens. The goals of prophylaxis are to decrease the risk of active HSV disease at the time of delivery and to reduce asymptomatic viral shedding, thus minimizing maternal morbidity and peripartum MTCT. A meta-analysis of randomized clinical trials concluded that prophylactic acyclovir beginning at 36 weeks' gestation reduced clinical HSV recurrence at delivery by 75%, cesarean deliveries for recurrent genital HSV by 70%, and the risk of HSV viral shedding and total HSV detection at delivery by 91% and 89%, respectively.[9] A similar meta-analysis that included valacyclovir reported similar overall results and effect sizes.[10] No cases of neonatal herpes occurred in either group of data sets, thus the effect of antepartum antiviral prophylaxis on neonatal outcomes could not be determined. However, prophylaxis does not eliminate HSV viral shedding or lesions at the time of delivery[11] nor does it absolutely prevent neonatal transmission of disease.[12]

Nucleoside Analogues

The mainstays of HSV treatment are nucleoside analogues including acyclovir, its prodrug valacyclovir, and less commonly, famciclovir. The pharmacokinetics of acyclovir is similar in nonpregnant and term pregnant patients.[13,14] Compared with acyclovir, valacyclovir has the benefit of better oral bioavailability and a longer half-life and thus requires less frequent and more convenient oral dosing, but it is more expensive than acyclovir.

Nucleoside analogues have not been shown to be teratogenic and are safe for use in pregnancy. Although acyclovir crosses the placenta and concentrates in amniotic fluid, it does not concentrate in the fetus, as measured by cord blood drug concentrations.[14,15] The teratogenicity of acyclovir, valacyclovir, and famciclovir was investigated in a large, population-based retrospective cohort study in Denmark.[16] Among 1804 pregnancies exposed to these antivirals during the first trimester, rates of birth defects were similar to unexposed population-based rates (2.2% vs 2.4% in exposed and unexposed infants, respectively). Individually, none of the drugs was associated with an increased rate of birth defects, but the data for famciclovir were limited. Furthermore, the international Acyclovir in Pregnancy Registry monitored outcomes of more than 1200 pregnancies exposed to oral or intravenous acyclovir from 1984 to 1998; 60% of exposures occurred during the first trimester. Acyclovir exposure in the first trimester or at any point during pregnancy was not associated with an increased rate of birth defects.[17]

CYTOMEGALOVIRUS

CMV is another member of the *Herpesviridae* family that is of concern to pregnant women because of its potential for congenital infection. In adults, CMV infection is usually asymptomatic or causes a mild flulike illness. As HSV, CMV then remains latent and can reactivate to cause an asymptomatic secondary infection and viral shedding; reinfection with a new CMV strain can also occur. Although CMV infection has limited maternal sequelae, vertical transmission of CMV can cause congenital CMV, the severity of which can vary widely but has the potential to be devastating.

The seroprevalence of CMV among pregnant women is high. In a population-wide study in the Unites States conducted from 1988 to 1994, the seroprevalence rate of CMV was 58.8%.[18] Among seronegative at-risk pregnant women, approximately 1% to 7% will develop a primary infection during pregnancy.[19] The overall birth prevalence of CMV is estimated at 0.6% to 1.08%; between 8% and 12% of these infections are symptomatic.[20–22] Vertical transmission is significantly more likely in cases of primary CMV than recurrent or reactivated CMV (32% vs 1.4%[22]); however, because of the high prevalence of CMV seropositivity and the overall low incidence rate of primary CMV during pregnancy, approximately 75% of cases of congenital CMV are due to nonprimary disease.[23] Fortunately, congenital CMV is generally less severe when due to recurrent or reactivated disease, and most neonates are asymptomatic at birth. Rarely, recurrent CMV infection can cause severe disease or even result in stillbirth.[24] When primary infection does occur during pregnancy, the risk of congenital infection depends on the gestational age of the fetus at the time of maternal infection and fetal transmission. Transmission rates range from 36% to 40% in the first and second trimesters to 65% in the third trimester[25]; earlier infections generally have more fetal implications than infections acquired during the third trimester.[25,26]

Congenital CMV has a variety of manifestations that can be identified on ultrasound including hepatosplenomegaly, echogenic bowel, ascites, intracranial calcifications, ventriculomegaly, microcephaly, growth restriction, and stillbirth.[27,28] In one study, approximately 43% of affected fetuses had abnormal ultrasound findings.[28] Infants with CMV are at risk for hyperbilirubinemia and jaundice, thrombocytopenia and petechial rashes, hepatitis, hearing loss, and death.[29] Up to 30% of severely affected infants will die of complications of CMV infection, and 80% of survivors will have major morbidity.[29] More commonly, infants are asymptomatic at birth, but they are still at risk for hearing loss, chorioretinitis, dental defects, seizures, intellectual disability, and death later in childhood.[29,30] Sensorineural hearing loss is the most common sequelae to develop in asymptomatic infants, and congenital CMV accounts for 15% to 20% of cases of sensorineural hearing loss.[31]

Treatment of Cytomegalovirus

Because of the potential for severe fetal and neonatal morbidity and mortality from CMV infection, research into treatments for CMV in pregnancy is geared toward preventing vertical transmission of the virus and improving outcomes when congenital infections occur. Several agents, including CMV hyperimmune globulin (HIG) and antiviral agents, have been investigated both as preventive agents and as treatments for congenital CMV. Data on the effects of these agents are reviewed later in this article, but at present, no treatment has proved definitively efficacious nor is currently recommended for treatment of CMV in pregnancy.

Early studies on passive immunization with CMV HIG were promising. It is hypothesized that HIG reduces maternal and placental viral loads to prevent fetal infection, and in cases where infection has already occurred, it likely reduces placental and fetal inflammation to improve outcomes.[32] In a prospective nonrandomized study, Nigro and colleagues[32] treated women with confirmed intraamniotic CMV infection with HIG and found a significant decrease from 50% to 3% in the presence of symptoms of congenital CMV at birth and at 2 years of age without adverse effects. A separate group of patients who were known to have primary CMV in the first half of pregnancy but who either had a negative amniocentesis or did not undergo amniocentesis were also treated with HIG. In this group, the rate of congenital CMV infection decreased significantly from 40% to 16%, again without adverse effects. Another observational study of pregnancies complicated by early primary CMV infection found that among infants born to women treated with HIG, the rate of poor childhood outcomes at 1 year of age decreased from 43% to 13%.[33] In a case-control study of young children with congenital CMV acquired before 20 weeks' gestation, HIG use during pregnancy was associated with lower rates of symptomatology, including psychomotor retardation and hearing impairment. Moreover, among children whose mothers had received HIG, the presence of symptoms was associated with a longer time lapse between occurrence of maternal infection and treatment with HIG.[34]

In contrast to these promising results, the phase II CHIP trial, which is the only published double-blinded, randomized controlled trial of HIG in women with primary CMV infection, failed to show a significant reduction in congenital CMV infection. In fact, women who received HIG had a trend toward a higher rate of obstetric complications including preterm birth, intrauterine growth restriction, and preeclampsia.[35] Although observational data do not support this increase in preterm birth and growth restriction,[36,37] a similar lack of efficacy has been seen in other small trials.[38,39] A multicenter phase III randomized trial investigating HIG recently completed enrollment (NCT01376778), but results are not yet available. The results of this trial should provide insight into the efficacy and safety of HIG.

Several studies have also evaluated the efficacy of antiviral agents in treating CMV during pregnancy. Drugs such as ganciclovir, foscarnet, and cidofovir, which are used to treat CMV in immunocompromised nonpregnant patients, are insufficiently studied or not considered safe in pregnancy. Valacyclovir and acyclovir are also used in immunocompromised patients as prophylaxis against CMV; given the aforementioned safety of these drugs in pregnancy, research into antiviral therapy for congenital CMV has used these agents. In a pilot study, patients with confirmed fetal infection were treated with valacyclovir, 8 g, daily and then underwent amniocentesis and fetal blood sampling. Therapeutic concentrations of drug were detected in amniotic fluid and in fetal blood with reductions in fetal viral load.[40] Subsequently, in an open-label phase II trial, patients with ultrasound findings of congenital CMV were treated with valacyclovir, 8 g, daily from the time of diagnosis until delivery; fetuses with severe brain anomalies and asymptomatic fetuses were both excluded given the low likelihood of a change in outcome with treatment. Women treated with valacyclovir were nearly twice as likely to deliver an asymptomatic neonate compared with a historical control. The treatment regimen required women to take 16 pills per day, but adherence was high, and the dosage was well tolerated.[41] A randomized phase II-III trial is underway in Israel to evaluate the efficacy of valacyclovir for preventing vertical transmission of CMV in cases of maternal primary infection (NCT02351102).

As a whole, the current published data on prevention and treatment of congenital CMV are inconclusive. No treatment has definitively been shown to be both safe and efficacious. At present, consensus guidelines from ACOG,[42] the Society for Maternal Fetal Medicine (SMFM),[43] and the International Congenital Cytomegalovirus Recommendations Group[44] all recommend that administration of HIG and antiviral agents for prevention and treatment of congenital CMV be restricted to research trial protocols. Data from the 2 randomized control trials that are in progress will elucidate the role of these agents in prevention and treatment of congenital CMV. Notably, vaccine development is another promising avenue of prevention for CMV.

VIRAL HEPATITIS

Viral hepatitis, including infections with HBV and HCV, is a global public health concern. Worldwide in 2015, there were 257 million and 71 million people living with HBV and HCV, respectively, and viral hepatitis was responsible for 1.34 million deaths in 2015.[45] The WHO has called for the elimination of viral hepatitis as a public health threat by 2030.[45] Children with vertically acquired viral hepatitis become chronic carriers at a high rate and represent an important viral reservoir. In addition, they can develop complications such as cirrhosis, liver failure, and hepatocellular carcinoma later in life and might require liver transplants. Treatment of pregnant women with HBV and HCV to prevent MTCT and its sequelae is a promising global health strategy to limit the viral reservoir and to prevent these sequelae of chronic disease.

Treatment of Hepatitis B Virus

Although widespread administration of the HBV vaccine to infants has significantly reduced the incidence of HBV,[46] most new cases still occur in children who acquire the virus via MTCT or through contact with other infected children.[45] For children born to HBV-positive mothers, it is standard of care to administer both HBV vaccine and HBV immunoglobulin within 12 hours of birth.[47–49] This strategy is effective but does not eliminate MTCT. Studies have demonstrated that the risk of failure of this passive-active immunization strategy is directly related to the presence of maternal e antigen (HBeAg) and to maternal viral load, with a viral load greater than 6 $\log_{10}$ copies/mL being the most important determinant of MTCT.[50–56] Targeting women with high viral loads for antiviral treatment could further reduce MTCT of HBV.

Among nonpregnant adults, first-line treatment for HBV is with the nucleoside or nucleotide analogue antivirals. These drugs inhibit viral reverse transcriptase to prevent DNA synthesis, thus decreasing viral DNA levels and preventing viral replication. Current recommendations from the WHO and the American Association of the Study of Liver Diseases (AASLD) support treatment with tenofovir or entecavir in the general population; lamivudine was used previously but is no longer recommended due to high levels of resistance.[46,57] Among pregnant women, HBV immunoglobulin, tenofovir, lamivudine, and telbivudine have been investigated as treatments to decrease the rate of MTCT. Antenatal administration of HBV immunoglobulin is not recommended due to the poor quality of data[58] and inefficacy.[59]

Data on the efficacy of the antiviral agents are more promising; these medications have favorable safety profiles and have not shown teratogenicity.[60] Two meta-analyses of the published RCTs investigating the effectiveness of lamivudine on MTCT have found beneficial effects with reductions in intrauterine transmission and overall MTCT, as demonstrated by levels of HBV DNA and the presence of the HBV s antigen (HBsAg) in neonates and infants at 6 to 12 months of age. Neither analysis identified higher rates of adverse effects or obstetric complications among women treated with lamivudine.[61,62]

Studies of tenofovir for treatment of HBV in pregnancy have also reported positive effects, although there are fewer data than for lamivudine. Observational studies of highly viremic mothers treated with tenofovir disoproxil fumarate (TDF) in the third trimester have reported decreases in maternal viremia and in MTCT.[63,64] In the first randomized controlled trial of TDF use,[65] mothers who were both HBeAg-positive and had an HBV DNA level greater than 200,000 IU/mL were randomly allocated to TDF (300 mg/d) or usual care from 30 to 32 weeks of gestation until 4 weeks postpartum. At delivery, maternal viremia decreased to less than 200,000 IU/mL in 69% of TDF-treated patients compared with 2% of controls, and at 28 weeks postpartum, MTCT decreased to 5% compared with 18% in controls. There were no teratogenic effects, but mothers in the TDF group had elevations in their creatine kinase and alanine aminotransferase levels after discontinuation of TDF. In a second randomized controlled trial,[66] women in Thailand with HBsAg and HBeAg, regardless of viremia, were treated with TDF or placebo from 28 weeks' gestation until 2 months postpartum. The median viral load in treated women decreased from 7.6 to 4.0 $\log_{10}$ IU/mL, whereas MTCT at 6 months of age decreased nonsignificantly from 2% in the placebo group to 0% in the TDF-treated group. The investigators had anticipated a 12% rate of transmission in the placebo group, and thus the study was underpowered to detect a significant difference at the observed effect size.[67] Moreover, infants received HBIG and the HBV vaccine more rapidly after birth than is typically accomplished outside of a clinical trial, and critics have questioned whether the early administration of passive-active immunization could have contributed to the overall low rate of MTCT observed in this trial.[67,68]

Given the promising results on the use of antivirals to decrease MTCT and analyses that suggest such an approach is cost-effective,[69,70] several professional societies have recently recommended treatment in the third trimester of pregnancy. In the United States, the AASLD[57,71] recommends tenofovir as the first-line treatment for pregnant women with an HBV viral load greater than 6 $\log_{10}$ copies/mL or 200,000 IU/mL to decrease MTCT, given concerns of lamivudine resistance. The CDC,[72] ACOG,[73] and SMFM[47] now have similar recommendations or have endorsed the AASLD recommendations.

Treatment of Hepatitis C Virus

In general, women with chronic HCV infection tolerate pregnancy well. Pregnancy has not been shown to affect disease progression,[74] but in observational studies, HCV is associated with adverse obstetric[75-79] and neonatal[75] outcomes. The risk of MTCT of HCV is approximately 5% and is essentially restricted to women with viremia; women who are coinfected with HIV have a higher rate of transmission.[74,80-84] Currently, there are no approved treatments to mitigate this risk.[85,86]

Before 2011, HCV in nonpregnant patients was treated with a cytokine, pegylated interferon-α, and a nucleoside inhibitor, ribavirin, for 24 to 48 weeks. This regimen had low efficacy in some populations and was poorly tolerated.[87,88] Importantly, both of these medications are contraindicated in pregnancy. Direct-acting antiviral drugs (DAAs) were introduced in 2011 and have revolutionized the treatment of HCV in the general population. This novel class of antiviral medications targets specific enzymes and proteins required for the viral lifecycle. The DAAs active against HCV are NS5A protein inhibitors, NS5B RNA-dependent RNA polymerase inhibitors, and NS3/4A protease inhibitors. These agents produce a sustained virologic response rate or a sustained undetectable viral load for 6 months after completion of treatment. In other words, DAAs can cure HCV infection.[86] Moreover, the specificity of DAAs for viral proteins limits their toxicity; they are administered orally; and most patients require only 8 to 12 weeks of therapy.[86,87]

From a global health perspective, pregnancy is an intriguing window of opportunity for treatment of HCV.[89] First, treatment of HCV during pregnancy might reduce the aforementioned obstetric and neonatal complications. Second, treatment of pregnant women theoretically might reduce MTCT. This reduction might limit the viral reservoir, prevent complications of chronic HCV infection in offspring of affected women, and reduce health care costs across the lifespan of these children. Third, pregnancy represents a unique time period to engage HCV-positive women in health care. Only 7.4% of people with HCV actually receive treatment,[45] despite recommendations from the AASLD and the WHO to assess everyone with chronic HCV infection for treatment. Young women are more likely to commit to health care during pregnancy, and with the short duration of therapy required to treat HCV with DAAs, full treatment and cure could be achieved during pregnancy. Thus far, the safety of DAAs has not been evaluated in pregnant women, but animal studies have not demonstrated fetal risk.[85] One ongoing phase I clinical trial (NCT02683005) is investigating the safety and pharmacokinetics of the combination of the NS5B polymerase inhibitor sofosbuvir and the NS5A inhibitor ledipasvir given orally once daily for 12 weeks during the second and third trimesters. If data from this trial demonstrate favorable safety and pharmacokinetic profiles, efficacy trials should be strongly considered. Currently, despite this promise, there are no recommendations for treatment of active HCV in pregnancy.

HUMAN IMMUNODEFICIENCY VIRUS

Worldwide, 36.9 million people were living with HIV at the end of 2017. In the United States, 235,004 women were living with HIV at the end of 2016,[90] and 8700 HIV-positive women give birth annually.[91] Nearly 25 years ago, the AIDS Clinical Trials Group 076 (ACTG 076) trial, published in 1994, first demonstrated a benefit of zidovudine in reducing MTCT of HIV. The effect size—a 68% reduction in relative risk of transmission—was so impressive that the trial was halted early so as not to withhold treatment from women randomized to placebo.[92] Since that time, combination antiretroviral therapy (ART) has become the standard of care for treatment of HIV during pregnancy, both to treat maternal disease and to minimize MTCT. Indeed, implementation of ART has reduced MTCT to less than 2% in high-income countries.[93–95] Although a full review of the pharmacology of ART and of treatment of HIV in pregnancy is beyond the scope of this review, the authors highlight several key features of ART in pregnancy.

Principles of Antiretroviral Therapy

ART should be administered to all pregnant women, regardless of viremia or CD4 count.[96] Several general principles guide the use of ART in pregnancy. First, antiretroviral agents work partly through a reduction in maternal viremia,[96] and the risk of MTCT of HIV depends on maternal HIV RNA level.[93,97,98] In one cohort, transmission decreased from 23.4% among women with a viral load greater than 30,000 copies/mL to 1% among women with a viral load less than 400 copies/mL with a 2.4-fold decrease in MTCT for every $\log_{10}$ decrease in viral load.[93] To maximize viral suppression, ART should be initiated before conception or as soon as pregnancy is diagnosed in an HIV-positive woman because perinatal transmission rates correlate with the duration of ART.[98] Women on ART before conception have a 0.2% to 0.7% risk of transmission,[95,99] and the risk of transmission increases with every trimester delay in initiation of ART.[95] In a South African cohort, each additional week of ART decreased MTCT by 8%.[99] Importantly, women who present late in gestation do still benefit from short-course therapy.[100] Next, studies show that combination therapy is superior to monotherapy, with multiagent therapy yielding the lowest rates of MTCT, compared with single- or dual-agent therapy.[93,99–101] In one study, the odds ratio of MTCT was 0.27 (95% confidence interval , 0.08–0.94) in women on ART compared with women treated with zidovudine alone.[93] In addition, ART should be administered antenatally, intrapartum, and to infants postnatally. The ACTG 076 trial relied on this 3-pronged approach.[92] Women with viral suppression near delivery should continue their oral ART intrapartum. Among women with unsuppressed viral loads (HIV RNA >1000 copies/mL), retrospective data suggest that intrapartum or precesarean intravenous zidovudine reduces perinatal HIV transmission.[102]

Finally, the transplacental passage of antiretroviral drugs is a key consideration when selecting an ART regimen for a pregnant woman because of the need for fetal preexposure prophylaxis. Suppressed maternal plasma viremia does not ensure protection of the fetus from infection. Indeed, in the French Perinatal Cohort between 1997 and 2006, 20% of infected children were born to mothers with plasma viral loads less than 500 copies/mL.[103] Genital viral shedding can persist despite initiation of ART[104] and despite undetectable maternal viral loads[105,106]; in some studies, HIV was detected in the genital tract of nearly 40% of women with undetectable plasma viral loads.[107,108] Moreover, genital viral shedding is an independent risk factor for MTCT.[109] Preexposure prophylaxis of the fetus is thought to be protective against exposure to these genital secretions and to reduce intrapartum HIV transmission. Therefore, ART regimens should include drugs that cross the placenta and reach therapeutic levels in the fetus. Evaluation of drug concentration in paired maternal plasma and umbilical cord blood samples collected at delivery is one method of assessing transplacental passage of drugs. A systematic review of such studies[110] indicates that the nucleoside/nucleotide reverse transcriptase inhibitors (NRTIs) such as abacavir, lamivudine, stavudine, and emtricitabine have high placental transfer and achieve approximately equal or higher concentrations in cord blood compared with maternal plasma. Data for tenofovir and zidovudine are more varied but also demonstrate high transplacental passage with ratios ranging from 0.8 to 6.0 for tenofovir and 0.81 to 1.6 for zidovudine. The NRTI didanosine, which is not recommended in pregnancy,[96] has limited transplacental passage. Among the nonnucleoside reverse transcriptase inhibitors (NNRTIs), measured cord blood to maternal plasma ratios for nevirapine range from 0.59 to 1.0, but other NNRTIs have limited to moderate transplacental passage or a paucity of data. Protease inhibitors are poorly transported across the placenta. National guidelines for ART in pregnant women recommend that the regimen include at least one NRTI with high transplacental passage (cord blood to maternal plasma ratio >0.6) to provide fetal preexposure prophylaxis.[96]

In addition to the aforementioned principles, the choice of specific ART components must take into consideration the efficacy, toxicity and associated adverse effects, and interactions of drugs; the HIV genotype and resistance profile; prior ART exposure; patient adherence; and pharmacokinetic changes of pregnancy. With few exceptions, women entering pregnancy on ART with suppression of viremia should continue their current regimen. Recommended treatment regimens to initiate in pregnancy consist of a dual NRTI backbone and either an NNRTI, a protease inhibitor, or an integrase inhibitor as a third drug; first-line drugs in each class are listed in **Table 2**. Detailed guidelines for prescribing and managing ART in pregnancy are available from the Department of Health and Human Services[96] and from the WHO.[111] When caring

Table 2
Preferred and alternative first-line agents for initiation of antiretroviral therapy for HIV in pregnant women

Drug Class	Drug
Nucleotide/nucleoside reverse transcriptase inhibitors (NRTIs)	Tenofovir Emtricitabine Lamivudine Zidovudine
Nonnucleoside reverse transcriptase inhibitors (NNRTIs)	Efavirenz Nevirapine Rilpivirine
Integrase inhibitors	Raltegravir
Protease inhibitors	Atazanavir/ritonavir Lopinavir/ritonavir

Data from Panel on treatment of pregnant women with HIV infection and prevention of perinatal transmission. Recommendations for use of antiretroviral drugs in transmission in the United States. Available at: http://aidsinfo.nih.gov/contentfiles/lvguidelines/PerinatalGL.pdf. Accessed November 21, 2018.

for HIV-infected pregnant women, it is recommended to work collaboratively with (and/or transfer care to) infectious disease providers with extensive clinical experience with selection and use of ARTs.

Teratogenicity and Adverse Obstetric Outcomes Associated with Antiretrovirals

Overall, data support the short-term safety of ART in pregnancy. The Antiretroviral Pregnancy Registry (APR), a prospective study of pregnancies exposed to ART, now contains outcome data on more than 19,000 pregnancies between 1989 and 2018. The rate of birth defects among women exposed to ART in the first trimester is 2.8%, which is not significantly different from the rate among women initially exposed later in gestation or from United States population-based comparator rates. The APR contains sufficient power to exclude a 1.5- to 2.0-fold increase in the rate of birth defects with first-trimester exposure to individual ART agents recommended for use in pregnancy.[112] Although there have been individual reports of associations between dolutegravir and neural tube defects,[113] first-trimester exposure to efavirenz and overall rates of birth defects,[114,115] atazanavir and musculoskeletal and skin defects,[116] and zidovudine and congenital heart disease,[117,118] these associations have not been replicated in other published studies or in data from the APR. The APR Advisory Committee Consensus states, "In reviewing all reported defects from the prospective registry, informed by clinical studies and retrospective reports of antiretroviral exposure, the Registry finds no apparent increases in frequency of birth defects with first trimester exposures compared to exposures starting later in pregnancy and no pattern to suggest a common cause. While the Registry population exposed and monitored to date is not sufficient to detect an increase in the risk of relatively rare defects, these findings should provide some assurance when counseling patients. However, potential limitations of registries such as this should be recognized. The Registry is ongoing. Given the use of new therapies about which data are still insufficient, health care providers are strongly encouraged to report eligible patients to the Registry at SM_APR@INCResearch.com via the data forms available at www. APRegistry.com/."

Some evidence suggests that ART might be associated with adverse obstetric outcomes including preterm birth and low birth weight of infants, but the data are contradictory. For example, although some studies have shown that multiagent ART is associated with increased odds of preterm birth compared with dual- or single-agent therapy[101,119] and that preconception and first-trimester ART exposure slightly increased the risk of preterm birth compared with later initiation,[120] other studies have shown that untreated HIV infection is itself associated with an increase in preterm birth[121] and that ART might be protective against preterm birth.[122] Longitudinal data from a large American cohort spanning 1989 to 2004 demonstrate that as ART administration to HIV-positive pregnant women increased from 2% to 84%, preterm birth declined from 35% to 22%.[123] Some studies have particularly implicated protease inhibitors in preterm birth.[120,124] In one randomized trial, treatment with ART including a protease inhibitor was associated with a 24% incidence of preterm birth compared with 11% for treatment with triple-NRTI ART.[125] Data are similarly conflicting for infant birth weight, with some studies finding an association between ART and low birth weight[126,127] and other studies failing to identify such an association.[124,128–130]

Despite these concerns regarding adverse obstetric outcomes, the benefit of ART in treating maternal disease and reducing MTCT of HIV are clear and currently outweigh any demonstrated or theoretic risks. As experience with ART in pregnancy grows, data on longer-term follow-up of children exposed to ART in utero will emerge that will hopefully reassure patients and providers as to the safety of antiviral agents.

Antiretroviral Therapy in Breastfeeding Women

HIV is transmissible through breast milk at rates as high as 24%.[131] Therefore, in the United States and other high-income countries where safe and nutritious alternatives to maternal breast milk are available (eg, formula, donor breast milk), avoidance of breastfeeding is the standard of care. In some low-resource settings, particularly where malnutrition and diarrhea are common, alternative feeding strategies are often not safe or feasible, either due to the cost and availability of formula or due to the lack of clean water with which to constitute the formula. In these settings, infant mortality is lower among breastfed infants,[132] and the risk of HIV transmission through breast milk is often outweighed by the potential benefits of breastfeeding. The transmission risk for breastfed infants depends on maternal viral load, CD4 cell count, and the viral load of breast milk.[133] Both maternal ART and infant antiretroviral treatment reduce the transmission of HIV to breastfed infants and are similarly efficacious and safe approaches.[134–139] Given the maternal health benefits of ART, the current recommendations for lifelong ART in adults, the comparable efficacy of maternal and infant treatment approaches, and the simpler approach of maternal compared with infant therapy, the WHO recommends use of maternal ART for prevention of HIV transmission through breast milk, in addition to a total of 6 to 12 weeks of infant therapy.[111]

It is unclear whether drug penetration into breast milk is important in determining the efficacy of ART in reducing transmission to breastfed infants. Several pharmacokinetic studies have measured and correlated concentrations of antiretroviral drugs in breast milk and in the blood of breastfed infants in comparison to maternal plasma drug concentrations. The NRTIs as a general class accumulate in breast milk but are variably detected in infant blood.[140–142] The exception is tenofovir, which enters breast milk in very low quantities and is undetectable in most breastfed infants who are exposed to it.[141,143] Similarly, low relative concentrations of protease inhibitors are measured in breast milk, and their levels are undetectable in breastfed infants.[140,142] The NNRTIs have good penetration but do not concentrate in breast milk; breast milk concentrations range from 71% to 94% of maternal plasma levels.[140,144] Notably, there is concern that the low-level exposure of breastfed infants to antiretrovirals could promote drug resistance,[145,146] but this concern is not sufficient to discourage ART use

Table 3
Recommended, acceptable, and contraindicated vaccines during pregnancy

Universally Recommended	Acceptable if Indicated	Contraindicated
Inactivated influenza	Hepatitis A	Live-attenuated (intranasal) influenza
Tetanus toxoid, diphtheria toxoid, and acellular pertussis (TdaP)	Hepatitis B	Measles-mumps-rubella (MMR)
	Inactivated poliovirus	Live-inactivated (oral) poliovirus
	Meningococcal	Varicella
	Pneumococcal	Smallpox
	Rabies	
	Yellow fever	

Data from ACOG committee opinion no. 741. Maternal immunization. Obstet Gynecol 2018;131(6):e214–7; and Kroger AT, Duchin J, Vázquez M. General best practice guidelines for immunization. Best practices guidance of the advisory committee on immunization practices (ACIP). Available at: http://www.cdc.gov/vaccines/hcp/acip-recs/general-recs/index.html. Accessed December 18, 2018.

in conjunction with breastfeeding in low-resource settings. The mainstay of prevention of MTCT is reduction of the maternal viral load, thus the varying passage of antiretrovirals into breast milk and the low infant drug levels do not imply inefficacy. In the Mma Bana cohort in Botswana, in which 97% of women breastfed while on ART, the overall HIV transmission risk at 6 months of infant life was 1.1%, and breastfeeding did not affect viral suppression or the efficacy of ART for the women.[147] In another cohort study of breastfeeding mothers on ART from Mozambique, cumulative MTCT of HIV at 12 months of infant life was 2.8%.[137] Thus, the risk of HIV transmission through breastfeeding is low for women on ART. The WHO recommends that health authorities decide on a national or subnational level whether to primarily support breastfeeding and use of ART to reduce transmission through breast milk or whether to primarily support avoidance of breastfeeding and alternative infant feeding strategies.[111]

VACCINATION IN PREGNANCY

A discussion of viral infections in pregnancy would not be complete without attention to the importance of currently recommended vaccines as well as developing immunizations that offer both proof (for approved vaccines) and the promise (vaccines under development) for prevention of disease in both mothers and their infants. A listing of pregnancy-specific, current vaccine recommendations is included in **Table 3**.

All pregnant women (lacking contraindication) should receive an inactivated influenza vaccine as well as the current tetanus, diphtheria, and pertussis vaccine (Tdap) during each pregnancy, for both maternal and neonatal disease prevention.[148,149] Given the proven benefits of influenza and Tdap vaccines for both maternal and neonatal disease prevention, this should be endorsed by all obstetrics care providers.

Importantly, there has been a resurgence of interest in recent years in the time-recognized concept of maternal immunization (immunizing pregnant mothers, with subsequent transplacental transfer of protective maternal antibody, primarily for neonatal benefit) in development of various vaccines that have such promise. These include but are not limited to respiratory syncytial virus, group B streptococcus (a bacterium), potentially CMV, and Zika virus. The optimal window for use of the latter 2 are still under deliberation; nevertheless, this renewed interest and active investigation during pregnancy is likely to generate important new advances in this rapidly changing field in the near future.

SUMMARY

The authors have reviewed some of the practice guidelines and recent advances in the treatment of crucial viral infections that affect pregnancy. For the infections described herein, maternal treatment during pregnancy has as the primary goal prevention of perinatal transmission and its sequelae, in addition to offering improved maternal health. The management of viral infections in pregnancy is a constantly evolving field. Despite the challenges of conducting research during pregnancy, numerous studies are ongoing with both medications and immunizations that will fill in current knowledge gaps and improve medical care for pregnant women and their unborn children. More definitive recommendations will await the outcomes of these ongoing important investigations for some of the relatively less-studied conditions.

Best Practices

What is the current practice?

- Identify pregnant women with specific viral infections through careful history taking, routine maternal serology assessment, and workup of fetal anomalies identified on screening ultrasound

- Assess maternal disease status through history, physical examination, and measurement of viral load and other laboratory parameters

- Initiate safe and effective antiviral treatments when indicated

Objective

To minimize the maternal symptoms and sequelae of viral infections and to prevent maternal-to-child transmission of such infections

What changes in current practice are likely to improve outcomes?

- Clarification of the role of CMV hyperimmune globulin and nucleoside analogue antiviral therapy for CMV infection during pregnancy could enable treatment and prevention of congenital CMV

- Identification of safe and effective direct-acting antivirals for the treatment of HCV in pregnancy could reduce maternal-to-child transmission of the virus and could cure maternal disease

- Continued research into antiretroviral therapy for HIV during pregnancy will allow selection of the best regimens to treat maternal disease; prevent maternal-to-child transmission of HIV; and minimize maternal, obstetric, and fetal complications of antiretroviral therapy

Major Recommendations

- Active maternal HSV during pregnancy should be treated with acyclovir or valacyclovir. Pregnant women with a history of genital HSV should receive prophylactic acyclovir or valacyclovir after 36 weeks' gestation.

- Pregnant women with HBV who have high levels of viremia should receive tenofovir in the third trimester to reduce maternal-to-child transmission of HBV.

- Combination antiretroviral therapy should be initiated as soon as pregnancy is diagnosed in a woman with HIV and should be continued intrapartum and postpartum.

- Women in low-resource settings who are HIV-positive and engage in breastfeeding should remain on antiretroviral therapy, whereas those women in resource-rich settings should not breastfeed.

- During pregnancy, CMV and chronic HCV should not be treated except within the context of a clinical trial.

Summary Statement

Treatment of viral infections during pregnancy can improve maternal health, reduce maternal-to-child viral transmission, and prevent long-term sequelae of perinatally acquired infections.

REFERENCES

1. Looker KJ, Magaret AS, Turner KME, et al. Global estimates of prevalent and incident herpes simplex virus type 2 infections in 2012. PLoS One 2015;10(1): e114989.
2. Looker KJ, Magaret AS, May MT, et al. Global and regional estimates of prevalent and incident herpes simplex virus type 1 infections in 2012. PLoS One 2015; 10(10):e0140765.
3. Mcquillan G, Kruszon-Moran D, Flagg EW, et al. Prevalence of herpes simplex virus type 1 and type 2 in persons aged 14-49: United States, 2015-2016. NCHS data brief, no 304. Hyattsville (MD): National Center for Health Statistics; 2018.
4. Brown ZA, Selke S, Zeh J, et al. The acquisition of herpes simplex virus during pregnancy. N Engl J Med 1997;337(8):509–16.
5. Bernstein DI, Bellamy AR, Hook EW, et al. Epidemiology, clinical presentation, and antibody response to primary infection with herpes simplex virus type 1 and type 2 in young women. Clin Infect Dis 2013;56(3):344–51.
6. Brown ZA, Benedetti J, Ashley R, et al. Neonatal herpes simplex virus infection in relation to asymptomatic maternal infection at the time of labor. N Engl J Med 1991;324(18):1247–52.
7. Workowski KA, Bolan GA. Sexually transmitted diseases treatment guidelines, 2015. MMWR Recomm Rep 2015;64(RR-03):1–137.
8. ACOG Committee on Practice Bulletins. ACOG practice bulletin. Clinical management guidelines for obstetrician-gynecologists. no. 82 June 2007. Management of herpes in pregnancy. Obstet Gynecol 2007;109(6):1489–98.
9. Sheffield JS, Hollier LM, Hill JB, et al. Acyclovir prophylaxis to prevent herpes simplex virus recurrence at delivery: a systematic review. Obstet Gynecol 2003;102(6):1396–403.
10. Hollier LM, Wendel GD. Third trimester antiviral prophylaxis for preventing maternal genital herpes simplex virus (HSV) recurrences and neonatal infection. Cochrane Database Syst Rev 2008;(1):CD004946.
11. Watts DH, Brown ZA, Money D, et al. A double-blind, randomized, placebo-controlled trial of acyclovir in late pregnancy for the reduction of herpes simplex virus shedding and cesarean delivery. Am J Obstet Gynecol 2003;188(3): 836–43.
12. Pinninti SG, Angara R, Feja KN, et al. Neonatal herpes disease following maternal antenatal antiviral suppressive therapy: a multicenter case series. J Pediatr 2012;161(1):134–8.e1-3.
13. Haddad J, Langer B, Astruc D, et al. Oral acyclovir and recurrent genital herpes during late pregnancy. Obstet Gynecol 1993;82(1):102–4.
14. Frenkel LM, Brown ZA, Bryson YJ, et al. Pharmacokinetics of acyclovir in the term human pregnancy and neonate. Am J Obstet Gynecol 1991;164(2): 569–76.

15. Kimberlin DF, Weller S, Whitley RJ, et al. Pharmacokinetics of oral valacyclovir and acyclovir in late pregnancy. Am J Obstet Gynecol 1998;179(4):846–51.
16. Pasternak B, Hviid A. Use of acyclovir, valacyclovir, and famciclovir in the first trimester of pregnancy and the risk of birth defects. JAMA 2010;304(8):859.
17. Stone KM, Reiff-Eldridge R, White AD, et al. Pregnancy outcomes following systemic prenatal acyclovir exposure: conclusions from the international acyclovir pregnancy registry, 1984-1999. Birth Defects Res A Clin Mol Teratol 2004; 70(4):201–7.
18. Staras SAS, Dollard SC, Radford KW, et al. Seroprevalence of cytomegalovirus infection in the United States, 1988-1994. Clin Infect Dis 2006;43(9):1143–51.
19. Hyde TB, Schmid DS, Cannon MJ. Cytomegalovirus seroconversion rates and risk factors: implications for congenital CMV. Rev Med Virol 2010;20(5):311–26.
20. Dollard SC, Grosse SD, Ross DS. New estimates of the prevalence of neurological and sensory sequelae and mortality associated with congenital cytomegalovirus infection. Rev Med Virol 2007;17(5):355–63.
21. Mussi-Pinhata MM, Yamamoto AY, Moura Brito RM, et al. Birth prevalence and natural history of congenital cytomegalovirus infection in a highly seroimmune population. Clin Infect Dis 2009;49(4):522–8.
22. Kenneson A, Cannon MJ. Review and meta-analysis of the epidemiology of congenital cytomegalovirus (CMV) infection. Rev Med Virol 2007;17(4):253–76.
23. Wang C, Zhang X, Bialek S, et al. Attribution of congenital cytomegalovirus infection to primary versus non-primary maternal infection. Clin Infect Dis 2011;52(2):e11–3.
24. Gaytant MA, Rours GIJG, Steegers EAP, et al. Congenital cytomegalovirus infection after recurrent infection: case reports and review of the literature. Eur J Pediatr 2003;162(4):248–53.
25. Picone O, Vauloup-Fellous C, Cordier AG, et al. A series of 238 cytomegalovirus primary infections during pregnancy: description and outcome. Prenat Diagn 2013;33(8):751–8.
26. Enders G, Daiminger A, Bäder U, et al. Intrauterine transmission and clinical outcome of 248 pregnancies with primary cytomegalovirus infection in relation to gestational age. J Clin Virol 2011;52(3):244–6.
27. Guerra B, Simonazzi G, Puccetti C, et al. Ultrasound prediction of symptomatic congenital cytomegalovirus infection. Am J Obstet Gynecol 2008;198(4): 380.e1-7.
28. Picone O, Teissier N, Cordier AG, et al. Detailed in utero ultrasound description of 30 cases of congenital cytomegalovirus infection. Prenat Diagn 2014;34(6): 518–24.
29. Stagno S, Whitley RJ. Herpesvirus infections of pregnancy. N Engl J Med 1985; 313(20):1270–4.
30. Fowler KB, Stagno S, Pass RF, et al. The outcome of congenital cytomegalovirus infection in relation to maternal antibody status. N Engl J Med 1992;326(10): 663–7.
31. Grosse SD, Ross DS, Dollard SC. Congenital cytomegalovirus (CMV) infection as a cause of permanent bilateral hearing loss: a quantitative assessment. J Clin Virol 2008;41(2):57–62.
32. Nigro G, Adler SP, La Torre R, et al. Passive immunization during pregnancy for congenital cytomegalovirus infection. N Engl J Med 2005;353(13):1350–62.
33. Visentin S, Manara R, Milanese L, et al. Early primary cytomegalovirus infection in pregnancy: maternal hyperimmunoglobulin therapy improves outcomes among infants at 1 year of age. Clin Infect Dis 2012;55(4):497–503.

34. Nigro G, Adler SP, Parruti G, et al. Immunoglobulin therapy of fetal cytomegalovirus infection occurring in the first half of pregnancy–a case-control study of the outcome in children. J Infect Dis 2012;205(2):215–27.

35. Revello MG, Lazzarotto T, Guerra B, et al. A randomized trial of hyperimmune globulin to prevent congenital cytomegalovirus. N Engl J Med 2014;370(14): 1316–26.

36. Nigro G, Capretti I, Manganello A-M, et al. Primary maternal cytomegalovirus infections during pregnancy: association of CMV hyperimmune globulin with gestational age at birth and birth weight. J Matern Fetal Neonatal Med 2015; 28(2):168–71.

37. Chiaie LD, Neuberger P, Vochem M, et al. No evidence of obstetrical adverse events after hyperimmune globulin application for primary cytomegalovirus infection in pregnancy: experience from a single centre. Arch Gynecol Obstet 2018;297(6):1389–95.

38. Minsart A-F, Smiljkovic M, Renaud C, et al. Use of cytomegalovirus-specific hyperimmunoglobulins in pregnancy: a retrospective cohort. J Obstet Gynaecol Can 2018;40(11):1409–16.

39. Blázquez-Gamero D, Galindo Izquierdo A, Del Rosal T, et al. Prevention and treatment of fetal cytomegalovirus infection with cytomegalovirus hyperimmune globulin: a multicenter study in Madrid. J Matern Fetal Neonatal Med 2019; 32(4):617–25.

40. Jacquemard F, Yamamoto M, Costa J-M, et al. Maternal administration of valaciclovir in symptomatic intrauterine cytomegalovirus infection. BJOG 2007; 114(9):1113–21.

41. Leruez-Ville M, Ghout I, Bussières L, et al. In utero treatment of congenital cytomegalovirus infection with valacyclovir in a multicenter, open-label, phase II study. Am J Obstet Gynecol 2016;215(4):462.e1–10.

42. American College of Obstetricians and Gynecologists. ACOG practice bulletin no. 151: cytomegalovirus, parvovirus B12, varicella zoster, and toxoplasmosis in pregnancy. Obstet Gynecol 2015;125(6):1510–25.

43. Hughes BL, Gyamfi-Bannerman C, Gyamfi-Bannerman C. Diagnosis and antenatal management of congenital cytomegalovirus infection. Am J Obstet Gynecol 2016;214(6):B5–11.

44. Rawlinson WD, Boppana SB, Fowler KB, et al. Congenital cytomegalovirus infection in pregnancy and the neonate: consensus recommendations for prevention, diagnosis, and therapy. Lancet Infect Dis 2017;17(6):e177–88.

45. World Health Organization. Global hepatitis report 2017. Geneva (Switzerland): World Health Organization; 2017. Available at: http://www.who.int/hepatitis/publications/global-hepatitis-report2017/en/. Accessed August 22, 2018.

46. World Health Organization. Guidelines for the prevention, care and treatment of persons with chronic hepatitis B infection. Geneva (Switzerland): World Health Organization; 2015. Available at: http://www.who.int/hepatitis/publications/hepatitis-b-guidelines/en/. Accessed August 22, 2018.

47. Dionne-Odom J, Tita ATN, Silverman NS. #38: Hepatitis B in pregnancy screening, treatment, and prevention of vertical transmission. Am J Obstet Gynecol 2016;214(1):6–14.

48. ACOG practice bulletin no. 86: viral hepatitis in pregnancy. Obstet Gynecol 2007;110(4):941–56.

49. Mast EE, Margolis HS, Fiore AE, et al. A comprehensive immunization strategy to eliminate transmission of hepatitis B virus infection in the United States: recommendations of the advisory committee on immunization practices (ACIP) part

1: immunization of infants, children, and adolescents. MMWR Recomm Rep 2005;54(RR-16):1–31.

50. Burk RD, Hwang LY, Ho GY, et al. Outcome of perinatal hepatitis B virus exposure is dependent on maternal virus load. J Infect Dis 1994;170(6):1418–23.

51. del Canho R, Grosheide PM, Mazel JA, et al. Ten-year neonatal hepatitis B vaccination program, The Netherlands, 1982-1992: protective efficacy and long-term immunogenicity. Vaccine 1997;15(15):1624–30.

52. Wiseman E, Fraser MA, Holden S, et al. Perinatal transmission of hepatitis B virus: an Australian experience. Med J Aust 2009;190(9):489–92.

53. Lin X, Guo Y, Zhou A, et al. Immunoprophylaxis failure against vertical transmission of hepatitis B virus in the Chinese population. Pediatr Infect Dis J 2014; 33(9):897–903.

54. Kubo A, Shlager L, Marks AR, et al. Prevention of vertical transmission of hepatitis B. Ann Intern Med 2014;160(12):828.

55. Pan CQ, Duan Z, Bhamidimarri KR, et al. An algorithm for risk assessment and intervention of mother to child transmission of hepatitis B virus. Clin Gastroenterol Hepatol 2012;10(5):452–9.

56. Zou H, Chen Y, Duan Z, et al. Virologic factors associated with failure to passive-active immunoprophylaxis in infants born to HBsAg-positive mothers. J Viral Hepat 2012;19(2):e18–25.

57. Terrault NA, Lok ASF, McMahon BJ, et al. Update on prevention, diagnosis, and treatment of chronic hepatitis B: AASLD 2018 hepatitis B guidance. Hepatology 2018;67(4):1560–99.

58. Eke AC, Eleje GU, Eke UA, et al. Hepatitis B immunoglobulin during pregnancy for prevention of mother-to-child transmission of hepatitis B virus. Cochrane Database Syst Rev 2017;(2):CD008545.

59. Yuan J, Lin J, Xu A, et al. Antepartum immunoprophylaxis of three doses of hepatitis B immunoglobulin is not effective: a single-centre randomized study. J Viral Hepat 2006;13(9):597–604.

60. Brown RS, Verna EC, Pereira MR, et al. Hepatitis B virus and human immunodeficiency virus drugs in pregnancy: findings from the antiretroviral pregnancy registry. J Hepatol 2012;57(5):953–9.

61. Han L, Zhang H-W, Xie J-X, et al. A meta-analysis of lamivudine for interruption of mother-to-child transmission of hepatitis B virus. World J Gastroenterol 2011; 17(38):4321.

62. Shi Z, Yang Y, Ma L, et al. Lamivudine in late pregnancy to interrupt in utero transmission of hepatitis B virus. Obstet Gynecol 2010;116(1):147–59.

63. Greenup A-J, Tan PK, Nguyen V, et al. Efficacy and safety of tenofovir disoproxil fumarate in pregnancy to prevent perinatal transmission of hepatitis B virus. J Hepatol 2014;61(3):502–7.

64. Chen H-L, Lee C-N, Chang C-H, et al. Efficacy of maternal tenofovir disoproxil fumarate in interrupting mother-to-infant transmission of hepatitis B virus. Hepatology 2015;62(2):375–86.

65. Pan CQ, Duan Z, Dai E, et al. Tenofovir to Prevent hepatitis B transmission in mothers with high viral load. N Engl J Med 2016;374(24):2324–34.

66. Jourdain G, Ngo-Giang-Huong N, Harrison L, et al. Tenofovir versus placebo to prevent perinatal transmission of hepatitis B. N Engl J Med 2018;378(10): 911–23.

67. Terrault NA, Feld JJ, Lok ASF. Tenofovir to prevent perinatal transmission of hepatitis B. N Engl J Med 2018;378(24):2348–50.

68. Dusheiko G. A shift in thinking to reduce mother-to-infant transmission of hepatitis B. N Engl J Med 2018;378(10):952–3.
69. Lee D, Shin H-Y, Park SM. Cost-effectiveness of antiviral prophylaxis during pregnancy for the prevention of perinatal hepatitis B infection in South Korea. Cost Eff Resour Alloc 2018;16(1):6.
70. Nayeri UA, Werner EF, Han CS, et al. Antenatal lamivudine to reduce perinatal hepatitis B transmission: a cost-effectiveness analysis. Am J Obstet Gynecol 2012;207(3):231.e1-7.
71. Terrault NA, Bzowej NH, Chang K-M, et al. AASLD guidelines for treatment of chronic hepatitis B. Hepatology 2016;63(1):261–83.
72. Schillie S, Vellozzi C, Reingold A, et al. Prevention of hepatitis B virus infection in the United States: recommendations of the advisory committee on immunization practices. MMWR Recomm Rep 2018;67(1):1–31.
73. ACOG practice advisory: hepatitis B prevention. Available at: http://www.acog.org/Clinical-Guidance-and-Publications/Practice-Advisories/Practice-Advisory-Hepatitis-B-Prevention. Accessed November 14, 2018.
74. Conte D, Fraquelli M, Prati D, et al. Prevalence and clinical course of chronic hepatitis C virus (HCV) infection and rate of HCV vertical transmission in a cohort of 15,250 pregnant women. Hepatology 2000;31(3):751–5.
75. Pergam SA, Wang CC, Gardella CM, et al. Pregnancy complications associated with hepatitis C: data from a 2003-2005 Washington state birth cohort. Am J Obstet Gynecol 2008;199(1):38.e1-9.
76. Reddick KLB, Jhaveri R, Gandhi M, et al. Pregnancy outcomes associated with viral hepatitis. J Viral Hepat 2011;18(7):e394–8.
77. Huang Q-T, Hang L-L, Zhong M, et al. Maternal HCV infection is associated with intrauterine fetal growth disturbance: a meta-analysis of observational studies. Medicine (Baltimore) 2016;95(35):e4777.
78. Connell LE, Salihu HM, Salemi JL, et al. Maternal hepatitis B and hepatitis C carrier status and perinatal outcomes. Liver Int 2011;31(8):1163–70.
79. Wijarnpreecha K, Thongprayoon C, Sanguankeo A, et al. Hepatitis C infection and intrahepatic cholestasis of pregnancy: a systematic review and meta-analysis. Clin Res Hepatol Gastroenterol 2017;41(1):39–45.
80. Benova L, Mohamoud YA, Calvert C, et al. Vertical transmission of hepatitis C virus: systematic review and meta-analysis. Clin Infect Dis 2014;59(6):765–73.
81. Resti M, Azzari C, Mannelli F, et al. Mother to child transmission of hepatitis C virus: prospective study of risk factors and timing of infection in children born to women seronegative for HIV-1. Tuscany study group on hepatitis C virus infection. BMJ 1998;317(7156):437–41.
82. Zanetti AR, Paccagnini S, Principi N, et al. Mother-to-infant transmission of hepatitis C virus. Lancet 1995;345(8945):289–91.
83. Gibb DM, Goodall RL, Dunn DT, et al. Mother-to-child transmission of hepatitis C virus: evidence for preventable peripartum transmission. Lancet 2000;356(9233):904–7.
84. Yeung L, King SM, Roberts EA. Mother-to-infant transmission of hepatitis C virus. Hepatology 2001;34(2):223–9.
85. Hughes BL, Page CM, Kuller JA. Hepatitis C in pregnancy: screening, treatment, and management. Am J Obstet Gynecol 2017;217(5):B2–12.
86. AASLD-IDSA. Recommendations for testing, managing, and treating hepatitis C. Available at: http://www.hcvguidelines.org. Accessed August 29, 2018.

87. World Health Organization. Guidelines for the care and treatment of persons diagnosed with chronic hepatitis C virus infection. Geneva (Switzerland): World Health Organization; 2018. Available at: http://www.who.int/hepatitis/publications/hepatitis-c-guidelines-2018/en/. Accessed August 22, 2018.

88. Jazwinski AB, Muir AJ. Direct-acting antiviral medications for chronic hepatitis C virus infection. Gastroenterol Hepatol (N Y) 2011;7(3):154–62.

89. Barritt AS, Jhaveri R. Treatment of hepatitis C during pregnancy-weighing the risks and benefits in contrast to HIV. Curr HIV/AIDS Rep 2018;15(2):155–61.

90. Centers for Disease Control and Prevention. HIV surveillance report, 2017, vol. 29, 2018. Available at: http://www.cdc.gov/hiv/library/reports/hiv-surveillance.html. Accessed November 21, 2018.

91. Whitmore SK, Zhang X, Taylor AW, et al. Estimated number of infants born to HIV-infected women in the United States and five dependent areas, 2006. J Acquir Immune Defic Syndr 2011;57(3):218–22.

92. Connor EM, Sperling RS, Gelber R, et al. Reduction of maternal-infant transmission of human immunodeficiency virus type 1 with zidovudine treatment. N Engl J Med 1994;331(18):1173–80.

93. Cooper ER, Charurat M, Mofenson L, et al. Combination antiretroviral strategies for the treatment of pregnant HIV-1-infected women and prevention of perinatal HIV-1 transmission. J Acquir Immune Defic Syndr 2002;29(5):484–94.

94. Forbes JC, Alimenti AM, Singer J, et al. A national review of vertical HIV transmission. AIDS 2012;26(6):757–63.

95. Mandelbrot L, Tubiana R, Le Chenadec J, et al. No perinatal HIV-1 transmission from women with effective antiretroviral therapy starting before conception. Clin Infect Dis 2015;61(11):1715–25.

96. Panel on treatment of pregnant women with HIV infection and prevention of perinatal transmission. Recommendations for use of antiretroviral drugs in transmission in the United States. Available at: http://aidsinfo.nih.gov/contentfiles/lvguidelines/PerinatalGL.pdf. Accessed November 21, 2018.

97. Mofenson LM, Lambert JS, Stiehm ER, et al. Risk factors for perinatal transmission of human immunodeficiency virus type 1 in women treated with zidovudine. N Engl J Med 1999;341(6):385–93.

98. Townsend CL, Byrne L, Cortina-Borja M, et al. Earlier initiation of ART and further decline in mother-to-child HIV transmission rates, 2000-2011. AIDS 2014;28(7):1049–57.

99. Hoffman RM, Black V, Technau K, et al. Effects of highly active antiretroviral therapy duration and regimen on risk for mother-to-child transmission of HIV in Johannesburg, South Africa. J Acquir Immune Defic Syndr 2010;54(1):35–41.

100. Siegfried N, van der Merwe L, Brocklehurst P, et al. Antiretrovirals for reducing the risk of mother-to-child transmission of HIV infection. Cochrane Database Syst Rev 2011;(7):CD003510.

101. Fowler MG, Qin M, Fiscus SA, et al. Benefits and risks of antiretroviral therapy for perinatal HIV prevention. N Engl J Med 2016;375(18):1726–37.

102. Briand N, Warszawski J, Mandelbrot L, et al. Is intrapartum intravenous zidovudine for prevention of mother-to-child HIV-1 transmission still useful in the combination antiretroviral therapy era? Clin Infect Dis 2013;57(6):903–14.

103. Tubiana R, Le Chenadec J, Rouzioux C, et al. Factors associated with mother-to-child transmission of HIV-1 despite a maternal viral load <500 Copies/mL at delivery: a case-control study nested in the French perinatal cohort (EPF-ANRS CO1). Clin Infect Dis 2010;50(4):585–96.

104. Graham SM, Holte SE, Peshu NM, et al. Initiation of antiretroviral therapy leads to a rapid decline in cervical and vaginal HIV-1 shedding. AIDS 2007;21(4):501–7.
105. Fiore JR, Suligoi B, Saracino A, et al. Correlates of HIV-1 shedding in cervicovaginal secretions and effects of antiretroviral therapies. AIDS 2003;17(15): 2169–76.
106. King CC, Ellington SR, Davis NL, et al. Prevalence, magnitude, and correlates of HIV-1 genital shedding in women on antiretroviral therapy. J Infect Dis 2017; 216(12):1534–40.
107. Cu-Uvin S, DeLong AK, Venkatesh KK, et al. Genital tract HIV-1 RNA shedding among women with below detectable plasma viral load. AIDS 2010;24(16): 2489–97.
108. Launay O, Tod M, Tschöpe I, et al. Residual HIV-1 RNA and HIV-1 DNA production in the genital tract reservoir of women treated with HAART: the prospective ANRS EP24 GYNODYN study. Antivir Ther 2011;16(6):843–52.
109. John GC, Nduati RW, Mbori-Ngacha DA, et al. Correlates of mother-to-child human immunodeficiency virus type 1 (HIV-1) transmission: association with maternal plasma HIV-1 RNA load, genital HIV-1 DNA shedding, and breast infections. J Infect Dis 2001;183(2):206–12.
110. McCormack SA, Best BM. Protecting the fetus against HIV infection: a systematic review of placental transfer of antiretrovirals. Clin Pharmacokinet 2014; 53(11):989–1004.
111. World Health Organization. Consolidated guidelines on the use of antiretroviral drugs for treating and preventing HIV infection: recommendations for a public health approach. Geneva (Switzerland): World Health Organization; 2016. Availabe at: http://www.who.int/hiv/pub/arv/arv-2016/en/. Accessed November 21, 2018.
112. Antiretroviral Pregnancy Registry Steering Committee. Antiretroviral pregnancy registry interim report for 1 January 1989 through 31 January 2018. Wilmington (NC): Registry Coordinating Center; 2017. Available at: www.APRegistry.com. Accessed September 24, 2018.
113. Zash R, Makhema J, Shapiro RL. Neural-tube defects with dolutegravir treatment from the time of conception. N Engl J Med 2018;379(10):979–81.
114. Knapp KM, Brogly SB, Muenz DG, et al. Prevalence of congenital anomalies in infants with in utero exposure to antiretrovirals. Pediatr Infect Dis J 2012;31(2): 164–70.
115. Brogly SB, Abzug MJ, Watts DH, et al. Birth defects among children born to human immunodeficiency virus-infected women: pediatric AIDS clinical trials protocols 219 and 219C. Pediatr Infect Dis J 2010;29(8):721–7.
116. Williams PL, Crain MJ, Yildirim C, et al. Congenital anomalies and in utero antiretroviral exposure in human immunodeficiency virus-exposed uninfected infants. JAMA Pediatr 2015;169(1):48–55.
117. Sibiude J, Mandelbrot L, Blanche S, et al. Association between prenatal exposure to antiretroviral therapy and birth defects: an analysis of the French perinatal cohort study (ANRS CO1/CO11). PLoS Med 2014;11(4):e1001635.
118. Sibiude J, Le Chenadec J, Bonnet D, et al. In Utero exposure to zidovudine and heart anomalies in the ANRS French perinatal cohort and the nested PRIMEVA randomized trial. Clin Infect Dis 2015;61(2):270–80.
119. Townsend C, Schulte J, Thorne C, et al. Antiretroviral therapy and preterm delivery-a pooled analysis of data from the United States and Europe. BJOG 2010;117(11):1399–410.

120. Kourtis AP, Schmid CH, Jamieson DJ, et al. Use of antiretroviral therapy in pregnant HIV-infected women and the risk of premature delivery: a meta-analysis. AIDS 2007;21(5):607–15.

121. Wedi CO, Kirtley S, Hopewell S, et al. Perinatal outcomes associated with maternal HIV infection: a systematic review and meta-analysis. Lancet HIV 2016;3(1):e33–48.

122. Chagomerana MB, Miller WC, Pence BW, et al. PMTCT option B+ does not increase preterm birth risk and may prevent extreme prematurity: a retrospective cohort study in Malawi. J Acquir Immune Defic Syndr 2017;74(4):367–74.

123. Schulte J, Dominguez K, Sukalac T, et al. Pediatric spectrum of HIV disease consortium. Declines in low birth weight and preterm birth among infants who were born to HIV-infected women during an era of increased use of maternal antiretroviral drugs: pediatric spectrum of HIV disease, 1989-2004. Pediatrics 2007;119(4):e900–6.

124. Cotter AM, Garcia AG, Duthely ML, et al. Is antiretroviral therapy during pregnancy associated with an increased risk of preterm delivery, low birth weight, or stillbirth? J Infect Dis 2006;193(9):1195–201.

125. Powis KM, Kitch D, Ogwu A, et al. Increased risk of preterm delivery among HIV-infected women randomized to protease versus nucleoside reverse transcriptase inhibitor-based HAART during pregnancy. J Infect Dis 2011;204(4):506–14.

126. Ekouevi DK, Coffie PA, Becquet R, et al. Antiretroviral therapy in pregnant women with advanced HIV disease and pregnancy outcomes in Abidjan, Côte d'Ivoire. AIDS 2008;22(14):1815–20.

127. Njom Nlend AE, Nga Motazé A, Moyo Tetang S, et al. Preterm birth and low birth weight after in utero exposure to antiretrovirals initiated during pregnancy in yaoundé, Cameroon. PLoS One 2016;11(3):e0150565.

128. Briand N, Mandelbrot L, Le Chenadec J, et al. No relation between in-utero exposure to HAART and intrauterine growth retardation. AIDS 2009;23(10):1235–43.

129. Tuomala RE, Shapiro DE, Mofenson LM, et al. Antiretroviral therapy during pregnancy and the risk of an adverse outcome. N Engl J Med 2002;346(24):1863–70.

130. Szyld EG, Warley EM, Freimanis L, et al. Maternal antiretroviral drugs during pregnancy and infant low birth weight and preterm birth. AIDS 2006;20(18):2345–53.

131. Read DJS. Late postnatal transmission of HIV-1 in breast-fed children: an individual patient data meta-analysis. J Infect Dis 2004;189(12):2154–66.

132. Arikawa S, Rollins N, Jourdain G, et al. Contribution of maternal antiretroviral therapy and breastfeeding to 24-month survival in human immunodeficiency virus-exposed uninfected children: an individual pooled analysis of African and Asian studies. Clin Infect Dis 2018;66(11):1668–77.

133. Rousseau CM, Nduati RW, Richardson BA, et al. Longitudinal analysis of human immunodeficiency virus type 1 RNA in breast milk and of its relationship to infant infection and maternal disease. J Infect Dis 2003;187(5):741–7.

134. Flynn PM, Taha TE, Cababasay M, et al. Prevention of HIV-1 transmission through breastfeeding. J Acquir Immune Defic Syndr 2018;77(4):383–92.

135. Chasela CS, Hudgens MG, Jamieson DJ, et al. Maternal or infant antiretroviral drugs to reduce HIV-1 transmission. N Engl J Med 2010;362(24):2271–81.

136. White AB, Mirjahangir JF, Horvath H, et al. Antiretroviral interventions for preventing breast milk transmission of HIV. Cochrane Database Syst Rev 2014;(10):CD011323.

137. Marazzi MC, Nielsen-Saines K, Buonomo E, et al. Increased infant human immunodeficiency virus-type one free survival at one year of age in sub-saharan Africa with maternal use of highly active antiretroviral therapy during breastfeeding. Pediatr Infect Dis J 2009;28(6):483–7.

138. Dinh T-H, Mushavi A, Shiraishi RW, et al. Impact of timing of antiretroviral treatment and birth weight on mother-to-child human immunodeficiency virus transmission: findings from an 18-month prospective cohort of a nationally representative sample of mother-infant pairs during the transition from option A to option B+ in Zimbabwe. Clin Infect Dis 2018;66(4):576–85.

139. Kesho Bora Study Group, de Vincenzi I. Triple antiretroviral compared with zidovudine and single-dose nevirapine prophylaxis during pregnancy and breastfeeding for prevention of mother-to-child transmission of HIV-1 (Kesho Bora study): a randomised controlled trial. Lancet Infect Dis 2011;11(3):171–80.

140. Waitt CJ, Garner P, Bonnett LJ, et al. Is infant exposure to antiretroviral drugs during breastfeeding quantitatively important? A systematic review and meta-analysis of pharmacokinetic studies. J Antimicrob Chemother 2015;70(7):1928–41.

141. Waitt C, Olagunju A, Nakalema S, et al. Plasma and breast milk pharmacokinetics of emtricitabine, tenofovir and lamivudine using dried blood and breast milk spots in nursing African mother-infant pairs. J Antimicrob Chemother 2018;73(4):1013–9.

142. Corbett AH, Kayira D, White NR, et al. Antiretroviral pharmacokinetics in mothers and breastfeeding infants from 6 to 24 weeks post partum: results of the BAN Study. Antivir Ther 2014;19(6):587–95.

143. Mugwanya KK, Hendrix CW, Mugo NR, et al. Pre-exposure prophylaxis use by breastfeeding HIV-uninfected women: a prospective short-term study of antiretroviral excretion in breast milk and infant absorption. PLoS Med 2016;13(9):e1002132.

144. Palombi L, Pirillo MF, Marchei E, et al. Concentrations of tenofovir, lamivudine and efavirenz in mothers and children enrolled under the option B-plus approach in Malawi. J Antimicrob Chemother 2016;71(4):1027–30.

145. Zeh C, Weidle PJ, Nafisa L, et al. HIV-1 drug resistance emergence among breastfeeding infants born to HIV-infected mothers during a single-arm trial of triple-antiretroviral prophylaxis for prevention of mother-to-child transmission: a secondary analysis. PLoS Med 2011;8(3):e1000430.

146. Fogel J, Li Q, Taha TE, et al. Initiation of antiretroviral treatment in women after delivery can induce multiclass drug resistance in breastfeeding HIV-infected infants. Clin Infect Dis 2011;52(8):1069–76.

147. Shapiro RL, Hughes MD, Ogwu A, et al. Antiretroviral regimens in pregnancy and breast-feeding in Botswana. N Engl J Med 2010;362(24):2282–94.

148. ACOG committee opinion no. 741. Maternal immunization. Obstet Gynecol 2018;131(6):e214–7.

149. Kroger AT, Duchin J, Vázquez M. General best practice guidelines for immunization. best practices guidance of the advisory committee on immunization practices (ACIP). Available at: http://www.cdc.gov/vaccines/hcp/acip-recs/general-recs/index.html. Accessed December 18, 2018.

Drugs to Control Diabetes During Pregnancy

Maisa N. Feghali, MD[a],*, Jason G. Umans, MD[b,c], Patrick M. Catalano, MD[d]

KEYWORDS

- Diabetes • Glucose • Insulin • Pregnancy

KEY POINTS

- Diabetes is a common complication of pregnancy, and the prevalence of all types of the disease is increasing worldwide in parallel with the increase in overweight and obesity.
- Despite ongoing research on treatment of diabetes in pregnancy for decades, changes in the characteristics of the patient population and increasing evidence of heterogeneous pathophysiology have highlighted the limited effectiveness of different therapies.
- While diabetes is associated with long-term outcomes for the offspring, there is limited data on long-term outcomes following exposure to different diabetes treatments.
- Further research is needed to develop novel and individualized treatment strategies to address the increasing frequency and complexity of diabetes in pregnancy.

INTRODUCTION

Diabetes complicates 6% to 9% of pregnancies with the vast majority (90%) of cases due to gestational diabetes (GDM).[1–4] The overall prevalence of all forms of diabetes in pregnancy is increasing, likely due to increases in obesity,[3,5–7] along with changes in diagnostic criteria for GDM.[8] The main goal of treating diabetes in pregnancy is to minimize maternal and fetal adverse events related to hyperglycemia (**Table 1**). Outside of pregnancy, options for the management of diabetes include lifestyle interventions, including weight loss, oral glucose-lowering agents, and various forms of insulin. During pregnancy, weight loss and most oral glucose-lowering agents are not

[a] Department of Obstetrics, Gynecology and Reproductive Sciences, Magee Women's Research Institute, University of Pittsburgh School of Medicine, 300 Halket Street, Pittsburgh, PA 15213, USA; [b] Department of Medicine, Georgetown-Howard Universities Center for Clinical and Translational Science, Georgetown University, 3800 Reservoir Rd NW, Washington, DC 20007, USA; [c] Department of Obstetrics and Gynecology, Georgetown-Howard Universities Center for Clinical and Translational Science, Georgetown University, 3800 Reservoir Rd NW, Washington, DC 20007, USA; [d] Maternal Infant Research Institute, Obstetrics and Gynecology Research, Tufts University School of Medicine, Friedman School of Nutrition Science and Policy, 800 Washington Street, Box 394, Boston, MA 02111, USA
* Corresponding author.
E-mail address: maisafeghali@gmail.com

Clin Perinatol 46 (2019) 257–272
https://doi.org/10.1016/j.clp.2019.02.005
0095-5108/19/© 2019 Elsevier Inc. All rights reserved.

Table 1
Professional guidelines for diabetes pharmacologic management during pregnancy

	ACOG[1,2]	ADA[4]	SMFM[55]	NICE UK[64]
Glucose targets for gestational and pregestational diabetes	Fasting <95 mg/dL 1-h postprandial <140 mg/dL 2-h postprandial <120 mg/dL	Fasting <95 mg/dL 1-h postprandial <140 mg/dL 2-h postprandial <120 mg/dL	Not specified	Fasting <95 mg/dL 1-h postprandial <140 mg/dL 2-h postprandial <115 mg/dL
HbA1c targets for pregestational diabetes	<6%	6%–6.5%; <6% if without significant hypoglycemia and <7% if necessary to prevent hypoglycemia	Not specified	If no hypoglycemia <6.5%
Drug therapy	Insulin—preferred agent for diabetes in pregnancy	Insulin—preferred agent for diabetes in pregnancy	Metformin—reasonable and safe first-line alternative to insulin	Pregestational: • NPH—first choice for long-acting insulin therapy GDM: • Metformin—first-line • Add insulin if blood glucose targets are not met

options.[1,2,4] Also, although effective, insulin does not eliminate adverse maternal and fetal outcomes. In addition, patients and providers have demonstrated a clear preference for oral glucose-lowering agents.[9]

The compressed timeline of pregnancy and of opportunities for achieving glucose control are significant hurdles to effectively treating diabetes in pregnancy, especially GDM. The physiologic changes of pregnancy, including a progressive increase in insulin resistance, gestational weight gain, and changes in body composition can further complicate the treatment of diabetes in pregnancy. More recently, it has become clear that the patient population of diabetes in pregnancy is heterogeneous with respect to pathophysiology, possibly limiting the effectiveness of standardized therapies, thus demanding continued research. In this review, the authors focus on recent studies that have evaluated treatment options for women with diabetes in pregnancy and recently updated professional guidelines.

GLUCOSE METABOLISM DURING PREGNANCY

Optimal pharmacotherapy of diabetes during pregnancy depends on an understanding of the physiologic changes in glucose metabolism during normal pregnancy. During pregnancy, there are both increases and decreases in insulin sensitivity and β-cell function with advancing gestation in women with normal glucose tolerance. In early pregnancy (12–14 weeks), insulin sensitivity can either increase or decrease compared with preconception measures when assessed using the hyperinsulinemic-euglycemic clamp method. However, by late gestation (34–36 weeks), insulin sensitivity decreases by 40% to 50% virtually in all women,[10] albeit with significant interindividual variation (**Fig. 1**). These changes in insulin sensitivity are more extreme in women developing GDM, because of their underlying subclinically altered glucose metabolism before pregnancy.[11]

It is generally thought that the changes in insulin response mirror the changes in insulin sensitivity. For example, decreased insulin sensitivity leads to an increased insulin response in order to maintain normoglycemia. The situation in early pregnancy, however, is quite different than in late pregnancy. In early pregnancy, insulin response is increased regardless of changes in insulin sensitivity (**Fig. 2**). In women with type 1 diabetes in excellent control before conception, an increase in insulin sensitivity in early pregnancy may decrease insulin requirements in early gestation.[12] However, starting at approximately 18 to 20 weeks, insulin requirements increase progressively through the late third trimester. Insulin requirements may plateau, increase, or

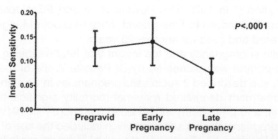

Fig. 1. Longitudinal changes in insulin sensitivity. Changes in insulin sensitivity in the pregravid, early pregnancy (12–14 weeks), and late pregnancy (34–36 weeks) period are shown in women with normal glucose tolerance based on hyperinsulinemic-euglycemic clamps (mean ± SD; *P* values are shown based on ANOVA).

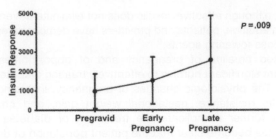

Fig. 2. Longitudinal changes in insulin response. Changes in insulin response in the pregravid, early pregnancy (12–14 weeks), and late pregnancy (34–36 weeks) period are shown in women with normal glucose tolerance based on first-phase insulin response to an intravenous glucose tolerance test (0–10 min) (mean ± SD; P values are shown based on ANOVA).

decrease in the late third trimester. Decreases may signal poor placental function and increasing risk of perinatal morbidity,[13] whereas increased requirements may be due to late gestational increases in insulin clearance.[14]

Although there are multiple formulae to estimate insulin requirements in pregnancy, their use requires care, even in women with type 1 diabetes, because of variable insulin sensitivity both before and during pregnancy.[15] Further, women with either type 2 diabetes or GDM requiring insulin therapy manifest both greater insulin resistance compared with matched normoglycemic women during pregnancy and widely varying impairment of β-cell function.[16] Together, these physiologic variables suggest that optimizing glucose control before conception would provide an easier transition to maintaining optimal glucose control during pregnancy.

DIABETES IN PREGNANCY BEFORE AND AFTER THE DISCOVERY OF INSULIN

Before discussing the pharmacology of current drug management of diabetes in pregnancy, it is helpful to recount the history of diabetes in pregnancy. An excellent review by Dr Steven Gabbe,[17] which the authors commend to all readers, is summarized here. Before the discovery of insulin in 1921 by Banting, Best, Macleod, and Collip, most women of reproductive age died shortly after the onset of what we now refer to as type 1 diabetes. The primary treatment at that time was a ketogenic diet, resulting in the wasted phenotype previously associated with type 1 diabetes. The cause of death was diabetes-related ketoacidosis, which was more likely to occur during pregnancy.[18] In the small number of pregnancies reported before the use of insulin, maternal mortality was approximately 50%. Hence many obstetricians encouraged pregnancy termination.[19] In 1922, Drs Howard Root and Elliot Joslin administered the first dose of purified insulin to their patient, Miss Elizabeth Mudge, a 37-year-old nurse, who recovered and lived for another 25 years.

The use of insulin in pregnancy and the insight that fetal wellbeing depended critically on glycemic control was pioneered by Dr Priscilla White of the Joslin Clinic in Boston.[20] In 1932, she described 3 successful pregnancies in women with type 1 diabetes.[21] Insulin treatment decreased maternal mortality significantly, but perinatal mortality, stillbirths, and prematurity all remained common.[22] In 1949, Dr White classified diabetes in pregnancy by her schema, which included the age of onset, duration, and vascular complications, all affecting fetal survival.[23] Advances in the use of insulin, insulin analogues, and self-monitoring of blood glucose have further decreased perinatal mortality so that it now approaches that observed in women with normal glucose tolerance. Further refinements in the management of diabetes in pregnancy over the last 20 years have steadily decreased maternal and perinatal morbidity. Further advances are awaited in the management of diabetes in pregnancy, such as closed loop systems, to further improve the perinatal outcomes of women with diabetes in pregnancy and their children.

INSULIN

Insulin remains the preferred therapy for pregnant women with pre-GDM and several professional societies endorse its use as a first-line therapy in GDM.[1,2,4] Treatment decisions regarding the type of insulin, timing of administration, and dose frequency are based on individual glycemic patterns. A comprehensive exploration of insulin formulations is beyond the scope of this review and the discussion is limited to novel insulin analogues and technological devices.

The goal of exogenous insulin therapy in pregnancy is to mimic the physiologic profile of insulin in response to diet and metabolic demands in order to achieve and maintain euglycemia. The changes in glucose metabolism that characterize advancing pregnancy require corresponding changes in dose and timing of insulin administration.[12,24,25] To improve treatment compliance and patient satisfaction, newer rapid-acting analogues were developed to limit the inconvenience of regular insulin administration half an hour before meals and "peakless" slow-acting analogues to limit the risk of hypoglycemia between meals and during sleep. The use of most insulin analogues in pregnancy is often extrapolated from experience in nonpregnant patients rather than studies in pregnant women. Although the 3 rapidly acting insulin analogues (ie, lispro, aspart, glulisine) are comparable in immunogenicity to human regular insulin, only lispro and aspart have been investigated in pregnancy. They seem to have acceptable safety profiles, minimal transplacental transfer, and no evidence of teratogenicity.[26–28] In one study, the use of short-acting insulin analogues reduced the risk of postprandial glycemic excursion and limited the risk of delayed postprandial hypoglycemia when compared with regular human insulin.[29] In an observational study, there were no differences in pregnancy outcome between pregnant women who used lispro and those who used regular insulin, but the former reported increased treatment satisfaction.[26] The long-acting insulin analogue, insulin detemir (Food and Drug Administration pregnancy category B by old nomenclature), was compared with NPH insulin in 310 pregnant women with type 1 diabetes mellitus, resulting in similar glycemic control (assessed as hemoglobin A1c [HbA1c] levels) and incidence of hypoglycemia.[30] Like detemir, insulin glargine can similarly provide a stable basal insulin during pregnancy. Likewise, the safety of glargine as a basal insulin during pregnancy was addressed in a systematic review of 8 observational studies involving a total 702 women with pre-GDM or GDM treated with either insulin glargine (n = 331) or NPH (n = 371) revealing similar maternal and neonatal outcomes between treatments.[31] However, there is a lack of adequate data for any insulin analogue to ensure fetal safety equivalence with insulin and large studies are still needed to explore potential mechanisms of teratogenicity.

More recently, studies have focused on novel advances in insulin delivery and continuous glucose monitoring technologies. Continuous subcutaneous insulin infusion (CSII) devices can be programmed to deliver basal and subcutaneous insulin without any abrupt changes and limiting the need for additional subcutaneous injections. In nonpregnant individuals, CSII use results in lower HbA1c levels and fewer hypoglycemic episodes.[32] By comparison, the benefit of CSII use during pregnancy is less clear.[33–35] Some studies have noted lower HbA1c levels and lower insulin requirements at the time of delivery with CSII use in women with type 1 diabetes compared with multiple daily injections (MDI).[36] Yet, maternal and neonatal outcomes did not differ significantly when comparing CSII use with MDI regimens in studies of pregnant women with type 1 diabetes.[34,36,37] In parallel with CSII devices, continuous glucose monitors (CGMs) were developed to increase the frequency of glucose measurements while limiting the need for timed, self-collected capillary glucose values. The utility of CGMs was recently evaluated in the CONCEPTT study, which randomized 325 pregnant women with type 1 diabetes to real-time CGM technology or capillary glucose monitoring.[38] CGM users were within glucose target values more frequently (68% vs 61%, P = .003) and exceeded glycemic goals less often (27% vs 32%, P = .028) compared with women who monitored their capillary glucose by intermittent self-sampling.[38] The study also noted a 50% reduction in rates of large-for-gestational age (LGA) infants, newborn intensive care unit (NICU) admission and neonatal hypoglycemia in women randomized to CGM use.[38] Interestingly, these results were independent of the mode of insulin delivery, CSII or MDI. Recently, sensor-augmented insulin pump devices have been developed to combine CSII and CGM technologies by automatically adjusting the CSII basal rate to create a closed-loop therapy system. In a proof of principle crossover trial performed in 16 pregnant women with type 1 diabetes, closed-loop therapy resulted in a higher percentage of time within glycemic goals (75% vs 60%, P = .002) than did sensor-augmented pump therapy (ie, separate CGM and CSII).[39] However, there was no clear benefit for closed-loop therapy on adverse pregnancy outcomes, because 13 of the 16 newborns in this small crossover study with open extension following the randomized comparison had a birth weight greater than the 90th percentile.[39] Also, 2 recent Cochrane database reviews found no evidence to support one type of insulin or insulin regimen over another and no evidence to suggest CGM over intermittent monitoring.[40,41] Despite the significant advances in CSII and CGM technologies, overall rates of adverse pregnancy outcomes remain high, especially in women with type 1 diabetes, and further studies are needed to explore the use of these novel technologies to reduce maternal and fetal risks further.

ORAL AGENTS
Glyburide

Sulfonylureas stimulate insulin secretion primarily by interacting with adenosine triphosphate–sensitive K^+ channels to mimic effects of glucose metabolism coupling to insulin release in pancreatic β cells. For approximately 50 years, until the recent introduction of alternative oral hypoglycemic drugs, sulfonylureas were the mainstay of type 2 diabetes treatment.[42] Glyburide is the sulfonylurea most commonly used and studied in pregnancy, as early studies had suggested minimal transplacental transfer and thus presumption of fetal safety. This led to a landmark clinical trial in which glyburide outcomes compared favorably with those with insulin in women with GDM.[43–45] Glyburide use in pregnancy increased dramatically; by 2011, it had become the most frequently used treatment for women with GDM.[46] With its widespread use, data emerged on increased glyburide clearance due to its biotransformation during pregnancy and the potential need for higher or more frequent doses to mimic pharmacokinetics in nonpregnant patients. As well, more sensitive analytical methods revealed previously unsuspected placental transfer of glyburide to the fetus, with cord blood concentrations of glyburide 50% to 70% of those in maternal plasma, albeit at very low levels and with very limited sampling.[47,48] These findings were soon followed by various reports comparing pregnancy outcomes in women with GDM treated with glyburide or insulin. In a retrospective cohort study comparing outcomes in 4982 women treated with glyburide and 4191 women treated with insulin, glyburide treatment was associated with increased risks for NICU admission, respiratory distress, hypoglycemia, birth injury, and LGA birth weight.[49] These data highlighted potential concerns with glyburide use, but the study was unable to conclude whether its findings were related to direct drug effects in the fetus. The study lacked any information about potential confounders, including pre-pregnancy body mass index (BMI), and details about glycemic control were missing. Several meta-analyses added to concerns about the appropriate use of glyburide in GDM.[49–53] A meta-analysis by Balsells and colleagues[54] described higher birth weight infants, more macrosomia, and more neonatal hypoglycemia following treatment with glyburide compared with insulin. Together, these led to recent changes in professional guidelines; the American College of Obstetrics and Gynecology now recommends insulin as the first-line agent for GDM treatment[2] and the Society for Maternal-Fetal Medicine endorses metformin as an alternative first-line agent to insulin.[55] Both the observational studies and meta-analyses of randomized controlled studies (RCTs) raise questions about the appropriate use of glyburide. However, the initial glyburide clinical trial, the largest to date, suggests that, as long as glycemic control is comparable, outcomes do not differ between groups.[45] The other trials included in these meta-analyses all had small sample sizes and differed in their approach to glyburide dosing. In addition, the observational studies demonstrating increased risk each have methodological inadequacies, including an inability to account for variation in glycemic control, often (6%–20%) failing to achieve the excellent control observed in the original large randomized trial.[54] Several factors have been associated with higher rates of glyburide failure, including fasting plasma glucose greater than 110 mg/dL (on the oral glucose tolerance test), older maternal age, multiparity, and GDM diagnosis before 25 weeks. Despite this, we still lack prediction tools to aid providers in selecting the women with GDM most likely to achieve optimal glycemic control with glyburide (or with other oral or parenteral hypoglycemic agents) or in tailoring dosing regimens so as to achieve glycemic control rapidly.[56–59] Glyburide concentrations increase within 30 to 60 minutes of dosing, peak in 2 to 3 hours, and return to baseline by 8 hours,[47] which suggests, by contrast with usual practice, that optimal effect might be achieved with glyburide administration 30 to 60 minutes before meals to adequately target postprandial excursions and that more frequent, perhaps thrice daily dosing, may be needed to maintain glucose control throughout the day. It remains unclear if glyburide use increases the risk for fetal overgrowth independent of glycemic control. As well, the studies needed to critically examine new, pharmacokinetically driven glyburide dosing strategies have not been reported.

Metformin

Metformin is recommended as first-line therapy for type 2 diabetes outside of pregnancy.[60,61] Its glucose-lowering effect is thought to be related to its action on mitochondrial metabolism and cellular pathways reducing hepatic gluconeogenesis.[62] Metformin likewise lowers glucose by improving insulin sensitivity, particularly in the liver, without excess weight gain or significant hypoglycemia. Results from the United Kingdom Prospective Diabetes Study showed that it reduced both macrovascular events and mortality in obese individuals with type 2 diabetes.[62,63] Metformin was recently endorsed as an alternative to insulin for the treatment of GDM.[55,64] Given its popularity outside of pregnancy and the absence of excess congenital anomalies with first-trimester use, metformin use was explored for the treatment of GDM later in pregnancy.[65,66] The Metformin in Gestational Diabetes (MiG) study remains the largest RCT to compare metformin with insulin therapy in women with GDM.[67] Glycemic control was similar between groups in MiG, yet 46% of women randomized to metformin required supplemental insulin.[67] Even though metformin improves insulin resistance, it primarily acts on hepatic insulin resistance while the increase in insulin resistance during pregnancy is mostly peripheral.[11,16] Similar to glyburide, metformin failure is more likely to occur in older women, those with higher fasting glucose and those with GDM diagnosis earlier in pregnancy.[68] Furthermore, metformin clearance is increased during pregnancy.[69] The high rate of metformin failure in achieving glycemic control has raised questions about appropriate dosing. However, its concentration-effect relationship has not been determined and may reach a plateau, making it unclear if higher doses would overcome increases in renal clearance to improved glycemic control in pregnancy.[70]

Neonatal outcomes in MiG were similar between groups except for lower rates of neonatal hypoglycemia in women treated with metformin.[67] Maternal outcomes were mixed; metformin therapy was associated with lower gestational weight gain (0.4 ± 2.9 kg vs 2.0 ± 3.3 kg, $P<.001$) but higher rates of preterm birth (12.1 vs 7.6%, $P = .04$).[67] Recent meta-analyses and systematic reviews have suggested favorable pregnancy outcomes with metformin use in women with GDM. A recent network meta-analysis that included unpublished trials found lower risks of LGA births, macrosomia, NICU admission, neonatal hypoglycemia, and preeclampsia in women treated with metformin compared with insulin.[54] Furthermore, recent meta-analyses did not find any difference in preterm delivery between metformin and insulin treatment.[71,72]

Several studies have also suggested a biologically plausible association between metformin use and decreased risk of hypertensive disorders of pregnancy. Metformin lowers soluble fms-like tyrosine kinase 1 and soluble endoglin secretion from primary human tissues in vitro, perhaps mediated by its effect on mitochondrial electron transport and downstream inhibition of hypoxia-inducible factor-1α. These studies also demonstrated improvements in endothelial dysfunction, vasodilation, and angiogenesis, all impaired in the pathophysiology of preeclampsia.[73] Metformin was evaluated in a study of 400 obese women (BMI >35 kg/m^2) without diabetes who were randomized to metformin or placebo and its use was associated with less maternal weight gain and a lower incidence of preeclampsia (3.0 vs 11.3%; odds ratio, 0.24; 95% confidence interval [CI], 0.10–0.61; $P = .001$).[74] This association was also described in a meta-analysis comparing metformin with placebo or insulin in pregnant women with insulin resistance, whether related to GDM, type 2 diabetes mellitus, or polycystic ovary syndrome (PCOS).[75]

Despite these recent findings and professional guidelines endorsing the use of metformin, several concerns remain regarding its use in women with GDM, including inadequate glycemic control requiring supplemental insulin in approximately half of women, its extensive transplacental transfer to the fetus, and unexplored concerns regarding long-term outcomes following in utero exposure to a drug that seems to inhibit the mechanistic target of rapamycin pathway.[76,77] Although metformin treatment failure in GDM may be influenced by its increased (renal) clearance in pregnancy,[69] it remains unclear whether higher doses would improve glycemic control. As well, metformin pharmacokinetics is complex, with slow accumulation in the liver and red blood cells, limiting our ability to determine the relevance of plasma drug concentrations to glycemic control.[78] Furthermore, this slow accumulation and thus lag between changes in dosing, plasma drug concentrations, and pharmacologic effect limit the speed and confidence with which quick dose titration can translate into improved glycemic control.

Metformin's extensive transplacental passage is unsurprising, because it is a small hydrophilic molecule with low protein binding. Metformin umbilical cord serum concentrations may approximate or even exceed maternal concentrations.[69,79] However, there is no significant increase in neonatal complications when metformin is used in women with GDM.[54,67,71,72] Although there is no evidence of perinatal risk, long-term observations of children exposed to metformin in utero are concerning. Several studies have examined offspring of women with PCOS treated with metformin during pregnancy and found that the offspring of mothers randomized to metformin weighed more at 1 year of age compared with those who received placebo.[80,81] Another follow-up study of women with PCOS treated with metformin during pregnancy noted higher offspring weight and BMI z-scores at 4 years of age, with twice as many overweight and obese children in the metformin-exposed group compared with placebo.[82] In women with GDM, offspring data following metformin exposure are limited to the MiG study cohort. At 2 years of age, offspring exposed to metformin in utero had higher subcutaneous fat mass without a decrease in visceral fat.[83] A subset of offspring was also followed-up at 7 and 9 years of age.[84] In this subset from New Zealand, offspring exposed to metformin in utero were heavier, had higher arm and waist circumferences and waist:height ratios ($P<.05$), and trended toward higher BMI and abdominal fat volume by magnetic resonance imaging (all $P = .05$).[84] There were no differences in glucose, lipids, insulin resistance, or liver function test measures in the metformin- compared with insulin-exposed offspring.[84] By contrast, follow-up of the subset from Australia found no differences comparing the offspring exposed to metformin or insulin.[84] Although these observations are limited to only the subset of original MiG study cohort who had long term follow-up and are unable to support a direct link between drug exposure and adverse long-term outcomes, they raise the concern of potential long-term harm following exposure to metformin in utero. These data were included in a meta-analysis of 10 follow-up studies from RCTs that compared metformin with placebo or insulin used in pregnant women with GDM or insulin,[85] suggesting that metformin increased offspring weight (mean difference 0.26 kg, 95% CI, 0.11–0.41), albeit without changes in height or BMI.[85]

In addition to RCT data, our improved understanding of metformin effects, including its suppression of mitochondrial respiration, cellular growth inhibition, and gluconeogenic impact, suggests a possible impact on childhood development and support the need for further investigations regarding its use in pregnancy.[86,87] Collectively, these findings support the need for long-term offspring follow-up in studies evaluating GDM treatment and suggest a need for discretion in the use of metformin during pregnancy.

OTHER AGENTS
Myo-Inositol

Myo-inositol is a nutritional supplement also present in foods such as melons, citrus fruits, various vegetables, and legumes. Myo-inositol is hypothesized to function as an insulin sensitizer by acting through complex pathways that ultimately shift glucose intracellularly and then into fatty acid synthesis.[88,89] An ongoing study (NCT02149992) is assessing myo-inositol as a treatment for GDM, despite negative previous results.[90] By contrast, a mixed but encouraging literature has evaluated myo-inositol supplementation for GDM prevention in women at elevated risk.[91–93] Myo-inositol (1100 mg, in combination with D-chiro-inositol) failed to show benefit in an RCT including 240 pregnant women with a family history of diabetes,[94] whereas a pooled analysis of 3 RCTs, using 2000 mg myo-inositol and including 595 women, demonstrated greater than 60% reduced risk of GDM in gravidas at increased risk due to overweight, obesity, or parental history of type 2 diabetes mellitus.[95] Larger studies with varying doses of myo-inositol are needed to evaluate its potential role in pregnancy.

Acarbose

Acarbose, an alpha-glucosidase inhibitor, inhibits the conversion of polysaccharides into monosaccharides, thus reducing postprandial glucose excursions. Data regarding acarbose use in women with GDM are limited. Two initial reports, totaling 11 women, did not reveal any safety concerns.[96,97] Another small study from Brazil randomized 70 women with GDM to insulin (n = 27), glyburide (n = 24), or acarbose (n = 29), with similar fasting and postprandial glucose levels and average newborn weights across treatment groups.[98] However, glycemic goals were achieved more often with glyburide than acarbose (79% and 58%, respectively) and incidence of LGA infants were 3.7%, 25.0%, and 10.5% of the infants born to mothers treated with insulin, glyburide, and acarbose, respectively. None of these apparent differences were statistically significant due to heterogeneity and small sample size.[98]

FUTURE DIRECTIONS

Diabetes in pregnancy is a public health problem associated with both adverse pregnancy outcomes and long-term maternal and offspring risks. Diabetes prevalence is increasing in the setting of the obesity epidemic, increasing maternal age, and, for GDM, a change in diagnostic criteria. Although treatment of diabetes in pregnancy mitigates some of the perinatal risks, many questions about the management of diabetes in pregnancy remain unanswered. In women with pre-GDM, recent efforts have focused on improved glucose monitoring and insulin delivery. However, although these efforts have improved the rates of hypoglycemia and control of HbA1c levels, these benefits have not translated into improved pregnancy outcomes. In women with GDM, the optimal timing and method for diagnosis as well as our ability to individually predict responses to each of the available drug treatments, individually or in combination, are still undetermined. There is also evidence of significant metabolic and pathophysiologic heterogeneity in women with GDM, which may translate into variation in pregnancy outcomes.[99] Given the higher failure rate with metformin in women with GDM and the data on long-term childhood outcomes, further research is needed to address a potential role for glyburide to treat women with GDM. Overall, there is a need to (1) determine the long-term offspring outcomes associated with different drug treatments, (2) explore novel treatment strategies, including therapies that do not focus on glycemic control, but rather on decreasing prepregnancy weight in overweight and obese women, and (3) design and evaluate individualized therapies that would match the mechanisms of diabetes drugs or drug combinations, with the heterogeneous and distinct pathophysiologic mechanisms contributing to hyperglycemia and to adverse pregnancy outcomes. Individualized and gestation-specific strategies based on underlying maternal pathophysiology are needed to address the increasing frequency and complexity of diabetes in pregnancy.

ACKNOWLEDGMENTS

Maisa N. Feghali is supported by the National Institutes of Health through grant number K23HD092893. The funding source had no involvement in the preparation, analysis, and interpretation of the data or submission of this report.

REFERENCES

1. ACOG Committee on Practice Bulletins. ACOG Practice Bulletin. Clinical management guidelines for obstetrician-gynecologists. Number 60, March 2005. Pregestational diabetes mellitus. Obstet Gynecol 2005;105(3):675–85.
2. ACOG practice bulletin no. 190: gestational diabetes mellitus. Obstet Gynecol 2018;131(2):e49–64.
3. American Diabetes Association. 2. classification and diagnosis of diabetes: standards of medical care in diabetes-2018. Diabetes Care 2018;41(Suppl 1): S13–27.
4. American Diabetes A. 13. management of diabetes in pregnancy: standards of medical care in diabetes-2018. Diabetes care 2018;41(Suppl 1):S137–43.
5. Coton SJ, Nazareth I, Petersen I. A cohort study of trends in the prevalence of pregestational diabetes in pregnancy recorded in UK general practice between 1995 and 2012. BMJ Open 2016;6(1):e009494.
6. Fadl HE, Simmons D. Trends in diabetes in pregnancy in Sweden 1998-2012. BMJ Open Diabetes Res Care 2016;4(1):e000221.
7. Sacks DA, Hadden DR, Maresh M, et al. Frequency of gestational diabetes mellitus at collaborating centers based on IADPSG consensus panel-recommended criteria: the Hyperglycemia and Adverse Pregnancy Outcome (HAPO) Study. Diabetes care 2012;35(3):526–8.
8. Metzger BE, Gabbe SG, Persson B, et al. International association of diabetes and pregnancy study groups recommendations on the diagnosis and classification of hyperglycemia in pregnancy. Diabetes care 2010;33(3):676–82.
9. Finneran MM, Landon MB. Oral agents for the treatment of gestational diabetes. Curr Diab Rep 2018;18(11):119.
10. Catalano PM, Tyzbir ED, Roman NM, et al. Longitudinal changes in insulin release and insulin resistance in nonobese pregnant women. Am J Obstet Gynecol 1991; 165(6 Pt 1):1667–72.
11. Catalano PM, Tyzbir ED, Wolfe RR, et al. Carbohydrate metabolism during pregnancy in control subjects and women with gestational diabetes. Am J Physiol 1993;264(1 Pt 1):E60–7.
12. Garcia-Patterson A, Gich I, Amini SB, et al. Insulin requirements throughout pregnancy in women with type 1 diabetes mellitus: three changes of direction. Diabetologia 2010;53(3):446–51.
13. Padmanabhan S, McLean M, Cheung NW. Falling insulin requirements are associated with adverse obstetric outcomes in women with preexisting diabetes. Diabetes care 2014;37(10):2685–92.
14. Catalano PM, Drago NM, Amini SB. Longitudinal changes in pancreatic beta-cell function and metabolic clearance rate of insulin in pregnant women with normal and abnormal glucose tolerance. Diabetes care 1998;21(3):403–8.
15. Roeder HA, Moore TR, Ramos GA. Insulin pump dosing across gestation in women with well-controlled type 1 diabetes mellitus. Am J Obstet Gynecol 2012;207(4):324.e1-5.
16. Catalano PM, Huston L, Amini SB, et al. Longitudinal changes in glucose metabolism during pregnancy in obese women with normal glucose tolerance and gestational diabetes mellitus. Am J Obstet Gynecol 1999;180(4):903–16.
17. Gabbe SG. A story of two miracles: the impact of the discovery of insulin on pregnancy in women with diabetes mellitus. Obstet Gynecol 1992;79(2):295–9.
18. Joslin EP. Pregnancy and diabetes mellitus. Bost Med Surg J 1915;23:841–9.

19. DeLee JB, editor. The principles and practice of obstetrics. 1st edition. Philadelphia: Saunders; 1913. p. 502–3.
20. White P. Diabetes in pregnancy. In: Joslin EP, editor. The treatment of diabetes mellitus. 4th edition. Philadelphia: Lea & Febiger; 1928. p. 870–2.
21. White P. Diabetes in childhood and adolescence. Philadelphia: Lea & Febiger; 1932. p. 224.
22. Walker A. Diabetes mellitus and pregnancy. Proc R Soc Med 1928;21:337–83.
23. White P. Pregnancy complicating diabetes. Am J Med 1949;7:609–16.
24. Jovanovic L, Knopp RH, Brown Z, et al. Declining insulin requirement in the late first trimester of diabetic pregnancy. Diabetes care 2001;24(7):1130–6.
25. Steel JM, Johnstone FD, Hume R, et al. Insulin requirements during pregnancy in women with type I diabetes. Obstet Gynecol 1994;83(2):253–8.
26. Bhattacharyya A, Brown S, Hughes S, et al. Insulin lispro and regular insulin in pregnancy. QJM 2001;94(5):255–60.
27. Hirsch IB. Insulin analogues. N Engl J Med 2005;352(2):174–83.
28. Hod M, Damm P, Kaaja R, et al. Fetal and perinatal outcomes in type 1 diabetes pregnancy: a randomized study comparing insulin aspart with human insulin in 322 subjects. Am J Obstet Gynecol 2008;198(2):186.e1-7.
29. Mathiesen ER, Kinsley B, Amiel SA, et al. Maternal glycemic control and hypoglycemia in type 1 diabetic pregnancy: a randomized trial of insulin aspart versus human insulin in 322 pregnant women. Diabetes care 2007;30(4):771–6.
30. Mathiesen ER, Hod M, Ivanisevic M, et al. Maternal efficacy and safety outcomes in a randomized, controlled trial comparing insulin detemir with NPH insulin in 310 pregnant women with type 1 diabetes. Diabetes care 2012;35(10):2012–7.
31. Lepercq J, Lin J, Hall GC, et al. Meta-analysis of maternal and neonatal outcomes associated with the use of insulin glargine versus NPH insulin during pregnancy. Obstet Gynecol Int 2012;2012:649070.
32. Cummins E, Royle P, Snaith A, et al. Clinical effectiveness and cost-effectiveness of continuous subcutaneous insulin infusion for diabetes: systematic review and economic evaluation. Health Technol Assess 2010;14(11):iii–iv, xi–xvi, 1–181.
33. Farrar D, Tuffnell DJ, West J, et al. Continuous subcutaneous insulin infusion versus multiple daily injections of insulin for pregnant women with diabetes. Cochrane Database Syst Rev 2016;(6):CD005542.
34. Mukhopadhyay A, Farrell T, Fraser RB, et al. Continuous subcutaneous insulin infusion vs intensive conventional insulin therapy in pregnant diabetic women: a systematic review and metaanalysis of randomized, controlled trials. Am J Obstet Gynecol 2007;197(5):447–56.
35. Ranasinghe PD, Maruthur NM, Nicholson WK, et al. Comparative effectiveness of continuous subcutaneous insulin infusion using insulin analogs and multiple daily injections in pregnant women with diabetes mellitus: a systematic review and meta-analysis. J Womens Health (Larchmt) 2015;24(3):237–49.
36. Bruttomesso D, Bonomo M, Costa S, et al. Type 1 diabetes control and pregnancy outcomes in women treated with continuous subcutaneous insulin infusion (CSII) or with insulin glargine and multiple daily injections of rapid-acting insulin analogues (glargine-MDI). Diabetes Metab 2011;37(5):426–31.
37. Gonzalez-Romero S, Gonzalez-Molero I, Fernandez-Abellan M, et al. Continuous subcutaneous insulin infusion versus multiple daily injections in pregnant women with type 1 diabetes. Diabetes Technol Ther 2010;12(4):263–9.
38. Feig DS, Donovan LE, Corcoy R, et al. Continuous glucose monitoring in pregnant women with type 1 diabetes (CONCEPTT): a multicentre international randomised controlled trial. Lancet 2017;390(10110):2347–59.

39. Stewart ZA, Wilinska ME, Hartnell S, et al. Closed-loop insulin delivery during pregnancy in women with type 1 diabetes. N Engl J Med 2016;375(7):644–54.

40. Moy FM, Ray A, Buckley BS, et al. Techniques of monitoring blood glucose during pregnancy for women with pre-existing diabetes. Cochrane Database Syst Rev 2017;(6):CD009613.

41. O'Neill SM, Kenny LC, Khashan AS, et al. Different insulin types and regimens for pregnant women with pre-existing diabetes. Cochrane Database Syst Rev 2017;(2):CD011880.

42. Nathan DM, Buse JB, Davidson MB, et al. Medical management of hyperglycaemia in type 2 diabetes mellitus: a consensus algorithm for the initiation and adjustment of therapy: a consensus statement from the American Diabetes Association and the European Association for the Study of Diabetes. Diabetologia 2009;52(1):17–30.

43. Elliott BD, Langer O, Schenker S, et al. Insignificant transfer of glyburide occurs across the human placenta. Am J Obstet Gynecol 1991;165(4 Pt 1):807–12.

44. Elliott BD, Schenker S, Langer O, et al. Comparative placental transport of oral hypoglycemic agents in humans: a model of human placental drug transfer. Am J Obstet Gynecol 1994;171(3):653–60.

45. Langer O, Conway DL, Berkus MD, et al. A comparison of glyburide and insulin in women with gestational diabetes mellitus. N Engl J Med 2000;343(16):1134–8.

46. Camelo Castillo W, Boggess K, Sturmer T, et al. Trends in glyburide compared with insulin use for gestational diabetes treatment in the United States, 2000-2011. Obstet Gynecol 2014;123(6):1177–84.

47. Hebert MF, Ma X, Naraharisetti SB, et al. Are we optimizing gestational diabetes treatment with glyburide? The pharmacologic basis for better clinical practice. Clin Pharmacol Ther 2009;85(6):607–14.

48. Schwartz RA, Rosenn B, Aleksa K, et al. Glyburide transport across the human placenta. Obstet Gynecol 2015;125(3):583–8.

49. Camelo Castillo W, Boggess K, Sturmer T, et al. Association of adverse pregnancy outcomes with glyburide vs insulin in women with gestational diabetes. JAMA Pediatr 2015;169(5):452–8.

50. Brown J, Martis R, Hughes B, et al. Oral anti-diabetic pharmacological therapies for the treatment of women with gestational diabetes. Cochrane Database Syst Rev 2017;(1):CD011967.

51. Dhulkotia JS, Ola B, Fraser R, et al. Oral hypoglycemic agents vs insulin in management of gestational diabetes: a systematic review and metaanalysis. Am J Obstet Gynecol 2010;203(5):457.e1-9.

52. Poolsup N, Suksomboon N, Amin M. Efficacy and safety of oral antidiabetic drugs in comparison to insulin in treating gestational diabetes mellitus: a meta-analysis. PLoS One 2014;9(10):e109985.

53. Zeng YC, Li MJ, Chen Y, et al. The use of glyburide in the management of gestational diabetes mellitus: a meta-analysis. Adv Med Sci 2014;59(1):95–101.

54. Balsells M, Garcia-Patterson A, Sola I, et al. Glibenclamide, metformin, and insulin for the treatment of gestational diabetes: a systematic review and meta-analysis. BMJ 2015;350:h102.

55. SMFM Publications Committee. SMFM Statement: pharmacological treatment of gestational diabetes. Am J Obstet Gynecol 2018;218(5):B2–4.

56. Chmait R, Dinise T, Moore T. Prospective observational study to establish predictors of glyburide success in women with gestational diabetes mellitus. J Perinatol 2004;24(10):617–22.

57. Conway DL, Gonzales O, Skiver D. Use of glyburide for the treatment of gestational diabetes: the San Antonio experience. J Matern Fetal Neonatal Med 2004;15(1):51–5.
58. Kahn BF, Davies JK, Lynch AM, et al. Predictors of glyburide failure in the treatment of gestational diabetes. Obstet Gynecol 2006;107(6):1303–9.
59. Nachum Z, Zafran N, Salim R, et al. Glyburide versus metformin and their combination for the treatment of gestational diabetes mellitus: a randomized controlled study. Diabetes care 2017;40(3):332–7.
60. 14. diabetes care in the hospital: standards of medical care in diabetes-2018. Diabetes care 2018;41(Suppl 1);S144–s151.
61. Garber AJ, Abrahamson MJ, Barzilay JI, et al. Consensus statement by the American association of clinical endocrinologists and American college of endocrinology on the comprehensive type 2 diabetes management algorithm - 2018 executive summary. Endocr Pract 2018;24(1):91–120.
62. Foretz M, Guigas B, Bertrand L, et al. Metformin: from mechanisms of action to therapies. Cell Metab 2014;20(6):953–66.
63. Effect of intensive blood-glucose control with metformin on complications in overweight patients with type 2 diabetes (UKPDS 34). UK Prospective Diabetes Study (UKPDS) Group. Lancet 1998;352(9131):854–65.
64. National institute for health and care excellence: clinical guidelines. Diabetes in pregnancy: management of diabetes and its complications from preconception to the postnatal period. London: National Institute for Health and Care Excellence (UK) Copyright (c) 2015 National Collaborating Centre for Women's and Children's Health; 2015.
65. Lautatzis ME, Goulis DG, Vrontakis M. Efficacy and safety of metformin during pregnancy in women with gestational diabetes mellitus or polycystic ovary syndrome: a systematic review. Metabolism 2013;62(11):1522–34.
66. Scherneck S, Schlinke N, Beck E, et al. Pregnancy outcome after first-trimester exposure to metformin: a prospective cohort study. Reprod Toxicol 2018;81: 79–83.
67. Rowan JA, Hague WM, Gao W, et al. Metformin versus insulin for the treatment of gestational diabetes. N Engl J Med 2008;358(19):2003–15.
68. Khin MO, Gates S, Saravanan P. Predictors of metformin failure in gestational diabetes mellitus (GDM). Diabetes Metab Syndr 2018;12(3):405–10.
69. Eyal S, Easterling TR, Carr D, et al. Pharmacokinetics of metformin during pregnancy. Drug Metab Dispos 2010;38(5):833–40.
70. Chung H, Oh J, Yoon SH, et al. A non-linear pharmacokinetic-pharmacodynamic relationship of metformin in healthy volunteers: an open-label, parallel group, randomized clinical study. PLoS One 2018;13(1):e0191258.
71. Butalia S, Gutierrez L, Lodha A, et al. Short- and long-term outcomes of metformin compared with insulin alone in pregnancy: a systematic review and meta-analysis. Diabet Med 2017;34(1):27–36.
72. Farrar D, Simmonds M, Bryant M, et al. Treatments for gestational diabetes: a systematic review and meta-analysis. BMJ Open 2017;7(6):e015557.
73. Brownfoot FC, Hastie R, Hannan NJ, et al. Metformin as a prevention and treatment for preeclampsia: effects on soluble fms-like tyrosine kinase 1 and soluble endoglin secretion and endothelial dysfunction. Am J Obstet Gynecol 2016; 214(3):356.e1-15.
74. Syngelaki A, Nicolaides KH, Balani J, et al. Metformin versus placebo in obese pregnant women without diabetes mellitus. N Engl J Med 2016;374(5):434–43.

75. Alqudah A, McKinley MC, McNally R, et al. Risk of pre-eclampsia in women taking metformin: a systematic review and meta-analysis. Diabet Med 2018;35(2): 160–72.
76. Howell JJ, Hellberg K, Turner M, et al. Metformin inhibits hepatic mTORC1 signaling via dose-dependent mechanisms involving AMPK and the TSC complex. Cell Metab 2017;25(2):463–71.
77. Rena G, Hardie DG, Pearson ER. The mechanisms of action of metformin. Diabetologia 2017;60(9):1577–85.
78. Lalau JD, Lacroix C. Measurement of metformin concentration in erythrocytes: clinical implications. Diabetes Obes Metab 2003;5(2):93–8.
79. Vanky E, Zahlsen K, Spigset O, et al. Placental passage of metformin in women with polycystic ovary syndrome. Fertil Steril 2005;83(5):1575–8.
80. Vanky E, Stridsklev S, Heimstad R, et al. Metformin versus placebo from first trimester to delivery in polycystic ovary syndrome: a randomized, controlled multicenter study. J Clin Endocrinol Metab 2010;95(12):E448–55.
81. Carlsen SM, Martinussen MP, Vanky E. Metformin's effect on first-year weight gain: a follow-up study. Pediatrics 2012;130(5):e1222–6.
82. Hanem LGE, Stridsklev S, Juliusson PB, et al. Metformin use in PCOS pregnancies increases the risk of offspring overweight at 4 years of age: follow-up of two RCTs. J Clin Endocrinol Metab 2018;103(4):1612–21.
83. Rowan JA, Rush EC, Obolonkin V, et al. Metformin in gestational diabetes: the offspring follow-up (MiG TOFU): body composition at 2 years of age. Diabetes care 2011;34(10):2279–84.
84. Rowan JA, Rush EC, Plank LD, et al. Metformin in gestational diabetes: the offspring follow-up (MiG TOFU): body composition and metabolic outcomes at 7-9 years of age. BMJ Open Diabetes Res Care 2018;6(1):e000456.
85. van Weelden W, Wekker V, de Wit L, et al. Long-term effects of oral antidiabetic drugs during pregnancy on offspring: a systematic review and meta-analysis of follow-up studies of RCTs. Diabetes Ther 2018;9(5):1811–29.
86. Bridges HR, Jones AJ, Pollak MN, et al. Effects of metformin and other biguanides on oxidative phosphorylation in mitochondria. Biochem J 2014;462(3): 475–87.
87. Sacco F, Calderone A, Castagnoli L, et al. The cell-autonomous mechanisms underlying the activity of metformin as an anticancer drug. Br J Cancer 2016; 115(12):1451–6.
88. Croze ML, Soulage CO. Potential role and therapeutic interests of myo-inositol in metabolic diseases. Biochimie 2013;95(10):1811–27.
89. Croze ML, Vella RE, Pillon NJ, et al. Chronic treatment with myo-inositol reduces white adipose tissue accretion and improves insulin sensitivity in female mice. J Nutr Biochem 2013;24(2):457–66.
90. Brown J, Crawford TJ, Alsweiler J, et al. Dietary supplementation with myo-inositol in women during pregnancy for treating gestational diabetes. Cochrane Database Syst Rev 2016;(9):CD012048.
91. D'Anna R, Di Benedetto A, Scilipoti A, et al. Myo-inositol supplementation for prevention of gestational diabetes in obese pregnant women: a randomized controlled trial. Obstet Gynecol 2015;126(2):310–5.
92. D'Anna R, Di Benedetto V, Rizzo P, et al. Myo-inositol may prevent gestational diabetes in PCOS women. Gynecol Endocrinol 2012;28(6):440–2.
93. Santamaria A, Di Benedetto A, Petrella E, et al. Myo-inositol may prevent gestational diabetes onset in overweight women: a randomized, controlled trial. J Matern Fetal Neonatal Med 2016;29(19):3234–7.

94. Farren M, Daly N, McKeating A, et al. The prevention of gestational diabetes mellitus with antenatal oral inositol supplementation: a randomized controlled trial. Diabetes care 2017;40(6):759–63.

95. Santamaria A, Alibrandi A, Di Benedetto A, et al. Clinical and metabolic outcomes in pregnant women at risk for gestational diabetes mellitus supplemented with myo-inositol: a secondary analysis from 3 RCTs. Am J Obstet Gynecol 2018; 219(3):300.e1-6.

96. Zarate A, Ochoa R, Hernandez M, et al. Effectiveness of acarbose in the control of glucose tolerance worsening in pregnancy. Ginecol Obstet Mex 2000;68:42–5 [in Spanish].

97. Wilton LV, Pearce GL, Martin RM, et al. The outcomes of pregnancy in women exposed to newly marketed drugs in general practice in England. Br J Obstet Gynaecol 1998;105(8):882–9.

98. Bertini AM, Silva JC, Taborda W, et al. Perinatal outcomes and the use of oral hypoglycemic agents. J Perinat Med 2005;33(6):519–23.

99. Powe CE, Allard C, Battista MC, et al. Heterogeneous contribution of insulin sensitivity and secretion defects to gestational diabetes mellitus. Diabetes care 2016;39(6):1052–5.

The Use of Cardiotonic Drugs in Neonates

Eugene Dempsey, MD[a,b,]*, Heike Rabe, MD[c,d]

KEYWORDS

- Low blood pressure • Inotrope • Inodilator • Vasopressor • Shock • Newborn

KEY POINTS

- There is a distinct lack of age-appropriate cardiotonic drugs, and adult formulations are administered without evidence-based knowledge on their dosing, safety, efficacy, and long-term effects.
- Dopamine remains the most commonly studied and prescribed cardiotonic drug in the neonatal intensive care unit (NICU), but evidence of its effect on end-organ perfusion is still lacking.
- Unlike adult and pediatric critical care, there are significant gaps in knowledge on the use of various cardiotonic drugs in various forms of circulatory failure in the NICU.
- Performing clinical trials in this area has been challenging and highlights the need for international collaborations, the importance of synergy between the Food and Drug Administration and European Medicines Agency, and the inclusion of industry in the conduct of such trials.

INTRODUCTION

Inotrope/vasopressors are commonly used in the neonatal intensive care unit (NICU) but with wide variations in practice regarding indications, duration, and dosing[1,2] (**Table 1**). Following delivery, neonates need to adapt their cardiorespiratory system from intrauterine to extrauterine life. During this transition phase, many additional

Funding: This research was partially funded by the European Commission within the 7th Framework Programme (EU FP7/2007-2013) under grant agreement no. 260777 (The HIP Trial) and NEO-CIRC FP7-HEALTH grant agreement no. 282533. Prof. E. Dempsey is supported by a Science Foundation Ireland Research Centre Award (INFANT-12/RC/2272).
Conflict of Interest: None.
a Department of Paediatrics and Child Health, Neonatal Intensive Care Unit, University College Cork, Wilton, Cork, Ireland; b Irish Centre for Fetal and Neonatal Translational Research (IN-FANT), University College Cork, Cork, Ireland; c Brighton and Sussex Medical School, University of Sussex, Brighton, UK; d Department of Neonatology, Brighton & Sussex University Hospitals NHS Trust, Brighton, UK
* Corresponding author. Department of Paediatrics and Child Health, Neonatal Intensive Care Unit, Wilton, Cork, Ireland.
E-mail address: gene.dempsey@hse.ie

Table 1
Overview of inotropes used for treatment of cardiovascular failure in neonates

Drug Name	Receptors	Proposed Physiologic Effects Related to Cardiovascular Failure	Dosing in Newborns	Administration
Dopamine	β1, β2 agonist, dopaminergic receptors	Increases in heart rate, BP, myocardial contractility, and variable effects on SVR	2–20 µg/kg/min	Continuous infusion through central venous line
Dobutamine	α and β1 agonist, weak effect on β2	Increases heart rate, myocardial contractility, and stroke volume	5–20 µg/kg/min	Continuous infusion via peripheral or central venous line
Epinephrine	α1, α2, β1, β2 agonist	Increases heart rate and stroke volume, variable effect on SVR	0.05–1.0 µg/kg/min	Continuous infusion through central venous line
Norepinephrine	α1, α2, β1 agonist	Increases heart rate, myocardial contractility, and vascular resistance causing vasoconstriction and increase in BP	0.02–1 µg/kg/min	Continuous infusion through central venous line
Levosimendon	Calcium sensitizer activating sarcolemmal K-sensitive adenosine triphosphate channel at cellular smooth muscle level	Increases cardiac output and cardiac index Vasodilatory effects, may cause decrease in heart rate and BP	0.1–0.2 µg/kg/min	Limited evidence after cardiac surgery
Milrinone	Type III phosphodiesterase inhibitor	Decrease of pulmonary and SVR, may cause increase in heart rate and decrease in BP	0.2–1 µg/kg/min A bolus of 50 µg/kg may be considered	Continuous infusion through central venous line
Vasopressin	Vasopressin 1 receptors for vasoconstriction in systemic arteries Vasopressin 2 receptors for vasodilation in cerebral, renal, and pulmonary circulation	Increase in BP, cardiac output; may decrease pulmonary vascular resistance	0.00001–0.003 units/kg/min	Continuous infusion through central venous line; used as rescue treatment in persistent cardiovascular failure during sepsis

factors can impact this process, including timing of umbilical cord clamping, chorioamnionitis, inadequate oxygenation, relative adrenal insufficiency, and infection, especially in the most extreme preterm neonates. These interrelated factors often result in a clinical picture characterized by low blood pressure (BP), which often is treated with agents such as dopamine, dobutamine, noradrenaline, and corticosteroids.[3]

None of these drugs are currently licensed for the use in preterm or term neonates despite the introduction of the Medicines in Children's Acts in several countries.[4] Because of the lack of age-appropriate formulations, many adult formulations are administered without evidence-based knowledge on their safety, efficacy, long-term effects of excipients, and age-appropriate dosing.[5,6] Recently, efforts have been initiated to address these deficiencies through funding large randomized trials of inotropes in newborns.[7,8]

Neonatal circulatory failure may occur in many settings. Hypovolemic shock, an infrequent cause of hypotension in the immediate transition period, may be minimized by providing enhanced placental transfusion.[9–12] A recent meta-analysis in preterm neonates receiving placental transfusion found an increased death rate (30%) if the cord was clamped immediately.[13] Long-term follow-up studies in preterm and term neonates have shown a good safety profile with improved neurodevelopmental outcomes up to 4 years of age.[9,14–16] In term neonates, circulatory failure may occur in the setting of early-onset sepsis, persistent pulmonary hypertension (PPHN) of the newborn, perinatal asphyxia, or as a result of complex congenital cardiac defects. Preterm neonates more often have difficulty in adapting their circulation to extrauterine life during the first 72 hours of birth. Additional causes for circulatory failure later during their hospital stay include sepsis, necrotizing enterocolitis, and patent ductus arteriosus (PDA).

Defining circulatory failure in the neonate poses many challenges for clinicians. Traditionally, BP has been the main criteria used to define the adequacy of circulatory well-being. Numerous BP reference ranges exist based on gestational age, birth weight, and postnatal age. Defining mean BP values below a particular centile, less than an absolute value, or less than a gestational age equivalent in millimeters of mercury has been the most popular definition[3,17] used, but this is too simplistic an approach. More recently, other surrogate markers of circulatory failure have been considered, such as base excess and blood lactate as markers of poor tissue perfusion.[18,19] Cardiac function and organ perfusion are now assessed by functional echocardiography, tissue Doppler, pulse plethysmography, or near-infrared spectroscopy (NIRS).[20] Treatment algorithms and guidelines often rely on preferences of local clinicians and their ability to use these additional assessment methods.[5] Although several groups continue to evaluate the role of additional monitoring tools in hemodynamic assessment,[21–24] further evaluation and clinical trials are necessary before they are routinely incorporated into clinical practice[25] (**Fig. 1**). In the following sections, the authors review some of the most commonly prescribed drugs and the conditions in which they are used.

INOTROPIC/VASOPRESSORS/INODILATORS
Dopamine

Dopamine is the most commonly used inotrope in the treatment of neonatal hypotension[26,27] and is certainly the most studied of all the cardiotonic drugs used in newborn care. There are numerous observational studies of its use in neonates, and there are now more than 20 randomized controlled trials comparing dopamine to other agents,

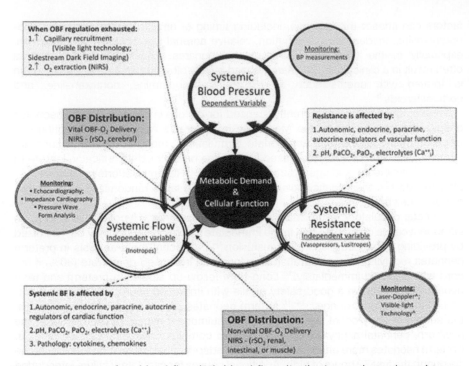

Fig. 1. Monitoring of BP, blood flow (BF), blood flow distribution, and vascular resistance. OBF, organ blood flow; rSO₂, regional tissue oxygen saturation. (*From* Soleymani S, Borzage M, Seri I. Hemodynamic monitoring in neonates: advances and challenges. J Perinatol 2010;30:S40; with permission.)

including placebo. Dopamine works through stimulation of α- and β-adrenergic receptors and dopaminergic receptors. The results of these numerous observational studies are several postulated effects, suggesting a dose-dependent effect on different organs systems.[28,29] The standard administration is by continuous infusion at doses of 2 to 20 µg/kg/min with the assumption being that the lower doses of 2 to 5 µg/kg/min mainly affect the dopaminergic receptors.[30,31] Further increasing the dose stimulates α-adrenergic receptors, causing vasoconstriction and increases in systemic vascular resistance (SVR).[32] Although this leads to an increase in cardiac contractility and output,[27,33] evidence from randomized controlled trials suggests that dopamine may have a negative impact on cardiac output through an inotrope/ vasopressor imbalance.[34–36] It would be too simple to state that above a certain level one effect is greater than the other, but certainly with increasing doses one is likely to see more vasopressor than inotrope effects; thus, the potential to impair end-organ perfusion becomes a reality. There is a great deal of overlap in these effects, particularly in critically ill neonates. The choice of an appropriate drug for a specific clinical condition depends on several complex interrelated factors, including determinants of cardiovascular function and the underlying disease process. There are several studies that have assessed the pharmacokinetic (PK) and pharmacodynamic (PD) properties of dopamine in the pediatric population, some of these in neonates.[37–45] The methods of analysis have differed, which may account for some of the variability across the studies. The effects on systemic, pulmonary, and cerebral hemodynamics can be monitored at the bedside. Echocardiographic assessment, in particular in the presence of a PDA,[46,47] has provided some insights into the systemic and pulmonary effects. NIRS has permitted a better understanding of the potential effects on cerebral oxygenation, blood flow, and autoregulation. It has been suggested that dopamine may have negative effects on the cerebrovascular autoregulatory capacity in very pre-term neonates,[48] which has not been seen by others.[49] In a follow-up study, neurode-velopmental outcome at 3 years may be worse in neonates treated with dopamine versus dobutamine.[50] In a meta-analysis of observational studies, dopamine increased not only BP but also cerebral blood flow.[51] There are no studies comparing dopamine versus placebo in neonates with low BP, including evaluating the effects on measures of cerebral perfusion/cerebral oxygenation. Such studies are warranted.

Dobutamine

Dobutamine is often used as a second-line inotropic agent if a maximum dose of dopamine has been reached.[26] It is a synthetic inotrope that directly stimulates α and β1 receptors in the myocardium. Dobutamine increases cardiac output by increasing contractility and heart rate. In addition, it can have a vasodilatory effect through stimulation of peripheral β2 receptors.[52,53] Dobutamine is administered by continuous infusion with recommended doses of 5 to 20 µg/kg/min. Several studies have compared dopamine with dobutamine for circulatory failure, and most have demonstrated a greater increase in mean BP with dopamine administration.[33,35,54]

However, dobutamine has been observed to increase right and left ventricular output in comparison to dopamine. Comparative studies reported a 21% increase in left ventricular outflow with dobutamine and observed a 14% decrease with dopa-mine.[34,35] Dobutamine has been shown to increase superior vena cava blood flow in comparison to both dopamine and placebo in neonates with low BP. As with all studies of cardiotonic drugs, very few long-term neurodevelopmental outcome data are available.

Epinephrine

Epinephrine (adrenaline) is secreted by the adrenal medulla as an endogenous cate-cholamine. It stimulates α and β receptors. It is typically used in protracted neonatal hypotension if dopamine and dobutamine do not achieve the desired effects.[6] How-ever, it is used as a first-line agent by some as determined from surveys of practice.[2,55] The effects on the circulation are generally dose dependent. At lower doses, the stim-ulated β receptors cause vasodilation in the systemic and pulmonary circulations. It also increases heart rate and cardiac stroke volume. At increasing doses, α receptor–mediated effects are seen resulting in vasoconstriction.[27] The infusion should be administered through a central venous line with a dosing range of 0.05 to 1.0 µg/kg/min. Higher doses have been used but are not recommended.[56,57]

There are very few randomized controlled studies of epinephrine in preterm neo-nates.[58] Valverde and colleagues[59] compared dopamine to epinephrine in preterm ne-onates with low BP. The clinical effects and the side-effect profile included a significant increase in heart rate, serum glucose concentration, and increase in lactate after 24 to 36 hours of continuous infusion compared with dopamine.

Norepinephrine

Norepinephrine is an endogenous catecholamine that is released from adrenergic nerve endings. It has strong stimulating effects on α and β1 receptors and weaker ef-fects on β2 receptors. Noradrenaline has more potent α-mediated effects compared with adrenaline, which results in vascular constriction with a subsequent increase in SVR and BP. It may be useful in septic shock, in order to correct the low SVR.[60] Although several cohort studies have reported the effects of norepinephrine in preterm neonates,[61,62] randomized controlled trials to confirm these findings are lacking. Norepinephrine might have a role in treating circulatory failure in severe PPHN of the newborn due to a reported pulmonary vasodilator effect.[61] Administration should be via central venous access at doses of 0.02 to 1 μg/kg/min.

Milrinone

Milrinone is a type III phosphodiesterase inhibitor that acts directly on the myocardium through its inotrope and lusitrope effects. In addition, it can cause vasodilation in the systemic and pulmonary circulation, which makes it a drug of choice for treatment of PPHN.[63] In a comparative study of levosimendan versus milrinone in neonates undergoing cardiac surgery, cerebral tissue oxygenation measurements were similar for both groups during the immediate 24-hour postoperative phase.[64] In contrast, peripheral oxygenation showed an increase in the levosimendan group and a decrease in the milrinone group together with an increase in lactate. Serial assessments of cardiac function by echocardiography did not demonstrate any differences between both groups.

There is limited evidence for use of milrinone in preterm neonates. It did not prevent the development of a low-flow state in high-risk preterm neonates when compared with placebo.[65,66] The evidence for prophylactic milrinone administration following PDA ligation is conflicting.[67–69] Dosing regimens vary, but milrinone is often started with a loading dose of 50 μg/kg followed by a continuous infusion. There is 1 PK study that recommends a bolus infusion of 0.73 μg/kg/min over 3 hours followed by a continuous infusion of 0.16 μg/kg/min in preterm neonates.[70] Side effects of tachycardia and hypotension have been described, so it should be used cautiously in the setting of low BP.

Vasopressin

Vasopressin is an endogenous peptide that is expressed in the hypothalamus. The initial prohormone preprovasopressin is converted to provasopressin and vasopressin in the pituitary gland.[71] It causes vasoconstriction through stimulation of vasopressin V1 receptors in smooth muscle. In addition, it has a vasodilatory effect on cerebral and renal arterioles by stimulation of vasopressin V2 receptors. Overall data on the use in preterm and term neonates are limited and mostly reported as case series.[72–77] Dosing is by continuous infusion of 0.00001 to 0.003 unit/kg/min. There is quite a variation in the literature regarding the appropriate dosing, and bolus administration of 2 to 20 μg/kg every 4 to 6 hours has been reported. Because of the short half-life of 5 to 15 minutes, the effects last only for about 30 to 60 minutes. A recent pilot study in 20 very preterm neonates compared vasopressin to dopamine during the first 24 hours of life. Both agents resulted in similar increases in BP but with less tachycardia in the vasopressin group.[78] However, more studies are needed before any recommendations can be made for its routine use in the preterm neonate.

Levosimendan

Levosimendan is used in adults with acute decompensated congestive heart failure. In neonates, it has mainly been used during cardiac surgery as an inodilator. Levosimendan acts as a calcium sensitizer. It binds to C cardiac troponin and enhances the sensitivity of contractile myofilaments to intracellular calcium in the cardiac muscle cells, thus improving myocardial contractility.[79,80] It activates sarcolemmal K-sensitive adenosine triphosphate channels of vascular smooth muscle cells, which has vasodilatory effects. It is thought to have protective effects on ischemia of brain and kidney tissue in neonates. Improved tissue oxygenation measured by NIRS has been reported in a cohort of neonates undergoing cardiac surgery.[81,82] Infusion doses for neonates range from 0.1 to 0.2 µg/kg/min. The potential benefits include increased cardiac output and cardiac index as well as a decrease in heart rate and lactate levels.[82] The side effects include hypotension, which needs careful and continuous monitoring. There are no reliable data on the use of levosimendan in preterm neonates, and its use as such cannot be recommended at present.

Despite their ongoing use, there is surprisingly very little PK and PD data available on the drugs highlighted above. **Table 2** provides a summary of the PK/PD studies on dopamine in the neonate. What is evident is the lack of more recent PK/PD data, especially in the very preterm neonate. Smits and colleagues[83] propose an outline on how to use hemodynamic and cerebral monitoring to study PD in neonates. This sort of monitoring will aid in better understanding the effects of inotropes, especially on brain perfusion in very preterm neonates. **Fig. 2** provides an overview of these potential processes and mechanisms and the monitoring tools available.

TREATMENT SCENARIOS

There are several treatment categories in which cardiotonic drugs are administered to the neonate. These treatment categories include, but are not limited to, the clinical situations outlined in later discussion and listed in **Table 2**. These categories were chosen because these are common situations in which the agents are prescribed in the NICU.

Transitional Low Blood Pressure in the Preterm Neonate

The most common situation in which cardiotonic drugs are administered to neonates is in the first day of life, primarily in preterm neonates with evidence of low BP.[84,85] Uncertainty remains over criteria used to define low BP, criteria upon which to intervene,

Table 2
Some unanswered questions in the treatment of cardiovascular failure and how echocardiography may influence the choice of agent used

Conditions	Typical Echocardiography Findings	Possible Agents
Preterm transitional low BP	Normal Decreased myocardial contractility Presence of large PDA	Observation, low-dose epinephrine or dopamine Low-dose epinephrine or dobutamine Consider nonsteroidal anti-inflammatory drug
PPHN	Low systemic BP Decreased right ventricular function	Consider epinephrine Consider dobutamine or milrinone Monitor BP continuously
Cardiac dysfunction in the setting of sepsis	Decreased contractility Increased pulmonary artery Low systemic BP	Consider epinephrine Consider doutmaine or milrinone Consider epinephrine, norepinephrine
Cardiac dysfunction in the setting of therapeutic hypothermia	Decreased contractility Increased pulmonary artery Low systemic BP	Consider epinephrine Consider doutmaine or milrinone Consider epinephrine, norepinephrine

Note. Evidence supporting these interventions is limited, and future clinical studies are essential.

MODEL FOR BRAIN CIRCULATION

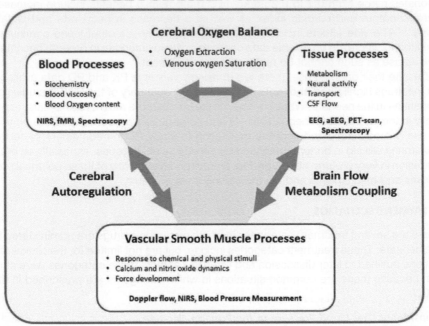

Fig. 2. The adapted brain circulation model: Overview of the hemodynamic effects on the brain. Interaction between the 3 processes (blood processes, vascular smooth muscle processes, and tissue processes) and 3 mechanisms (cerebral autoregulation, blood flow metabolism coupling, and cerebral oxygen balance) as well as value of the appropriate monitoring tools. aEEG, amplitude-integrated electroencephalography; CSF, cerebrospinal fluid; EEG, electroencephalography; fMRI, functional MRI. (*From* Thewissen L, Caicedo A, Lemmers P, et al. Measuring near-infrared spectroscopy derived cerebral autoregulation in neonates: from research tool toward bedside multimodal monitoring. Front Pediatr 2018;6:117; with permission.)

and what treatment strategy should be used.[86] Currently, most interventions occur when the BP is below a defined value for a certain period of time, with the most common cardiotonic drug administered being dopamine.[26] This approach is primarily based on familiarity; dopamine has been used as the primary inotrope since the 1970s and when administered will generally result in an increase in BP, which has been the main focus of cardiovascular stability. This approach is now being questioned by many groups, with the focus shifting toward assessment of flow rather than BP.[87,88] However, defining cardiovascular stability during transition remains a key challenge. In a recent observational study by Batton and colleagues,[84] which included more than 360 preterm neonates born at less than 27 weeks' gestation across 16 sites, almost 55% were treated for cardiovascular instability, with more than 30% of neonates receiving a cardiotonic drug (mostly dopamine).

Although dopamine has been the subject of several systematic reviews[51,89] and more than 20 randomized controlled trials in neonates, significant uncertainty remains.[90] Most studies have been characterized by small numbers, heterogenous inclusion criteria, and limited short- and long-term follow-up. Although data obtained from these studies are very informative, the limitations need to be acknowledged. A recent observational study by the Epipage group has highlighted the potential benefits of an interventional approach to low BP during the transitional phase of adaptation, suggesting that neonates who receive an intervention are less likely to sustain brain injury compared with neonates who have an observational approach to care only.[91] It is fair to say that this complex problem remains unresolved, but several ongoing or planned studies in this area may shed further light on the problem in the future.

Pulmonary Hypertension

Although the incidence of pulmonary hypertension (PH) seems to have decreased, and improved management strategies have resulted in fewer neonates requiring more extensive interventions, PH remains a significant problem. Supporting the cardiorespiratory system in the setting of PPHN is primarily based on the use of inhaled nitric oxide, with evidence suggesting that the number needed to treat to prevent one neonate requiring extracorporeal membrane oxygenation is low (eg, 5).[92] However, there are limited data on the use of various cardiotonic agents in the setting of PPHN.[93] The effect of each agent on systemic and pulmonary vascular resistance as well as ductal and atrial shunting needs to be considered. Finally, the effects on the peripheral vasculature, in particular cerebral vasculature, also need to be considered. There is currently no obvious first-line agent, and the appropriate choice of first-line inotropes/inodilators/lusitrope remains unclear.

The role of echocardiography in the setting of PPHN is crucial, both to determine the extent of the problem and also to determine the effect of various intervention strategies.[94] Animal data suggest that epinephrine may be a more suitable agent than dopamine because it has a relatively lower increase in pulmonary vascular resistance compared with dopamine.[95] However, norepinephrine may be a better alternative. The use of milrinone has increased significantly in the NICU,[96] primarily in the setting of PPHN. Although there are several case reports and case series, there are no randomized controlled trials addressing the use of milrinone in the setting of PPHN.[97–99] There is currently one small pilot trial enrolling and a larger planned study of milrinone in the setting of congenital diaphragmatic hernia. However, it should be noted that enrollment into such studies may prove difficult. A recent multisite randomized trial of bosentan in the setting of PPHN failed to enroll sufficient numbers of neonates.[100] The reasons included the changing clinical spectrum and difficulties in obtaining timely informed consent. These challenges have afflicted several other studies in the area of cardiovascular support and are discussed in a later section.

Cardiovascular Instability in the Setting of Sepsis

Sepsis remains a common problem in newborn care, predominantly in low-resource settings. Septic shock is a condition of inadequate tissue perfusion secondary to cardiovascular dysfunction occurring with suspected or certain systemic infection. It is interesting to note the recent guidance provided by the Surviving Sepsis Campaign. The algorithm addresses a goal-directed approach to therapy, and the initial inotrope suggested is dopamine. If resistant to therapy, epinephrine should be administered. However, there is very limited evidence to support such an approach, and the authors suggest than an alternative approach be given consideration. There have been several trials in the pediatric population, from 1 month of age upwards comparing dopamine with epinephrine in the setting of sepsis. The consistent finding in this age group is that epinephrine is associated with improved survival in fluid refractory hypotensive shock.[101] The effect of sepsis on drug PK/PD is not well understood in the neonate, and undoubtedly an individualized approach with particular dosing regimens needs to be carefully considered. One recent trial compared epinephrine and dopamine as a first-line vasoactive drug in 40 neonates with fluid-refractory septic shock in a low-resource setting.[102] The initial starting dose of epinephrine was 0.2 μg/kg/min and dopamine 10 μg/kg/min, with subsequent increases of each agent depending on the response. All-cause mortality by 28 days was very high (70%) in the epinephrine compared with the dopamine group (80%). The investigators concluded that epinephrine (0.2–0.4 μg/kg/min) and dopamine (10–20 μg/kg/min) had comparable efficacy and safety in neonatal septic shock. However mortality was extremely high, and generalizability of these findings needs to be interpreted cautiously.

Cardiovascular Instability in the Setting of Perinatal Asphyxia and Therapeutic Hypothermia

The definition of perinatal asphyxia is broad but typically characterized by evidence of metabolic acidosis, low Apgar scores, and the need for initial respiratory support. The primary insult can have implications for cardiovascular function, often in the setting of multiorgan dysfunction. Echocardiography findings after asphyxia include decreased contractility and cardiac output, impaired end diastolic filling, and increased pulmonary artery pressure. The presence of some cardiac biomarkers is associated with altered echocardiographic findings. For neonates with evidence of clinical encephalopathy in the setting of perinatal asphyxia, the primary therapy is therapeutic hypothermia. This intervention has been associated with a reduction in heart rate, stroke volume, and cardiac output and an increase in PH.[103–106] However, these changes do not seem to be associated with an increase in mortality or adverse neurodevelopmental outcome in a meta-analysis of various trials of cooling strategies compared with controls. Therapeutic strategies include use of various agents, such as dopamine, dobutamine, and epinephrine. There is no consensus as to which agent may be the most appropriate, and most of the current evidence available is derived from animal studies.[107,108]

ADMINISTRATION OF AGENTS

There are no neonatal-specific cardiotonic formulations, and this presents significant challenges, particularly in very preterm neonates, whereby effective and timely delivery of an inotrope infusion may be crucial. There are many problems with the current use of adult preparations. A ready-to-use neonatal formulation means avoidance of unnecessary delays in formulation preparation. It would also avoid unnecessary dilutions, which are both time consuming and also increase the likelihood of contamination or a drug error. Stability testing would be needed with neonatal-specific formulations to ensure that the solution has an equal distribution of the drug as opposed to the current method, which involves dilutions whereby there may be unequal distribution resulting in a risk of boluses of drug being administered. These problems can only be overcome with the use of specific ready-to-use neonatal formulations.

Even with the use of neonatal-specific formulations, other administration challenges include very low infusion rates and relatively large dead space considerations, which will result in long lag times before the drug gets to the desired location. The syringe size as well as the diameter and length of the tubing are other important factors that need to be considered. Upward displacement of the syringe pump results in a potential increase in the flow rate. The lower the infusion rates, the greater the relative bolus delivery of the drug.[109–112] Physicians need to be aware of these potential side effects and minimize their occurrence.

Inotropes as molecules can be quite unstable if exposed to oxygen and diluted in infusion mixtures. A study on the stability of typical dopamine and dobutamine infusions made from adult formulations used in the NICU demonstrated 2 time points of significant changes in the concentration of dopamine. Time point 1 was within the first 30 minutes of preparing the infusion, and the second time point was after approximately 12 hours after the dopamine infusion.[113] Drug concentrations dropped by more than 7%, which is outside the standard tolerance rate. It is therefore suggested to wait 30 minutes before connecting a new infusion mixture to the neonate for infusion and to change dopamine infusions after 12 hours rather than every 24 hours. However, more frequent changing of inotrope infusions carries their own unwanted side effects, and perhaps of more importance is the development of stable neonatal formulations.

FUTURE DIRECTIONS

The study of cardiotonic drugs in the neonate appears to be particularly challenging, especially in comparison to other areas of newborn care. There are no large randomized controlled trials evaluating the efficacy of various agents in the conditions outlined above. The lack of evidence is in stark contrast to the pediatric and adult population, whereby large randomized controlled trials have been performed and have helped to inform practice. There are many potential reasons to explain this dearth of studies. Because there are no neonatal-specific formulations available, it is more challenging to perform studies in time-sensitive situations. The incidence of the various conditions outlined seems to have decreased somewhat over time, which again makes it more challenging to enroll. Obtaining valid informed consent also remains a major hurdle to recruitment. Several trials have met challenges in enrollment. These trials include a study on neonatal hypotension in extreme preterm neonates,[114] a study of corticosteroid in cardiovascular instability in late preterm neonates,[115] and a study of bosentan use in PPHN.[100] These trials serve as a stark reminder of the challenges in conducting studies in this area and highlight the need for international collaborations, the importance of synergy between the Food and Drug Administration and European Medicines Agency, and the inclusion of industry in the conduct of such trials. The role of the International Neonatal Consortium is crucial to facilitating this engagement and ensuring the foundations are established to finally try and answer some of these age old questions with clear and concise evidence.

ACKNOWLEDGMENTS

The authors would like to acknowledge the support of both the Neocirculation (http://neocirculation.eu) and Hypotension in Preterm Infants (HIP) (https://www.hip-trial.com) consortia. The authors thank Igor Brbre, clinical librarian, for his help with the literature search.

REFERENCES

1. Batton BJ, Li L, Newman NS, et al. Feasibility study of early blood pressure management in extremely preterm infants. J Pediatr 2012;161(1):65–9.e1.
2. Dempsey EM, Barrington KJ. Diagnostic criteria and therapeutic interventions for the hypotensive very low birth weight infant. J Perinatol 2006;26(11):677–81.
3. Faust K, Hartel C, Preuss M, et al. Short-term outcome of very-low-birthweight infants with arterial hypotension in the first 24 h of life. Arch Dis Child Fetal Neonatal Ed 2015;100(5):F388–92.
4. Ruggieri L, Giannuzzi V, Baiardi P, et al. Successful private-public funding of paediatric medicines research: lessons from the EU programme to fund research into off-patent medicines. Eur J Pediatr 2015;174(4):481–91.

5. Ergenekon E, Rojas-Anaya H, Bravo MC, et al. Cardiovascular drug therapy for human newborn: review of pharmacodynamic data. Curr Pharm Des 2017; 23(38):5850–60.

6. Mahoney L, Crook D, Walter KN, et al. What is the evidence for the use of adrenaline in the treatment of neonatal hypotension? Cardiovasc Hematol Agents Med Chem 2012;10(1):50–98.

7. Dempsey EM. Under pressure to treat? Arch Dis Child Fetal Neonatal Ed 2015; 100(5):F380–1.

8. Rabe H, Rojas-Anaya H. Inotropes for preterm babies during the transition period after birth: friend or foe? Arch Dis Child Fetal Neonatal Ed 2017; 102(6):F547–50.

9. Katheria AC, Lakshminrusimha S, Rabe H, et al. Placental transfusion: a review. J Perinatol 2017;37(2):105–11.

10. Rabe H, Diaz-Rossello JL, Duley L, et al. Effect of timing of umbilical cord clamping and other strategies to influence placental transfusion at preterm birth on maternal and infant outcomes. Cochrane Database Syst Rev 2012;(8):CD003248.

11. McDonald SJ, Middleton P, Dowswell T, et al. Effect of timing of umbilical cord clamping of term infants on maternal and neonatal outcomes. Cochrane Database Syst Rev 2013;(7):CD004074.

12. Finn D, Roehr CC, Ryan CA, et al. Optimising intravenous volume resuscitation of the newborn in the delivery room: practical considerations and gaps in knowledge. Neonatology 2017;112(2):163–71.

13. Fogarty M, Osborn DA, Askie L, et al. Delayed vs early umbilical cord clamping for preterm infants: a systematic review and meta-analysis. Am J Obstet Gynecol 2018;218(1):1–18.

14. Al-Wassia H, Shah PS. Efficacy and safety of umbilical cord milking at birth: a systematic review and meta-analysis. JAMA Pediatr 2015;169(1):18–25.

15. Andersson O, Hellstrom-Westas L, Andersson D, et al. Effects of delayed compared with early umbilical cord clamping on maternal postpartum hemorrhage and cord blood gas sampling: a randomized trial. Acta Obstet Gynecol Scand 2013;92(5):567–74.

16. Ghavam S, Batra D, Mercer J, et al. Effects of placental transfusion in extremely low birthweight infants: meta-analysis of long- and short-term outcomes. Transfusion 2014;54(4):1192–8.

17. Farrugia R, Rojas H, Rabe H. Diagnosis and management of hypotension in neonates. Future Cardiol 2013;9(5):669–79.

18. de Boode WP. Clinical monitoring of systemic hemodynamics in critically ill newborns. Early Hum Dev 2010;86(3):137–41.

19. Osborn DA, Evans N, Kluckow M. Clinical detection of low upper body blood flow in very premature infants using blood pressure, capillary refill time, and central-peripheral temperature difference. Arch Dis Child Fetal Neonatal Ed 2004;89(2):F168–73.

20. Dempsey EM, El-Khuffash AF. Objective cardiovascular assessment in the neonatal intensive care unit. Arch Dis Child Fetal Neonatal Ed 2018;103(1): F72–7.

21. Van Laere D, Voeten M, O' Toole JM, et al. Monitoring circulation during transition in extreme low gestational age newborns: what's on the horizon? Front Pediatr 2018;6:74.

22. Rodriguez Sanchez de la Blanca A, Sanchez Luna M, Gonzalez Pacheco N, et al. Electrical velocimetry for non-invasive monitoring of the closure of the ductus arteriosus in preterm infants. Eur J Pediatr 2018;177(2):229–35.

23. Papadhima I, Louis D, Purna J, et al. Targeted neonatal echocardiography (TNE) consult service in a large tertiary perinatal center in Canada. J Perinatol 2018;38(8):1039–45.

24. de Boode WP, van der Lee R, Eriksen BH, et al. The role of Neonatologist Performed Echocardiography in the assessment and management of neonatal shock. Pediatr Res 2018;84(Suppl 1):57–67.

25. da Costa CS, Greisen G, Austin T. Is near-infrared spectroscopy clinically useful in the preterm infant? Arch Dis Child Fetal Neonatal Ed 2015;100(6):F558–61.

26. Stranak Z, Semberova J, Barrington K, et al. International survey on diagnosis and management of hypotension in extremely preterm babies. Eur J Pediatr 2014;173(6):793–8.

27. Subhedar NV. Treatment of hypotension in newborns. Semin Neonatol 2003; 8(6):413–23.

28. Hentschel R, Hensel D, Brune T, et al. Impact on blood pressure and intestinal perfusion of dobutamine or dopamine in hypotensive preterm infants. Biol Neonate 1995;68(5):318–24.

29. Lundstrom K, Pryds O, Greisen G. The haemodynamic effects of dopamine and volume expansion in sick preterm infants. Early Hum Dev 2000;57(2):157–63.

30. Seri I, Abbasi S, Wood DC, et al. Regional hemodynamic effects of dopamine in the sick preterm neonate. J Pediatr 1998;133(6):728–34.

31. Seri I, Rudas G, Bors Z, et al. Effects of low-dose dopamine infusion on cardiovascular and renal functions, cerebral blood flow, and plasma catecholamine levels in sick preterm neonates. Pediatr Res 1993;34(6):742–9.

32. Zhang J, Penny DJ, Kim NS, et al. Mechanisms of blood pressure increase induced by dopamine in hypotensive preterm neonates. Arch Dis Child Fetal Neonatal Ed 1999;81(2):F99–104.

33. Subhedar NV, Shaw NJ. Dopamine versus dobutamine for hypotensive preterm infants. Cochrane Database Syst Rev 2000;(2):CD001242.

34. Roze JC, Tohier C, Maingueneau C, et al. Response to dobutamine and dopamine in the hypotensive very preterm infant. Arch Dis Child 1993;69(1 Spec No): 59–63.

35. Osborn D, Evans N, Kluckow M. Randomized trial of dobutamine versus dopamine in preterm infants with low systemic blood flow. J Pediatr 2002;140(2): 183–91.

36. Phillipos EZ, Barrington KJ, Robertson MA. Dopamine versus epinephrine for inotropic support in the neonate: a randomised blinded trial. Pediatr Res 1996;(39):A238.

37. Bhatt-Mehta V, Nahata MC. Dopamine and dobutamine in pediatric therapy. Pharmacotherapy 1989;9(5):303–14.

38. Filippi L, Pezzati M, Poggi C, et al. Dopamine versus dobutamine in very low birthweight infants: endocrine effects. Arch Dis Child Fetal Neonatal Ed 2007; 92(5):F367–71.

39. Seri I, Abbasi S, Wood DC, et al. Regional hemodynamic effects of dopamine in the indomethacin-treated preterm infant. J Perinatol 2002;22(4):300–5.

40. Seri I, Tulassay T, Kiszel J, et al. Cardiovascular response to dopamine in hypotensive preterm neonates with severe hyaline membrane disease. Eur J Pediatr 1984;142(1):3–9.

41. Seri I, Tulassay T, Kiszel J, et al. Effect of low-dose dopamine infusion on prolactin and thyrotropin secretion in preterm infants with hyaline membrane disease. Biol Neonate 1985;47(6):317–22.

42. Driscoll DJ, Gillette PC, Duff DF, et al. The hemodynamic effect of dopamine in children. J Thorac Cardiovasc Surg 1979;78(5):765–8.

43. Williams DB, Kiernan PD, Schaff HV, et al. The hemodynamic response to dopamine and nitroprusside following right atrium-pulmonary artery bypass (Fontan procedure). Ann Thorac Surg 1982;34(1):51–7.

44. Driscoll DJ. Use of inotropic and chronotropic agents in neonates. Clin Perinatol 1987;14(4):931–49.

45. Eldadah MK, Schwartz PH, Harrison R, et al. Pharmacokinetics of dopamine in infants and children. Crit Care Med 1991;19(8):1008–11.

46. Liet JM, Boscher C, Gras-Leguen C, et al. Dopamine effects on pulmonary artery pressure in hypotensive preterm infants with patent ductus arteriosus. J Pediatr 2002;140(3):373–5.

47. Bouissou A, Rakza T, Klosowski S, et al. Hypotension in preterm infants with significant patent ductus arteriosus: effects of dopamine. J Pediatr 2008;153(6): 790–4.

48. Eriksen VR, Hahn GH, Greisen G. Dopamine therapy is associated with impaired cerebral autoregulation in preterm infants. Acta Paediatr 2014; 103(12):1221–6.

49. Wong FY, Barfield CP, Horne RS, et al. Dopamine therapy promotes cerebral flow-metabolism coupling in preterm infants. Intensive Care Med 2009;35(10): 1777–82.

50. Osborn DA, Evans N, Kluckow M, et al. Low superior vena cava flow and effect of inotropes on neurodevelopment to 3 years in preterm infants. Pediatrics 2007; 120(2):372–80.

51. Sassano-Higgins S, Friedlich P, Seri I. A meta-analysis of dopamine use in hypotensive preterm infants: blood pressure and cerebral hemodynamics. J Perinatol 2011;31(10):647–55.

52. Bravo MC, Lopez-Ortego P, Sanchez L, et al. Randomized, placebo-controlled trial of dobutamine for low superior vena cava flow in infants. J Pediatr 2015; 167(3):572–8.e1-2.

53. Mielgo VE, Valls ISA, Lopez-de-Heredia JM, et al. Hemodynamic and metabolic effects of a new pediatric dobutamine formulation in hypoxic newborn pigs. Pediatr Res 2017;81(3):511–8.

54. Klarr JM, Faix RG, Pryce CJ, et al. Randomized, blind trial of dopamine versus dobutamine for treatment of hypotension in preterm infants with respiratory distress syndrome. J Pediatr 1994;125(1):117–22.

55. Dempsey EM, Barrington KJ, Marlow N, et al. Management of hypotension in preterm infants (The HIP Trial): a randomised controlled trial of hypotension management in extremely low gestational age newborns. Neonatology 2014; 105(4):275–81.

56. Cheung PY, Barrington KJ. The effects of dopamine and epinephrine on hemodynamics and oxygen metabolism in hypoxic anesthetized piglets. Crit Care 2001;5(3):158–66.

57. Germanakis I, Bender C, Hentschel R, et al. Hypercontractile heart failure caused by catecholamine therapy in premature neonates. Acta Paediatr 2003; 92(7):836–8.

58. Paradisis M, Osborn DA. Adrenaline for prevention of morbidity and mortality in preterm infants with cardiovascular compromise. Cochrane Database Syst Rev 2004;(1):CD003958.

59. Valverde E, Pellicer A, Madero R, et al. Dopamine versus epinephrine for cardiovascular support in low birth weight infants: analysis of systemic effects and neonatal clinical outcomes. Pediatrics 2006;117(6):e1213–22.

60. Rizk MY, Lapointe A, Lefebvre F, et al. Norepinephrine infusion improves haemodynamics in the preterm infants during septic shock. Acta Paediatr 2017;107(3): 408–13.

61. Tourneux P, Rakza T, Abazine A, et al. Noradrenaline for management of septic shock refractory to fluid loading and dopamine or dobutamine in full-term newborn infants. Acta Paediatr 2008;97(2):177–80.

62. Rowcliff K, de Waal K, Mohamed AL, et al. Noradrenaline in preterm infants with cardiovascular compromise. Eur J Pediatr 2016;175(12):1967–73.

63. Fuloria M, Aschner JL. Persistent pulmonary hypertension of the newborn. Semin Fetal Neonatal Med 2017;22(4):220–6.

64. Pellicer A, Riera J, Lopez-Ortego P, et al. Phase 1 study of two inodilators in neonates undergoing cardiovascular surgery. Pediatr Res 2013;73(1):95–103.

65. Paradisis M, Evans N, Kluckow M, et al. Pilot study of milrinone for low systemic blood flow in very preterm infants. J Pediatr 2006;148(3):306–13.

66. Paradisis M, Evans N, Kluckow M, et al. Randomized trial of milrinone versus placebo for prevention of low systemic blood flow in very preterm infants. J Pediatr 2009;154(2):189–95.

67. Sehgal A. Haemodynamically unstable preterm infant: an unresolved management conundrum. Eur J Pediatr 2011;170(10):1237–45.

68. Jain A, Sahni M, El-Khuffash A, et al. Use of targeted neonatal echocardiography to prevent postoperative cardiorespiratory instability after patent ductus arteriosus ligation. J Pediatr 2012;160(4):584–9.e1.

69. El-Khuffash AF, Jain A, Weisz D, et al. Assessment and treatment of post patent ductus arteriosus ligation syndrome. J Pediatr 2014;165(1):46–52.e1.

70. Hallik M, Tasa T, Starkopf J, et al. Dosing of milrinone in preterm neonates to prevent postligation cardiac syndrome: simulation study suggests need for bolus infusion. Neonatology 2017;111(1):8–11.

71. Beaulieu MJ. Vasopressin for the treatment of neonatal hypotension. Neonatal Netw 2013;32(2):120–4.

72. Lechner E, Hofer A, Mair R, et al. Arginine-vasopressin in neonates with vasodilatory shock after cardiopulmonary bypass. Eur J Pediatr 2007;166(12):1221–7.

73. Bidegain M, Greenberg R, Simmons C, et al. Vasopressin for refractory hypotension in extremely low birth weight infants. J Pediatr 2010;157(3):502–4.

74. Ikegami H, Funato M, Tamai H, et al. Low-dose vasopressin infusion therapy for refractory hypotension in ELBW infants. Pediatr Int 2010;52(3):368–73.

75. Filippi L, Gozzini E, Daniotti M, et al. Rescue treatment with terlipressin in different scenarios of refractory hypotension in newborns and infants. Pediatr Crit Care Med 2011;12(6):e237–41.

76. Shivanna B, Rios D, Rossano J, et al. Vasopressin and its analogues for the treatment of refractory hypotension in neonates. Cochrane Database Syst Rev 2013;(3):CD009171.

77. Mohamed A, Nasef N, Shah V, et al. Vasopressin as a rescue therapy for refractory pulmonary hypertension in neonates: case series. Pediatr Crit Care Med 2014;15(2):148–54.

78. Rios DR, Kaiser JR. Vasopressin versus dopamine for treatment of hypotension in extremely low birth weight infants: a randomized, blinded pilot study. J Pediatr 2015;166(4):850–5.
79. Bhat BV, Plakkal N. Management of shock in neonates. Indian J Pediatr 2015; 82(10):923–9.
80. Egan JR, Clarke AJ, Williams S, et al. Levosimendan for low cardiac output: a pediatric experience. J Intensive Care Med 2006;21(3):183–7.
81. Esch J, Joynt C, Manouchehri N, et al. Differential hemodynamic effects of levosimendan in a porcine model of neonatal hypoxia-reoxygenation. Neonatology 2012;101(3):192–200.
82. Ricci Z, Garisto C, Favia I, et al. Levosimendan infusion in newborns after corrective surgery for congenital heart disease: randomized controlled trial. Intensive Care Med 2012;38(7):1198–204.
83. Smits A, Thewissen L, Dereymaeker A, et al. The use of hemodynamic and cerebral monitoring to study pharmacodynamics in neonates. Curr Pharm Des 2017;23(38):5955–63.
84. Batton B, Li L, Newman NS, et al. Use of antihypotensive therapies in extremely preterm infants. Pediatrics 2013;131(6):e1865–73.
85. Laughon M, Bose C, Allred E, et al. Factors associated with treatment for hypotension in extremely low gestational age newborns during the first postnatal week. Pediatrics 2007;119(2):273–80.
86. Dempsey EM, Barrington KJ. Treating hypotension in the preterm infant: when and with what: a critical and systematic review. J Perinatol 2007;27(8):469–78.
87. Giesinger RE, McNamara PJ. Hemodynamic instability in the critically ill neonate: an approach to cardiovascular support based on disease pathophysiology. Semin Perinatol 2016;40(3):174–88.
88. Noori S, Seri I. Evidence-based versus pathophysiology-based approach to diagnosis and treatment of neonatal cardiovascular compromise. Semin Fetal Neonatal Med 2015;20(4):238–45.
89. Osborn DA, Paradisis M, Evans N. The effect of inotropes on morbidity and mortality in preterm infants with low systemic or organ blood flow. Cochrane Database Syst Rev 2007;(1):CD005090.
90. Dempsey EM, Barrington KJ. Evaluation and treatment of hypotension in the preterm infant. Clin Perinatol 2009;36(1):75–85.
91. Durrmeyer X, Marchand-Martin L, Porcher R, et al. Abstention or intervention for isolated hypotension in the first 3 days of life in extremely preterm infants: association with short-term outcomes in the EPIPAGE 2 cohort study. Arch Dis Child Fetal Neonatal Ed 2017;102(6):490–6.
92. Barrington KJ, Finer N, Pennaforte T, et al. Nitric oxide for respiratory failure in infants born at or near term. Cochrane Database Syst Rev 2017;(1):CD000399.
93. Barrington KJ. Common hemodynamic problems in the neonate. Neonatology 2013;103(4):335–40.
94. Mukerji A, Diambomba Y, Lee SK, et al. Use of targeted neonatal echocardiography and focused cardiac sonography in tertiary neonatal intensive care units: time to embrace it? J Ultrasound Med 2016;35(7):1579–91.
95. Cheung PY, Barrington KJ, Pearson RJ, et al. Systemic, pulmonary and mesenteric perfusion and oxygenation effects of dopamine and epinephrine. Am J Respir Crit Care Med 1997;155(1):32–7.
96. Rios DR, Moffett BS, Kaiser JR. Trends in pharmacotherapy for neonatal hypotension. J Pediatr 2014;165(4):697–701.e1.

97. McNamara PJ, Shivananda SP, Sahni M, et al. Pharmacology of milrinone in neonates with persistent pulmonary hypertension of the newborn and suboptimal response to inhaled nitric oxide. Pediatr Crit Care Med 2013;14(1): 74–84.

98. James AT, Corcoran JD, McNamara PJ, et al. The effect of milrinone on right and left ventricular function when used as a rescue therapy for term infants with pulmonary hypertension. Cardiol Young 2016;26(1):90–9.

99. Giaccone A, Zuppa AF, Sood B, et al. Milrinone pharmacokinetics and pharmacodynamics in neonates with persistent pulmonary hypertension of the newborn. Am J Perinatol 2017;34(8):749–58.

100. Steinhorn RH, Fineman J, Kusic-Pajic A, et al. Bosentan as adjunctive therapy for persistent pulmonary hypertension of the newborn: results of the randomized multicenter placebo-controlled exploratory trial. J Pediatr 2016;177: 90–96 e93.

101. Ventura AM, Shieh HH, Bousso A, et al. Double-blind prospective randomized controlled trial of dopamine versus epinephrine as first-line vasoactive drugs in pediatric septic shock. Crit Care Med 2015;43(11):2292–302.

102. Baske K, Saini SS, Dutta S, et al. Epinephrine versus dopamine in neonatal septic shock: a double-blind randomized controlled trial. Eur J Pediatr 2019;178(1): 115–6.

103. Wu TW, Tamrazi B, Soleymani S, et al. Hemodynamic changes during rewarming phase of whole-body hypothermia therapy in neonates with hypoxic-ischemic encephalopathy. J Pediatr 2018;197:68–74.e2.

104. Forman E, Breatnach CR, Ryan S, et al. Non-invasive continuous cardiac output and cerebral perfusion monitoring in term infants with neonatal encephalopathy: assessment of feasibility and reliability. Pediatr Res 2017;82(5): 789–95.

105. Cavallaro G, Filippi L, Raffaeli G, et al. Heart rate and arterial pressure changes during whole-body deep hypothermia. ISRN Pediatr 2013;2013:140213.

106. Gebauer CM, Knuepfer M, Robel-Tillig E, et al. Hemodynamics among neonates with hypoxic-ischemic encephalopathy during whole-body hypothermia and passive rewarming. Pediatrics 2006;117(3):843–50.

107. Cheung PY, Abozaid S, Al-Salam Z, et al. Systemic and regional hemodynamic effects of high-dose epinephrine infusion in hypoxic piglets resuscitated with 100% oxygen. Shock 2007;28(4):491–7.

108. Cheung DC, Gill RS, Liu JQ, et al. Vasopressin improves systemic hemodynamics without compromising mesenteric perfusion in the resuscitation of asphyxiated newborn piglets: a dose-response study. Intensive Care Med 2012;38(3):491–8.

109. Schmidt N, Saez C, Seri I, et al. Impact of syringe size on the performance of infusion pumps at low flow rates. Pediatr Crit Care Med 2010;11(2):282–6.

110. Seyberth HW, Kauffman RE. Basics and dynamics of neonatal and pediatric pharmacology. Handb Exp Pharmacol 2011;205:3–49.

111. Sherwin CM, Medlicott NJ, Reith DM, et al. Intravenous drug delivery in neonates: lessons learnt. Arch Dis Child 2014;99(6):590–4.

112. van der Eijk AC, van Rens RM, Dankelman J, et al. A literature review on flow-rate variability in neonatal IV therapy. Paediatr Anaesth 2013;23(1):9–21.

113. Kirupakaran K, Mahoney L, Rabe H, et al. Understanding the stability of dopamine and dobutamine over 24 h in simulated neonatal ward conditions. Paediatr Drugs 2017;19(5):487–95.

114. Vain NE, Barrington KJ. Feasibility of evaluating treatment of early hypotension in extremely low birth weight infants. J Pediatr 2012;161(1):4–7.

115. Watterberg KL, Fernandez E, Walsh MC, et al. Barriers to enrollment in a randomized controlled trial of hydrocortisone for cardiovascular insufficiency in term and late preterm newborn infants. J Perinatol 2017;37(11):1220–3.

Drugs for the Prevention and Treatment of Bronchopulmonary Dysplasia

Erica W. Mandell, DO[a,b], Panagiotis Kratimenos, MD, PhD[c],
Steven H. Abman, MD[a,d], Robin H. Steinhorn, MD[c],*

KEYWORDS

- Bronchopulmonary dysplasia • Chronic pulmonary insufficiency of prematurity
- Pharmacology • Lungs

KEY POINTS

- Despite high rates of bronchopulmonary dysplasia, no new drugs have been approved for BPD prevention or therapy in the last 25 years, and most currently available drugs remain inadequately tested.
- A limitation in the development of new therapies for BPD prevention is uncertainty over meaningful clinical end points. Many preterm neonates do not have clinical diagnosis of BPD but go on to develop chronic pulmonary insufficiency later in childhood.
- Perinatal factors that increase the risk for BPD, such as maternal smoking, intrauterine growth restriction, preeclampsia, and chorioamnionitis should be considered as targets for new drug development.
- Of available postnatal interventions, only caffeine, Vitamin A, and corticosteroids reduce the risk for BPD. Off target effects of steroids on neurodevelopmental outcomes continue to drive investigation on specific agents and dosage regimens.
- Promising new investigational agents include mesenchymal stem cells and insulin-like growth factor 1 (IGF-1).

INTRODUCTION

In 1967, Northway and colleagues[1] described bronchopulmonary dysplasia (BPD) as a lung condition of prematurity that began with diffuse parenchymal lung disease and

[a] Pediatric Heart Lung Center, Section of Neonatology, University of Colorado Denver, Anschutz Medical Center and Children's Hospital Colorado, 12700 E 19th Ave, P14-4460A, MS8614, Aurora, CO 80045, USA; [b] Section of Pulmonary Medicine, University of Colorado Denver, Anschutz Medical Center and Children's Hospital Colorado, Aurora, CO 80045, USA; [c] Division of Neonatology, Neonatology and Hospital Based Specialties, Children's National Medical Center, 111 Michigan Ave NW, Washington, DC 20010, USA; [d] Department of Pediatrics, University of Colorado Denver, Anschutz Medical Center and Children's Hospital Colorado, Mail Stop B395, 13123 East 16th Avenue, Aurora, CO 80045, USA
* Corresponding author.
E-mail address: RSTEINHORN@childrensnational.org

Clin Perinatol 46 (2019) 291–310
https://doi.org/10.1016/j.clp.2019.02.011
0095-5108/19/© 2019 Elsevier Inc. All rights reserved.
perinatology.theclinics.com

low lung volumes and progressed into a chronic pattern of spongelike or cystic lesions dispersed among heterogeneous infiltrates and areas of severe hyperinflation. There was significant mortality associated with this diagnosis, with 59% of neonates developing BPD ultimately dying.[1] At autopsy, there was evidence of airways disease, distal lung inflammation, diffuse fibroproliferative changes, and hypertensive pulmonary vascular remodeling. In 1967, BPD was primarily seen in larger, moderately preterm neonates with severe respiratory failure after exposure to high concentrations of oxygen and ventilator pressures. The so-called new BPD seen in contemporary practice is a disease mostly seen in extremely preterm infants born at less than 29 weeks' gestation.[2] The new BPD is generally defined based on a severity spectrum, with a minimum requirement of having received supplemental oxygen therapy use for the first 28 days of life considered as mild BPD, whereas moderate and severe disease are defined as sustained need for varying levels of supplemental oxygen and respiratory support.[3] On histology, this new BPD is characterized by an arrest of alveolar development with fewer and larger alveoli, decreased pulmonary vascular development, and variable airway smooth muscle hyperplasia.[4–6]

Although the severity of BPD may have improved, its incidence has remained stable at ~40% for the last decade for preterm neonates born before 29 weeks' gestation.[2] This fixed incidence is in part caused by the improved survival of extremely low gestational age neonates who are at highest risk for developing BPD.[7] Over the past 25 years, there have been significant efforts to develop new therapies to prevent or improve outcomes for neonates at risk for BPD. These efforts include improved resuscitation at birth, the use of lower inspired oxygen concentrations, increased use of noninvasive ventilation strategies such as continuous positive airflow pressure, improved invasive ventilation strategies, prevention of postnatal infections, and improved early nutrition. Several pharmacologic interventions have also been studied to modulate the pathobiology of BPD, including antenatal steroids, surfactant, caffeine, vitamin A, and inhaled nitric oxide (NO). However, despite an increased understanding of the pathobiology of BPD, these attempts to develop medications and other nonpharmacologic interventions to decrease the development of BPD have been largely disappointing.

Recent epidemiologic studies have shown that the risk for BPD and chronic pulmonary insufficiency of prematurity (CPIP) in the first year of life are both strongly established within days of birth.[8–10] There are also numerous epidemiologic studies that show intrauterine growth restriction, preeclampsia, chorioamnionitis, and maternal smoking significantly increase the risk of BPD.[11] Another recent report showed that the lasting impact of antenatal factors on lung development may in part be caused by specific effects of placental dysfunction.[12] These findings speak to a growing recognition that antenatal mechanisms are critical determinants of BPD. However, the exact relationships between these antenatal exposures and early postnatal events and the development of CPIP during infancy still need to be clarified.

The concept that BPD begins during fetal life was the topic of a recent National Heart, Lung, and Blood Institute (NHLBI) workshop that highlighted the need to better understand mechanisms by which antenatal factors and placental dysfunction contribute to increased BPD risk.[13] Although BPD status at 36 weeks postmenstrual age (PMA) is a known risk factor for compromised late respiratory outcomes, perinatal factors have been shown to be strong predictors of CPIP and comparable with BPD status alone. This report also stressed the need to identify early pathologic pathways to allow the development of effective disease predictors and therapeutic targets. Despite strong epidemiologic work supporting fetal origins of BPD, the mechanisms by which antenatal exposures lead to BPD are significantly underexplored. Further preclinical studies using antenatal models of BPD may help the development of novel interventions for prevention of BPD and CPIP beyond the current use of postnatal interventions. Basic work is needed to better define interactions between genetic and epigenetic factors, antenatal stress, and postnatal factors that contribute to disruption of lung development. It is clear that the prevention of BPD will require more understanding of these antenatal mechanisms as well as earlier and more precise identification of neonates at risk for BPD.

Another limitation in the development of effective therapies for BPD prevention is continued controversy over meaningful clinical end points. A recent review from the International Neonatal Consortium highlighted that ongoing gaps in drug development are in part caused by difficulties with clinical trial design created by inconsistent definitions of BPD and a lack of long-term outcomes of clinical importance.[10] Moreover, many preterm neonates who may not carry a formal diagnosis of BPD continue to develop CPIP later in childhood.[10] Infants with CPIP have a range of disease severity characterized by frequent, repeated hospitalizations with high rates of emergency room or medical visits because of recurrent respiratory exacerbations, lower respiratory tract infections, reactive airways disease, and pulmonary hypertension (PH). These infants may also have sustained abnormalities of lung function, poor exercise tolerance, and a need for chronic respiratory medications throughout childhood and adolescence, as well as other nonpulmonary comorbidities such as neurocognitive impairment and retinopathy of prematurity.[14,15]

The current yes/no diagnosis of BPD at 36 weeks' PMA does not capture all infants who ultimately develop CPIP and does not adequately differentiate between phenotypes of alveolar, airways, and vascular disease. In addition, there are many neonates who die of severe respiratory failure before a formal diagnosis of BPD can be made. These are neonates who may benefit the most from novel therapeutic approaches. Clinicians are just beginning to understand the complexity of interactions between genetic predisposition, antenatal factors and exposures, preterm birth, and postnatal exposures that culminate in persistent and progressive CPIP in survivors of preterm birth.[10,12,16,17] Broader and more precise definitions of clinically meaningful outcomes are needed to facilitate the specific development of new therapies for high-risk neonates.

DRUGS FOR THE PREVENTION OF BRONCHOPULMONARY DYSPLASIA

The currently available preventive pharmacologic agents are summarized in **Table 1**. The time and effort behind development, preclinical testing, and ongoing research for each of these medications have been enormous and have positively shaped contemporary care of preterm neonates. However, although survival for preterm neonates has improved, there have been fewer advances in the prevention of BPD, which partly explains why rates of BPD have not decreased. Further progress in reducing BPD and enhancing late respiratory outcomes will require the early identification of those preterm neonates at greatest risk for severe disease, improved understanding of factors that modulate respiratory phenotypes and outcomes, and the ability to intervene selectively for disease prevention.[10,12,13]

A better understanding of the respiratory phenotypes and specific antenatal causes will help direct drug therapies. In addition, randomized clinical trials targeted at the highest risk populations may assist discovery of more efficacious drugs or guide the use of current therapies in a more targeted fashion. Current strategies for the prevention of BPD include antenatal pharmacologic interventions such as maternal progesterone and antenatal steroids.

Table 1
Current preventive pharmacologic agents available for the prevention of bronchopulmonary dysplasia

Medication	Biological Role/Possible Mechanisms to Decrease BPD	Major Supporting Clinical Studies
Maternal progesterone	• Antiinflammatory • Prevents withdrawal of progesterone	• Challis,[122] 2009 • Zakar,[123] 2011 • Pieber,[124] 2001 • Dodd et al,[19] 2013
Antenatal steroids	• Decreased need for early mechanical ventilation • Decreased respiratory distress syndrome	• NIH Consensus Panel,[125] 1995 • Roberts et al,[25] 2017
Surfactant	• Facilitates early extubation to less aggressive ventilation modes	• Stevens,[126] 2007 • Ribo,[127] 2016
Caffeine	• Decreased time on mechanical ventilation • Antiinflammatory • Diuretic effects	• Schmidt et al,[34] 2006
Vitamin A	• Cell growth and differentiation • Respiratory epithelial cell integrity	• Tyson,[128] 1999 • Darlow et al,[32] 2016
Inhaled nitric oxide	• Required for alveolar and vascular development • Treatment of acute hypoxic respiratory failure and persistent pulmonary hypertension	• Jakkula et al,[91] 2000 • Donohue et al,[95] 2011 • Kinsella et al,[98] 2016 • Krishnan et al,[103] 2017 • Askie et al,[100] 2018

Antenatal Pharmacologic Interventions

Maternal progesterone

As the era of contemporary neonatology has emerged, in which the risk and severity of BPD are inversely correlated with gestation age, preventing non–medically indicated preterm birth (particularly for women at <29 weeks' gestation) should decrease the incidence of BPD. Progesterone supplementation to prevent preterm birth has been used for decades but now has strong evidence for its efficacy.[18] In women with a past history of preterm birth, progesterone has been shown in the meta-analyses of randomized controlled trials to significantly reduce the risk of preterm birth at less than 34 weeks.[19] As a result of these findings, the American College of Obstetricians and Gynecologists recommends progesterone supplementation starting at 16 to 24 weeks of gestation to reduce the risk of recurrent spontaneous preterm birth.[20] Data from the Centers for Disease Control and Prevention (CDC) show that from 2007 to 2014, the preterm birth rate decreased from 10.41% to 9.54%.[21] This decrease in preterm birth rate was attributed to the decreased number of teen pregnancies. However, the preterm birth rate increased in 2017 for the third year in a row, questioning the impact of widespread progesterone use and highlighting the complexity of this problem.

Antenatal steroids

The administration of antenatal corticosteroids to women at risk for imminent preterm birth is strongly associated with decreases in severity of acute respiratory disease and neonatal morbidity and mortality. Neonates whose mothers received antenatal corticosteroids have significantly lower severity, frequency, or both of respiratory distress syndrome compared with neonates whose mothers did not receive antenatal corticosteroids.[22–24] However, a recent Cochrane Review did not show an overall decreased risk for BPD.[25] Although antenatal steroids may modify the risk factors for BPD, they have not been consistently shown to decrease the incidence of BPD.

Postnatal Pharmacologic Interventions: Prevention

The time and effort behind the development, preclinical testing, and evaluation of medications used to prevent BPD have been enormous and have positively shaped the current care of extremely preterm neonates. However, it is surprising and disappointing that these therapies have not had a more significant impact on BPD prevention. Although there is a need for new drug development, further progress in reducing BPD and adverse late respiratory outcomes will also require the early and accurate identification of preterm newborns who are at greatest risk for severe disease, a better understanding of factors that modulate respiratory phenotypes and outcomes, and the ability to intervene selectively for disease prevention.[10,12,13] In addition, randomized clinical trials targeted at high-risk populations may help to discover more efficacious drugs or to identify more targeted approaches for current therapies. It is likely that clear benefits of current drugs have not been shown in large clinical trials because the study groups of neonates have significantly varied physiology. This issue was highlighted most recently in a retrospective study examining the effects of inhaled NO (iNO) to improve the survival of extremely preterm neonates diagnosed with pulmonary hypoplasia. In neonates with pulmonary hypoplasia and PH, iNO improved survival by 33% (iNO, 47% survival vs no iNO, 35% survival), but did not reach statistical significance.[26] This finding may have been caused by the retrospective study design and the use of diagnostic billing codes (designations that are notoriously inaccurate) across many sites to identify which neonates had lung hypoplasia and PH. However, there was still a strong signal despite these limitations and the study being underpowered.[26] The authors suggest that a better understanding and accuracy in defining respiratory phenotypes and the use of specific antenatal determinants or early postnatal factors to assess risk will enhance clinical research, which may improve the use of currently available drug therapies and development of new drugs.

Oxygen

In preclinical models, exposure of neonatal animals to hyperoxia reliably produces lung injury. However, the data from human neonates, in whom oxygen saturations are specifically targeted to mitigate the impact of hyperoxia, are less clear. The recent Neonatal Oxygenation Prospective Meta-analysis (NeOProM) individual patient meta-analysis of high versus low saturation targets (91%–95% vs 85%–89%) for extremely preterm neonates showed that lower saturation targets were associated with a significant reduction in days on oxygen and on oxygen requirement at 36 weeks' PMA (relative risk [RR], 0.87; 95% confidence interval [CI], 0.81–0.94; 5 trials, 4175 neonates).[27] For those neonates who went home on supplemental oxygen (n = 237), hyperoxia did not affect total days on home oxygen. However, the lower target oxygen saturation range also significantly increased necrotizing enterocolitis (RR, 1.24; 95% CI, 1.05–1.47; 5 trials, 4929 neonates) and mortality at 18 to 24 months' corrected gestational age (RR, 1.16; 95% CI, 1.03–1.31; 5 trials, 4873 neonates).[27] Another recent meta-analysis of delivery room studies found that, compared with higher inspired oxygen concentrations (0.60–1.0), neonates randomized to receive lower inspired oxygen concentrations (0.21–0.30) for initial stabilization had lower mortality (RR, 0.62; 95% CI, 0.37–1.04) but no differences in the incidence of BPD.[28] In the SUPPORT trial, mortality associated with lower oxygen saturations was greatest in small-for-gestational-age preterm neonates relative to those who were appropriate for gestational age.[29]

These findings suggest that antenatal stress may play an important role in susceptibility to hypoxia and that it may be important to avoid even mild hypoxia in this subgroup.

Vitamin A

Past work has shown that vitamin A is essential for normal respiratory epithelium development and repair.[30,31] Large randomized studies found a small but beneficial effect in lowering rates of BPD in preterm neonates born before 29 weeks' gestation (RR, 0.87; 95% CI, 0.77–0.99; 5 studies, 986 infants)[32] and when given in combination with iNO in those weighing 750 to 100 g[33] However, neurodevelopmental assessment of surviving infants in the largest trial showed no difference between the groups at 18 to 22 months of age, although specific pulmonary outcomes were not recorded. The use of vitamin A has been adopted into fewer than half of the neonatal units in the United States given the lack of availability, expense, and frequent intramuscular injections. Post hoc analysis of one of the multicenter randomized trials of iNO suggested that neonates who received vitamin A in combination with iNO had better respiratory outcomes than preterm neonates who received either vitamin A or iNO alone.[33]

Caffeine

Although not part of the original hypothesis, a large randomized, placebo-controlled trial to study the late neurodevelopmental effects of caffeine for the treatment of apnea of prematurity reported the exciting findings of a reduction in BPD in addition to a reduction in the combined outcome of death or disability at 18 to 21 months' corrected gestational age.[34,35] There are numerous proposed mechanisms for these beneficial effects, including a shorter duration of mechanical ventilation and more specific anti-inflammatory and/or diuretic effects.[36,37] For instance, short-term effects of caffeine administration may include significant improvements in tidal volume and lung compliance and reductions in total lung resistance.[38] Nagatomo and colleagues[39] found that caffeine prevented hyperoxia-induced lung injury in a preterm rabbit model of BPD. On a molecular level, caffeine may attenuate lung injury by inhibiting Smad signaling and transforming growth factor-β1–regulated genes involved in airway remodeling.[40] These are key signaling pathways involved in lung development, airway inflammation, airway remodeling, and lung fibrosis.[41,42]

It is not clear whether early caffeine prophylaxis also benefits ventilated preterm neonates before they are ready for extubation. Taha and colleagues[43] reported a retrospective analysis of 2951 premature neonates and found that early use of caffeine (begun at <2 days of life) was associated with reduction in death or BPD relative to neonates who began caffeine between days 3 and 10 of life. However, early caffeine was also associated with increased rates of necrotizing enterocolitis. Another meta-analysis combined retrospective cohort studies and randomized trials and reported lower rates of BPD but higher rates of mortality in neonates who were treated with early caffeine.[44] A recent randomized trial of 83 extremely preterm ventilated neonates found that initiation of caffeine in the first 5 days of life did not reduce the time to the first successful extubation.[45] Moreover, a nonsignificant trend toward higher mortality was observed in the early caffeine group, which led to early closure of the trial. At present, caffeine should be reserved for those neonates with apnea of prematurity or those who are ready for extubation or with significant lung disease.[46]

Postnatal Pharmacologic Interventions: Prevention and/or Treatment

Corticosteroids

The currently available pharmacologic agents used to treat evolving or established BPD are summarized in **Table 2**. Cortisol synthesis is decreased in preterm neonates and is likely one of the factors that increases the risk of acute and chronic lung

Table 2
Pharmacologic agents frequently used for the treatment of established bronchopulmonary dysplasia

Medication	Mechanisms of Action	Major Supporting Clinical Studies
Postnatal steroids	• Promote pulmonary surfactant synthesis • Reduce pulmonary edema • Inhibition of inflammatory cell infiltration and fibroblast proliferation • Increase expression of lung antioxidant enzymes	• Onland et al,[47] 2017 • Ng et al,[50] 2012 • Laughon et al,[51] 2011 • Doyle et al,[52] 2014 • Doyle et al,[59] 2005; Doyle et al,[62] 2006 • Baud et al,[63] 2017 • Bassler et al,[68] 2015; Bassler et al,[69] 2018 • Yeh et al,[70] 2008 • Yeh et al,[71] 2016
Diuretics	• Reduce fluid overload and pulmonary edema	• Kao et al,[87] 1994 • Blaisdell et al,[83] 2018 • Thompson et al,[86] 2018r
Bronchodilators	• Decrease airway resistance and improve lung compliance • Improve lung mechanics following bronchospasm	• De Boeck et al,[77] 1998 • Brundage,[129] 1990 • Slaughter et al,[75] 2015
Sildenafil	• Selective inhibitor of cGMP-PDE5 • Promotes pulmonary vasodilation	• Mourani et al,[108] 2009 • Barst et al,[111] 2014 • Backes et al,[113] 2016 • Krishnan et al,[103] 2017

*Abbreviations:*cGMP, cyclic GMP; PDE5, phosphodiesterase type 5

disease. Corticosteroids, as major antiinflammatory agents, have been used in the prevention and treatment of BPD for decades. They promote the synthesis of pulmonary surfactant and the expression of lung antioxidant enzymes, reduce pulmonary edema and inflammation, inhibit inflammatory cell infiltration and fibroblast proliferation, and have a short-term clinical impact on established BPD.

Administration of systemic steroids within the first 2 weeks of life has been consistently associated with a reduction of the risk of BPD in preterm neonates.[47–50] However, the potential pulmonary benefits of corticosteroids must be weighed against the possible risk of harm, and considerable debate continues to this day. One important analysis showed a strong negative relationship between the risk of death or cerebral palsy (CP) and the rate of BPD, indicating that neonates with the highest risk of BPD (according to the National Institute of Child Health and Human Development [NICHD] calculator[51]) had the greatest benefit from treatment with postnatal steroids.[52]

Numerous studies have attempted to identify the optimal steroid and timing and route of administration to achieve the best outcome with the fewest complications and neurodevelopmental deficits. Most systematic reviews and meta-analysis studies differentiate early from late steroid administration, with most investigators drawing the line between early and late at 2 weeks' postnatal age.[53]

Dexamethasone

Dexamethasone treatment shortly after birth shortens the duration of mechanical ventilation and reduces the incidence of BPD.[54–56] However, there is increasing concern about the off-target effects of steroids, mainly on neurodevelopmental outcome and especially the risk for CP.[57–59] These risks are clearly complex and multi-factorial, requiring an understanding of the risks and benefits across the spectrum of clinical disease (**Fig. 1**). The proposed mechanism of glucocorticoid-induced brain injury is through interaction with the Sonic Hedgehog (Shh) protein, a regulator of brain organogenesis and development. Heine and Rowitch[60] reported that glucocorticoids can modulate the Shh pathway in postnatal mice and suppress Shh-induced proliferation of cerebellar progenitor cells. In contrast, Shh signaling is protective against glucocorticoid-induced neonatal cerebellar injury by inducing the enzyme 11βHSD2. Note that 11βHSD2 inhibits hydrocortisone and prednisolone but not dexamethasone, indicating that the former agents would be expected to have less neurotoxicity. In clinical cohorts, postnatal corticosteroid treatment has been associated with increased risk for gastrointestinal bleeding, spontaneous intestinal perforation (in combination with indomethacin), hyperglycemia, hypertension, hypertrophic cardiomyopathy, growth disorders, neurodevelopmental deficits, and CP.[53,59,61]

In 2017, a Cochrane database report assessed the effects of different dexamethasone treatment regimens on mortality, pulmonary morbidity, and neurodevelopmental outcome in very-low-birth-weight (VLBW) infants. Although some of the included studies suggested a beneficial effect of higher-dosage (cumulative dose of >4 mg/kg) versus lower-dosage (cumulative dose of <2 mg/kg) dexamethasone regimens in reducing BPD and neurodevelopmental impairment, the overall quality of evidence was low and definitive conclusions could not be drawn.[47] The Dexamethasone: A Randomized Trial (DART) study was an international multicenter, randomized controlled trial with the main aim to assess the effects of low-dose dexamethasone on long-term survival free of major neurologic disability. The study included extremely preterm neonates who were ventilator dependent after the first week of life that received either placebo or dexamethasone at a total dose of 0.89 mg/kg delivered over 10 days. Although dexamethasone was associated with decreased mortality, duration of intubation, and oxygen requirement, enrollment had to stop when recruitment decreased to a rate that was too low to complete the study.[62]

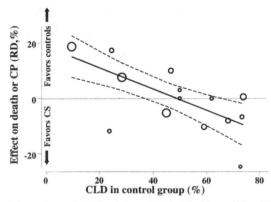

Fig. 1. The relationship of net benefit or net harm (death or CP) of corticosteroids (CS) against baseline BPD event rate (in control groups of infants) in randomized trials. Each study is shown by a circle whose area is proportional to that study's weight. CLD, chronic lung disease. RD, risk difference. (*From* Doyle LW, Halliday HL, Ehrenkranz RA, et al. Impact of postnatal systemic corticosteroids on mortality and cerebral palsy in preterm infants: effect modification by risk for chronic lung disease. Pediatrics 2005;115:655–61; with permission.)

Hydrocortisone

Hydrocortisone may be associated with fewer systemic adverse effects than dexamethasone, but the effect of early hydrocortisone treatment on survival without BPD remains unclear. In the large multicenter PREMILOC study conducted in France, low-dose hydrocortisone was administered within 24 hours after birth for a total of 3 days. Survival without BPD was better in the hydrocortisone versus placebo group (adjusted odds ratio [OR], 1.48; 95% CI, 1.02–2.16; P = .04). Rates of gastrointestinal perforation were similar between the two groups and neurodevelopmental outcomes were comparable at 2 years' corrected gestational age.[63] In a recent individual patient meta-analysis of 4 randomized trials, early low-dose hydrocortisone treatment for 10 to 15 days significantly increased survival without BPD (OR, 1.45; 95% CI, 1.11–1.90; P = .007).[64] Although rates of late-onset sepsis were increased in neonates exposed to hydrocortisone (OR, 1.34; 95% CI, 1.02–1.75; P = .04), no differences were reported for death or 2-year neurodevelopmental outcomes. Another ongoing trial in the Netherlands (Systemic Hydrocortisone to Prevent Bronchopulmonary Dysplasia in preterm infants [SToP-BPD]) will provide additional evidence on the efficacy and safety of postnatal hydrocortisone administration for the reduction of death or BPD in ventilator-dependent preterm neonates.[65]

Inhaled steroids

To reduce off-target effects, some investigators have proposed the use of inhaled steroids to provide local effect in the lungs while avoiding the high rate of complications observed with systemic steroid use. A 2010 survey of 223 European neonatal centers found that approximately 50% administered inhaled corticosteroids to preterm neonates either as prophylaxis or treatment of BPD.[66] In a retrospective study of neonates in the Canadian Neonatal Network, exposure to inhaled steroids reduced BPD but was not associated with increased odds of death or significant neurodevelopmental impairment. However, use of systemic steroids before 4 weeks of age was associated with significantly worse outcomes.[67]

Bassler and colleagues[68] randomized extremely preterm neonates to receive inhaled steroids or placebo within the first 24 hours after birth until they no longer needed oxygen or positive pressure ventilation and assessed mortality, risk of BPD, and neurodevelopmental outcome. Although the risk of BPD, reintubation rate, and the need for surgical closure of patent ductus arteriosus was lower in the budesonide group, mortalities were lower in the placebo group. The rate of neurodevelopmental disability at 2 years' corrected gestational age did not differ significantly between neonates who received early inhaled budesonide for the prevention of BPD and those who received placebo. However, the mortality continued to be higher among those who received budesonide.[69]

An intriguing study by Yeh and colleagues[70] showed that intratracheal instillation of budesonide mixed with surfactant (as a delivery vehicle) significantly improved pulmonary status in VLBW neonates with severe respiratory distress syndrome. These investigators randomized 265 neonates to receive intratracheal administration of surfactant/budesonide versus surfactant alone and found that budesonide with surfactant significantly decreased the incidence of BPD or death without immediate adverse effects.[71] Other respiratory assessments during the initial neonatal intensive care unit stay were not different, which makes the impact of the late effects more puzzling.

A subsequent meta-analysis of 25 studies and 3249 patients showed that airway-administered steroids (especially instillation of budesonide using surfactant as a vehicle) reduced the risk of death or BPD (RR, 0.81; 95% CI, 0.71–0.97).[72] However, a meta-analysis analyzed the effect of administration of inhaled corticosteroids to preterm neonates at high risk of developing BPD after the first week of life and assessed outcomes at 36 weeks' PMA. This study examined 8 trials and found that inhaled corticosteroids administered after 7 days of life did not reduce BPD or the duration of mechanical ventilation,[49] an effect that has previously been reported.[73,74]

Bronchodilators

Inhaled and systemic bronchodilators have been widely used over the years for the prevention and treatment of BPD, but large interhospital variation in their use suggests that there is little agreement on their efficacy.[75] Few trials have assessed the effect of bronchodilators on the prevention of BPD and no benefit has been reported for this indication.[50] Although the β2 agonist albuterol may improve pulmonary resistance and lung mechanics following bronchospasm, the use of chronic albuterol therapy for airway disease associated with BPD has not been supported by significant evidence.[50,76,77] Even so, data from the Pediatric Health Information System (PHIS) administrative database suggest that about a third of neonates with evolving BPD receive bronchodilators during their hospitalizations, with a prolonged course of mechanical ventilation the best predictor of receiving a bronchodilator.[75]

Ipratropium is a synthetic anticholinergic agent used for treatment of acute bronchospasm and to decrease airway resistance and improve compliance in preterm neonates with BPD. Its impact on the course and long-term prognosis of BPD has not been extensively studied. Although 1 study showed that ipratropium bromide in combination with albuterol did not alter pulmonary resistance in patients with BPD, another group reported that there was improvement in lung mechanics when a higher dose was used.[76–78] In 1–year-old former preterm infants with BPD, the response to albuterol and ipratropium was variable. However, pulmonary resistance worsened after albuterol in infants without BPD, possibly because of loss of smooth muscle tone in airways with resulting dynamic compression.[77]

Diuretics

Preterm neonates often require more intravenous fluids to ensure metabolic and nutritional needs, but excessive fluids may cause pulmonary edema and increased respiratory support, which contribute to the development of BPD.[79] Although diuretics are commonly used in acute respiratory failure and for neonates with established BPD, there is little evidence to support their long-term efficacy and safety.[80,81]

Data from the large clinical database of the Pediatrix Medical Group indicate that more than 51% of all extremely preterm neonates are treated with furosemide during hospitalization.[82] In the 835 extremely preterm neonates enrolled in the Prematurity and Respiratory Outcomes Program (PROP), 58% were exposed at least once to a diuretic (>85% of these received furosemide or bumetanide).[83] The use of diuretics was most common in the smallest neonates born at 23 to 24 weeks' gestation. Several studies have shown that daily or intermittent administration of furosemide results in short-term improvements in pulmonary mechanics and oxygenation and facilitates weaning from mechanical ventilation. Even though these effects are likely caused by the mobilization of interstitial lung fluid, long-term benefits have never been established in neonates with BPD. For instance, data from the PROP cohort suggested that neonates receiving diuretics achieved no more short-term respiratory improvement than those managed without diuretics.[83] In contrast, a retrospective analysis based on the Pediatrix database found that, for every 10% increase in the proportion of furosemide exposure days, there was a 4.6% decrease in the incidence of BPD.[82] Inhalational furosemide also improves respiratory symptoms and oxygenation and may reduce systemic toxicity, but long-term benefits have not been established.[80]

The risks of furosemide have not been well studied. Furosemide stimulates renal prostaglandin production, which may promote patency of the ductus arteriosus. In 1 prospective trial, early use of furosemide for respiratory failure was associated with higher rates of patent ductus arteriosus[84] and studies in rats showed that furosemide delays closure of ductus arteriosus.[85] However, a recent large retrospective cohort study in human neonates did not support this finding.[86] Hypochloremic metabolic alkalosis is a frequent short-term complication of furosemide, but little is known about its effect on long-term bone growth and mineralization.

The benefits of thiazide diuretics (with or without spironolactone) are even less compelling. In some studies, thiazide diuretics produced short-term improvements in pulmonary compliance and oxygen requirements, but did not improve long-term measures such as days on oxygen.[87] They seem to be used less than loop diuretics; for instance, only ~15% of the extremely preterm PROP cohort received a thiazide diuretic during hospitalization.[83]

The discordant evidence that diuretics improve early but not late outcomes in infants with BPD may explain the large variation in center-to-center usage of diuretics.[88] This variation highlights the need for future studies to gain a better understanding of which infants with BPD will respond to diuretic therapy. In particular, neonates with left ventricle dysfunction and PH may be good candidates for study.

Inhaled nitric oxide and sildenafil

Recent prospective studies indicate that early echocardiogram evidence of pulmonary vascular disease and the need for mechanical ventilation at 7 days of life are each strongly associated with development of BPD and also CPIP.[89,90] Endogenous production of NO is required for alveolar and vascular development.[91] Alterations in NO signaling have been observed in conjunction with, or perhaps as a cause of, the lung and vascular injury characteristic of BPD.[92] Extensive data from animal models confirmed that exogenous NO or iNO promotes lung angiogenesis and reduces inflammation, oxidative stress, and apoptosis.[93,94] However, based on large clinical studies, early prophylactic or rescue iNO in preterm neonates with respiratory failure did not reduce BPD.[95–99] Despite these findings, it is probable that specific subgroups of neonates will benefit from iNO. For instance, in an individual patient meta-analysis conducted by Askie and colleagues[100] (the Meta-analysis of Preterm Patients on Inhaled Nitric Oxide [MAPPiNO] Collaboration), African American neonates realized a clinically meaningful and statistically significant benefit from iNO treatment (RR for death or BPD of 0.77; 95% CI, 0.65–0.91; number needed to treat = 7). Racial differences in NO bioavailability and response caused by genetic variations have been described in key genes in the NO pathway, and this finding deserves more attention in the era of personalized medicine.

Pulmonary vascular disease is now recognized as a common precursor to and complication of BPD.[101] Early identification of high-risk neonates with early pulmonary vascular disease may allow selected clinical strategies to prevent or mitigate poor respiratory outcomes. Moreover, a recent meta-analysis of more than 1400 patients reported that PH is strongly associated with severity of pulmonary disease, with cumulative prevalence of PH in 6%, 12%, and 39% of neonates with mild, moderate, and severe BPD, respectively.[102] Although therapeutic options for BPD-associated PH were recently reviewed by the Pediatric Pulmonary Hypertension Network (PPHNet), few therapies have been rigorously studied in clinical trials.[103] Mourani and colleagues[104] showed that pulmonary pressures in neonates with established

BPD improved to near-normal levels with acute exposure to iNO during cardiac catheterization, with the effect greater than pulmonary vasodilation induced by oxygen alone. However, the benefit of prolonged exposure to iNO in BPD-associated PH has not been evaluated. The logistics of continuous inhalational treatment currently restrict the chronic use of iNO in the outpatient setting; instead, the drug is mainly used for acute PH exacerbations in hospitalized neonates.

Sildenafil is a selective cyclic GMP (cGMP) phosphodiesterase inhibitor that increases lung cGMP concentrations and promotes pulmonary vasodilation.[105,106] In animal models, sildenafil promotes alveolar development, reduces lung inflammation, attenuates PH, and reduces lung injury caused by hyperoxia.[107] Sildenafil is easily administered enterally and well tolerated, but clinical data are limited regarding its efficacy for BPD-associated PH. Small, retrospective studies of neonates with BPD have suggested improved right ventricular function and reduced mortality compared with historical controls.[108–110] However, the risks and benefits of chronic use of sildenafil are not well understood, particularly for older infants with CPIP. Based on the results of the STARTS-2 trial,[111] the European Medication Authority approved chronic use of low-dose sildenafil (≤ 2 mg/kg/d) for children, but the US Food and Drug Administration recommended that sildenafil not be prescribed for children aged 1 to 17 years.[112] One cohort study using data from the PHIS administrative database found that 17% of the 598 infants diagnosed with BPD-associated PH received sildenafil, with significant variability in use across institutions. Likelihood of treatment correlated with gestational age, small for gestational age, and severity of BPD.[113] There are reports that sildenafil may worsen gastroesophageal reflux, which is a common problem of preterm neonates with BPD. Longer-acting phosphodiesterase inhibitors, such as tadalafil, have not yet been evaluated in BPD.

INVESTIGATIONAL THERAPIES
Stem Cells

Mesenchymal stem cells (MSCs) play a significant role in lung development. Stem cell dysfunction may impede the self-repair of immature lung tissue, contributing to the development of BPD.[114] It has been shown that depletion and/or dysfunction of endogenous progenitor/stem cells can increase the risk of BPD.[114] In animal experiments, exogenous stem cells protect and repair lung injury, in part because of the preservation of endogenous stem cell pools. Bone marrow mesenchymal stem cells can ameliorate BPD by preventing lung inflammation.[115] The effect of MSCs is thought to be primarily paracrine rather than caused by the effects of engraftment. The discovery of MSCs in human umbilical cord tissue (Wharton jelly) and cord blood was an important advance that provided a clinically relevant and feasible source of these potent cells for the treatment of neonatal disease.[116] A phase I clinical trial of human cord blood–derived MSCs was successfully conducted in South Korea in 9 extremely preterm neonates[117] and 2-year outcomes did not reveal any safety concerns.[117,118] In the United States, another phase I clinical trial of human umbilical cord blood–derived MSCs has been completed, and a phase II trial is anticipated to begin soon (NCT03392467).

Other sources of cells are also under investigation. An Australian group has studied a population of stemlike cells derived from placental membranes, human amnion epithelial cells (hAECs), which has shown therapeutic promise in preclinical models of BPD. They conducted a first-in-human clinical trial of hAECs in neonates with BPD to assess the safety of these cells. With the exception of the first patient, who developed respiratory distress attributed to an embolic event, the investigators did not report any other adverse events related to cell administration.[119]

Insulinlike Growth Factor-1

Insulin-like growth factor-1 (IGF-1) is an important regulator of fetal growth and lung angiogenesis and development. IGF-1 levels increase rapidly during the last 2 trimesters of pregnancy, and then decrease rapidly after birth. Lower serum IGF-1 levels in extremely preterm neonates have been independently associated with increased risk of BPD and other morbidities, such as retinopathy of prematurity.[120] Administration of IGF-1 to neonatal rodent models seems to reduce lung injury in response to hyperoxia. In a recent phase II clinical trial, treatment with recombinant human IGF in combination with its binding protein (rhIGF-1/rhIGFBP-3) reduced the number of extremely preterm neonates with severe BPD and shifted the disease severity to milder BPD.[121]

SUMMARY

Despite many scientific advances, rates of BPD have continued to increase over the last decade. The pathobiology of BPD remains a rapidly evolving field of research and a picture is emerging that links the initial life course from conception through birth, as well as early neonatal events that affect the development of CPIP. After preterm birth, there are important developmental periods in which neonates are more vulnerable to stressful events. These periods are opportunities for pharmacologic interventions to reduce the impact of prematurity and postnatal lung injury. Despite the need, many currently available drugs remain inadequately tested and no new drugs have been approved in more than 25 years for BPD prevention or therapy. More progress is needed in defining appropriate end points based on the pathophysiology of BPD and postdischarge CPIP and to design, test, and gain approval for effective new drugs. In addition, much work is needed to better define perinatal factors, early postnatal findings, and physiologic phenotypes or endotypes that will enable more precise clinical interventions for research and care that can reduce CPIP in preterm neonates.

REFERENCES

1. Northway WH Jr, Rosan RC, Porter DY. Pulmonary disease following respirator therapy of hyaline-membrane disease. Bronchopulmonary dysplasia. N Engl J Med 1967;276:357–68.
2. Stoll BJ, Hansen NI, Bell EF, et al. Trends in care practices, morbidity, and mortality of extremely preterm neonates, 1993-2012. JAMA 2015;314:1039–51.
3. Jobe AH, Bancalari E. Bronchopulmonary dysplasia. Am J Respir Crit Care Med 2001;163:1723–9.
4. Jobe AJ. The new BPD: an arrest of lung development. Pediatr Res 1999;46: 641–3.
5. Husain AN, Siddiqui NH, Stocker JT. Pathology of arrested acinar development in postsurfactant bronchopulmonary dysplasia. Hum Pathol 1998;29:710–7.
6. Coalson JJ, Winter VT, Siler-Khodr T, et al. Neonatal chronic lung disease in extremely immature baboons. Am J Respir Crit Care Med 1999;160:1333–46.
7. Schmidt B, Roberts RS, Davis PG, et al. Prediction of late death or disability at age 5 years using a count of 3 neonatal morbidities in very low birth weight infants. J Pediatr 2015;167:982–6.e2.
8. Morrow LA, Wagner BD, Ingram DA, et al. Antenatal determinants of bronchopulmonary dysplasia and late respiratory disease in preterm infants. Am J Respir Crit Care Med 2017;196:364–74.
9. Keller RL, Feng R, DeMauro SB, et al. Bronchopulmonary dysplasia and perinatal characteristics predict 1-year respiratory outcomes in newborns born at

extremely low gestational age: a prospective cohort study. J Pediatr 2017;187: 89–97.e3.

10. Steinhorn R, Davis JM, Gopel W, et al. Chronic pulmonary insufficiency of prematurity: developing optimal endpoints for drug development. J Pediatr 2017; 191:15–21.e1.

11. Manuck TA, Levy PT, Gyamfi-Bannerman C, et al. Prenatal and perinatal determinants of lung health and disease in early life: a national heart, lung, and blood institute workshop report. JAMA Pediatr 2016;170:e154577.

12. Mestan KK, Check J, Minturn L, et al. Placental pathologic changes of maternal vascular underperfusion in bronchopulmonary dysplasia and pulmonary hypertension. Placenta 2014;35:570–4.

13. McEvoy CT, Jain L, Schmidt B, et al. Bronchopulmonary dysplasia: NHLBI workshop on the primary prevention of chronic lung diseases. Ann Am Thorac Soc 2014;11(Suppl 3):S146–53.

14. Islam JY, Keller RL, Aschner JL, et al. Understanding the short- and long-term respiratory outcomes of prematurity and bronchopulmonary dysplasia. Am J Respir Crit Care Med 2015;192:134–56.

15. Gunville CF, Sontag MK, Stratton KA, et al. Scope and impact of early and late preterm infants admitted to the PICU with respiratory illness. J Pediatr 2010;157: 209–14.e1.

16. Aschner JL, Bancalari EH, McEvoy CT. Can we prevent bronchopulmonary dysplasia? J Pediatr 2017;189:26–30.

17. Abman SH, Bancalari E, Jobe A. The evolution of bronchopulmonary dysplasia after 50 years. Am J Respir Crit Care Med 2017;195:421–4.

18. Newnham JP, Dickinson JE, Hart RJ, et al. Strategies to prevent preterm birth. Front Immunol 2014;5:584.

19. Dodd JM, Jones L, Flenady V, et al. Prenatal administration of progesterone for preventing preterm birth in women considered to be at risk of preterm birth. Cochrane Database Syst Rev 2013;(7):CD004947.

20. Committee on Practice Bulletins-Obstetrics TACoO, Gynecologists. Practice bulletin no. 130: prediction and prevention of preterm birth. Obstet Gynecol 2012;120:964–73.

21. Ferre C, Callaghan W, Olson C, et al. Effects of maternal age and age-specific preterm birth rates on overall preterm birth rates - United States, 2007 and 2014. MMWR Morb Mortal Wkly Rep 2016;65:1181–4.

22. Effect of corticosteroids for fetal maturation on perinatal outcomes. NIH consensus development panel on the effect of corticosteroids for fetal maturation on perinatal outcomes. JAMA 1995;273:413–8.

23. Crowley P, Chalmers I, Keirse MJ. The effects of corticosteroid administration before preterm delivery: an overview of the evidence from controlled trials. Br J Obstet Gynaecol 1990;97:11–25.

24. Van Marter LJ, Leviton A, Kuban KC, et al. Maternal glucocorticoid therapy and reduced risk of bronchopulmonary dysplasia. Pediatrics 1990;86:331–6.

25. Roberts D, Brown J, Medley N, et al. Antenatal corticosteroids for accelerating fetal lung maturation for women at risk of preterm birth. Cochrane Database Syst Rev 2017;(3):CD004454.

26. Ellsworth KR, Ellsworth MA, Weaver AL, et al. Association of early inhaled nitric oxide with the survival of preterm neonates with pulmonary hypoplasia. JAMA Pediatr 2018;172:e180761.

27. Askie LM, Darlow BA, Davis PG, et al. Effects of targeting lower versus higher arterial oxygen saturations on death or disability in preterm infants. Cochrane Database Syst Rev 2017;(4):CD011190.

28. Saugstad OD, Aune D, Aguar M, et al. Systematic review and meta-analysis of optimal initial fraction of oxygen levels in the delivery room at </=32 weeks. Acta Paediatr 2014;103:744–51.

29. Walsh MC, Di Fiore JM, Martin RJ, et al. Association of oxygen target and growth status with increased mortality in small for gestational age infants: further analysis of the surfactant, positive pressure and pulse oximetry randomized trial. JAMA Pediatr 2016;170:292–4.

30. Chytil F. The lungs and vitamin A. Am J Physiol 1992;262:L517–27.

31. Shenai JP, Rush MG, Stahlman MT, et al. Vitamin A supplementation and bronchopulmonary dysplasia–revisited. J Pediatr 1992;121:399–401.

32. Darlow BA, Graham PJ, Rojas-Reyes MX. Vitamin A supplementation to prevent mortality and short- and long-term morbidity in very low birth weight infants. Cochrane Database Syst Rev 2016;(8):CD000501.

33. Gadhia MM, Cutter GR, Abman SH, et al. Effects of early inhaled nitric oxide therapy and vitamin A supplementation on the risk for bronchopulmonary dysplasia in premature newborns with respiratory failure. J Pediatr 2014;164: 744–8.

34. Schmidt B, Roberts RS, Davis P, et al. Caffeine therapy for apnea of prematurity. N Engl J Med 2006;354:2112–21.

35. Schmidt B, Roberts RS, Davis P, et al. Long-term effects of caffeine therapy for apnea of prematurity. N Engl J Med 2007;357:1893–902.

36. Weichelt U, Cay R, Schmitz T, et al. Prevention of hyperoxia-mediated pulmonary inflammation in neonatal rats by caffeine. Eur Respir J 2013;41:966–73.

37. Endesfelder S, Zaak I, Weichelt U, et al. Caffeine protects neuronal cells against injury caused by hyperoxia in the immature brain. Free Radic Biol Med 2014;67: 221–34.

38. Davis JM, Bhutani VK, Stefano JL, et al. Changes in pulmonary mechanics following caffeine administration in infants with bronchopulmonary dysplasia. Pediatr Pulmonol 1989;6:49–52.

39. Nagatomo T, Jimenez J, Richter J, et al. Caffeine prevents hyperoxia-induced functional and structural lung damage in preterm rabbits. Neonatology 2016; 109:274–81.

40. Fehrholz M, Speer CP, Kunzmann S. Caffeine and rolipram affect Smad signalling and TGF-beta1 stimulated CTGF and transgelin expression in lung epithelial cells. PLoS One 2014;9:e97357.

41. Alejandre-Alcazar MA, Michiels-Corsten M, Vicencio AG, et al. TGF-beta signaling is dynamically regulated during the alveolarization of rodent and human lungs. Dev Dyn 2008;237:259–69.

42. Kunzmann S, Ottensmeier B, Speer CP, et al. Effect of progesterone on Smad signaling and TGF-beta/Smad-regulated genes in lung epithelial cells. PLoS One 2018;13:e0200661.

43. Taha D, Kirkby S, Nawab U, et al. Early caffeine therapy for prevention of bronchopulmonary dysplasia in preterm infants. J Matern Fetal Neonatal Med 2014; 27:1698–702.

44. Kua KP, Lee SW. Systematic review and meta-analysis of clinical outcomes of early caffeine therapy in preterm neonates. Br J Clin Pharmacol 2017;83: 180–91.

45. Amaro CM, Bello JA, Jain D, et al. Early caffeine and weaning from mechanical ventilation in preterm infants: a randomized, placebo-controlled trial. J Pediatr 2018;196:52–7.

46. Schmidt B, Davis PG, Roberts RS. Timing of caffeine therapy in very low birth weight infants. J Pediatr 2014;164:957–8.

47. Onland W, De Jaegere AP, Offringa M, et al. Systemic corticosteroid regimens for prevention of bronchopulmonary dysplasia in preterm infants. Cochrane Database Syst Rev 2017;(1):CD010941.

48. Shah SS, Ohlsson A, Halliday H, et al. Inhaled versus systemic corticosteroids for the treatment of chronic lung disease in ventilated very low birth weight preterm infants. Cochrane Database Syst Rev 2007;(4):CD002057.

49. Onland W, Offringa M, van Kaam A. Late (>/= 7 days) inhalation corticosteroids to reduce bronchopulmonary dysplasia in preterm infants. Cochrane Database Syst Rev 2017;(8):CD002311.

50. Ng G, da Silva O, Ohlsson A. Bronchodilators for the prevention and treatment of chronic lung disease in preterm infants. Cochrane Database Syst Rev 2012;(6):CD003214.

51. Laughon MM, Langer JC, Bose CL, et al. Prediction of bronchopulmonary dysplasia by postnatal age in extremely premature infants. Am J Respir Crit Care Med 2011;183:1715–22.

52. Doyle LW, Halliday HL, Ehrenkranz RA, et al. An update on the impact of postnatal systemic corticosteroids on mortality and cerebral palsy in preterm infants: effect modification by risk of bronchopulmonary dysplasia. J Pediatr 2014;165: 1258–60.

53. Doyle LW, Cheong JLY. Postnatal corticosteroids to prevent or treat bronchopulmonary dysplasia - who might benefit? Semin Fetal Neonatal Med 2017;22: 290–5.

54. Halliday HL, Ehrenkranz RA, Doyle LW. Early (< 8 days) postnatal corticosteroids for preventing chronic lung disease in preterm infants. Cochrane Database Syst Rev 2009;(1):CD001146.

55. Doyle LW, Ehrenkranz RA, Halliday HL. Postnatal hydrocortisone for preventing or treating bronchopulmonary dysplasia in preterm infants: a systematic review. Neonatology 2010;98:111–7.

56. Halliday HL, Ehrenkranz RA, Doyle LW. Early (< 8 days) postnatal corticosteroids for preventing chronic lung disease in preterm infants. Cochrane Database Syst Rev 2010;(1):CD001146.

57. Murphy BP, Inder TE, Huppi PS, et al. Impaired cerebral cortical gray matter growth after treatment with dexamethasone for neonatal chronic lung disease. Pediatrics 2001;107:217–21.

58. Yeh TF, Lin YJ, Lin HC, et al. Outcomes at school age after postnatal dexamethasone therapy for lung disease of prematurity. N Engl J Med 2004;350:1304–13.

59. Doyle LW, Halliday HL, Ehrenkranz RA, et al. Impact of postnatal systemic corticosteroids on mortality and cerebral palsy in preterm infants: effect modification by risk for chronic lung disease. Pediatrics 2005;115:655–61.

60. Heine VM, Rowitch DH. Hedgehog signaling has a protective effect in glucocorticoid-induced mouse neonatal brain injury through an 11betaHSD2-dependent mechanism. J Clin Invest 2009;119:267–77.

61. Malaeb SN, Stonestreet BS. Steroids and injury to the developing brain: net harm or net benefit? Clin Perinatol 2014;41:191–208.

62. Doyle LW, Davis PG, Morley CJ, et al. Low-dose dexamethasone facilitates extubation among chronically ventilator-dependent infants: a multicenter, international, randomized, controlled trial. Pediatrics 2006;117:75–83.

63. Baud O, Trousson C, Biran V, et al. Association between early low-dose hydrocortisone therapy in extremely preterm neonates and neurodevelopmental outcomes at 2 years of age. JAMA 2017;317:1329–37.

64. Shaffer ML, Baud O, Lacaze-Masmonteil T, et al. Effect of prophylaxis of early adrenal insufficiency using low-dose hydrocortisone in very preterm infants: an individual patient data meta-analysis. J Pediatr 2018. [Epub ahead of print].

65. Onland W, Merkus MP, Nuytemans DH, et al. Systemic Hydrocortisone to Prevent Bronchopulmonary Dysplasia in preterm infants (the SToP-BPD study): statistical analysis plan. Trials 2018;19:178.

66. Maas C, Poets CF, Bassler D. Survey of practices regarding utilization of inhaled steroids in 223 German neonatal units. Neonatology 2010;98:404–8.

67. Kelly EN, Shah VS, Levenbach J, et al. Inhaled and systemic steroid exposure and neurodevelopmental outcome of preterm neonates. J Matern Fetal Neonatal Med 2018;31:2665–72.

68. Bassler D, Plavka R, Shinwell ES, et al. Early inhaled budesonide for the prevention of bronchopulmonary dysplasia. N Engl J Med 2015;373:1497–506.

69. Bassler D, Shinwell ES, Hallman M, et al. Long-term effects of inhaled budesonide for bronchopulmonary dysplasia. N Engl J Med 2018;378:148–57.

70. Yeh TF, Lin HC, Chang CH, et al. Early intratracheal instillation of budesonide using surfactant as a vehicle to prevent chronic lung disease in preterm infants: a pilot study. Pediatrics 2008;121:e1310–8.

71. Yeh TF, Chen CM, Wu SY, et al. Intratracheal administration of budesonide/surfactant to prevent bronchopulmonary dysplasia. Am J Respir Crit Care Med 2016;193:86–95.

72. Zhang ZQ, Zhong Y, Huang XM, et al. Airway administration of corticosteroids for prevention of bronchopulmonary dysplasia in premature infants: a meta-analysis with trial sequential analysis. BMC Pulm Med 2017;17:207.

73. Shinwell ES, Portnov I, Meerpohl JJ, et al. Inhaled corticosteroids for bronchopulmonary dysplasia: a meta-analysis. Pediatrics 2016;138 [pii:e20162511].

74. Shah VS, Ohlsson A, Halliday HL, et al. Early administration of inhaled corticosteroids for preventing chronic lung disease in ventilated very low birth weight preterm neonates. Cochrane Database Syst Rev 2012;(5):CD001969.

75. Slaughter JL, Stenger MR, Reagan PB, et al. Inhaled bronchodilator use for infants with bronchopulmonary dysplasia. J Perinatol 2015;35:61–6.

76. Robin B, Kim YJ, Huth J, et al. Pulmonary function in bronchopulmonary dysplasia. Pediatr Pulmonol 2004;37:236–42.

77. De Boeck K, Smith J, Van Lierde S, et al. Response to bronchodilators in clinically stable 1-year-old patients with bronchopulmonary dysplasia. Eur J Pediatr 1998;157:75–9.

78. Brundage KL, Mohsini KG, Froese AB, et al. Bronchodilator response to ipratropium bromide in infants with bronchopulmonary dysplasia. Am Rev Respir Dis 1990;142:1137–42.

79. Oh W, Poindexter BB, Perritt R, et al. Association between fluid intake and weight loss during the first ten days of life and risk of bronchopulmonary dysplasia in extremely low birth weight infants. J Pediatr 2005;147:786–90.

80. Segar JL. Neonatal diuretic therapy: furosemide, thiazides, and spironolactone. Clin Perinatol 2012;39:209–20.

81. Donn SM. Bronchopulmonary dysplasia: Myths of pharmacologic management. Semin Fetal Neonatal Med 2017;22:354–8.

82. Greenberg RG, Gayam S, Savage D, et al. Furosemide exposure and prevention of bronchopulmonary dysplasia in premature infants. J Pediatr 2018. [Epub ahead of print].

83. Blaisdell CJ, Troendle J, Zajicek A, et al. Acute responses to diuretic therapy in extremely low gestational age newborns: results from the prematurity and respiratory outcomes program cohort study. J Pediatr 2018;197:42–7.e1.

84. Green TP, Thompson TR, Johnson DE, et al. Furosemide promotes patent ductus arteriosus in premature infants with the respiratory-distress syndrome. N Engl J Med 1983;308:743–8.

85. Toyoshima K, Momma K, Nakanishi T. In vivo dilatation of the ductus arteriosus induced by furosemide in the rat. Pediatr Res 2010;67:173–6.

86. Thompson EJ, Greenberg RG, Kumar K, et al. Association between furosemide exposure and patent ductus arteriosus in hospitalized infants of very low birth weight. J Pediatr 2018;199:231–6.

87. Kao LC, Durand DJ, McCrea RC, et al. Randomized trial of long-term diuretic therapy for infants with oxygen-dependent bronchopulmonary dysplasia. J Pediatr 1994;124:772–81.

88. Guaman MC, Gien J, Baker CD, et al. Point prevalence, clinical characteristics, and treatment variation for infants with severe bronchopulmonary dysplasia. Am J Perinatol 2015;32:960–7.

89. Mourani PM, Sontag MK, Younoszai A, et al. Early pulmonary vascular disease in preterm infants at risk for bronchopulmonary dysplasia. Am J Respir Crit Care Med 2015;191:87–95.

90. Mourani PM, Mandell EW, Meier M, et al. Early pulmonary vascular disease in preterm infants is associated with late respiratory outcomes in childhood. Am J Respir Crit Care Med 2018. [Epub ahead of print].

91. Jakkula M, Le Cras TD, Gebb S, et al. Inhibition of angiogenesis decreases alveolarization in the developing rat lung. Am J Physiol Lung Cell Mol Physiol 2000;279:L600–7.

92. Afshar S, Gibson LL, Yuhanna IS, et al. Pulmonary NO synthase expression is attenuated in a fetal baboon model of chronic lung disease. Am J Physiol Lung Cell Mol Physiol 2003;284:L749–58.

93. Tang JR, Seedorf G, Balasubramaniam V, et al. Early inhaled nitric oxide treatment decreases apoptosis of endothelial cells in neonatal rat lungs after vascular endothelial growth factor inhibition. Am J Physiol Lung Cell Mol Physiol 2007;293:L1271–80.

94. Balasubramaniam V, Maxey AM, Morgan DB, et al. Inhaled NO restores lung structure in eNOS-deficient mice recovering from neonatal hypoxia. Am J Physiol Lung Cell Mol Physiol 2006;291:L119–27.

95. Donohue PK, Gilmore MM, Cristofalo E, et al. Inhaled nitric oxide in preterm infants: a systematic review. Pediatrics 2011;127:e414–22.

96. Askie LM, Ballard RA, Cutter GR, et al. Inhaled nitric oxide in preterm infants: an individual-patient data meta-analysis of randomized trials. Pediatrics 2011;128: 729–39.

97. Abman SH, Hansmann G, Archer SL, et al. Pediatric pulmonary hypertension: guidelines from the American Heart Association and American Thoracic Society. Circulation 2015;132:2037–99.

98. Kinsella JP, Steinhorn RH, Krishnan US, et al. Recommendations for the use of inhaled nitric oxide therapy in premature newborns with severe pulmonary hypertension. J Pediatr 2016;170:312–4.

99. Cole FS, Alleyne C, Barks JD, et al. NIH Consensus Development Conference statement: inhaled nitric-oxide therapy for premature infants. Pediatrics 2011; 127:363–9.

100. Askie LM, Davies LC, Schreiber MD, et al. Race effects of inhaled nitric oxide in preterm infants: an individual participant data meta-analysis. J Pediatr 2018; 193:34–9.e2.

101. Mourani PM, Abman SH. Pulmonary hypertension and vascular abnormalities in bronchopulmonary dysplasia. Clin Perinatol 2015;42:839–55.

102. Arjaans S, Zwart EAH, Ploegstra MJ, et al. Identification of gaps in the current knowledge on pulmonary hypertension in extremely preterm infants: a systematic review and meta-analysis. Paediatr Perinat Epidemiol 2018;32:258–67.

103. Krishnan U, Feinstein JA, Adatia I, et al. Evaluation and management of pulmonary hypertension in children with bronchopulmonary dysplasia. J Pediatr 2017; 188:24–34.e1.

104. Mourani PM, Ivy DD, Gao D, et al. Pulmonary vascular effects of inhaled nitric oxide and oxygen tension in bronchopulmonary dysplasia. Am J Respir Crit Care Med 2004;170:1006–13.

105. Lakshminrusimha S, Konduri GG, Steinhorn RH. Considerations in the management of hypoxemic respiratory failure and persistent pulmonary hypertension in term and late preterm neonates. J Perinatol 2016;36(Suppl 2).S12–9.

106. Steinhorn RH. Advances in neonatal pulmonary hypertension. Neonatology 2016;109:334–44.

107. de Visser YP, Walther FJ, Laghmani el H, et al. Sildenafil attenuates pulmonary inflammation and fibrin deposition, mortality and right ventricular hypertrophy in neonatal hyperoxic lung injury. Respir Res 2009;10:30.

108. Mourani PM, Sontag MK, Ivy DD, et al. Effects of long-term sildenafil treatment for pulmonary hypertension in infants with chronic lung disease. J Pediatr 2009; 154:379–84, 384.e1-2.

109. Nyp M, Sandritter T, Poppinga N, et al. Sildenafil citrate, bronchopulmonary dysplasia and disordered pulmonary gas exchange: any benefits? J Perinatol 2012;32:64–9.

110. Wardle AJ, Wardle R, Luyt K, et al. The utility of sildenafil in pulmonary hypertension: a focus on bronchopulmonary dysplasia. Arch Dis Child 2013;98:613–7.

111. Barst RJ, Beghetti M, Pulido T, et al. STARTS-2: long-term survival with oral sildenafil monotherapy in treatment-naive pediatric pulmonary arterial hypertension. Circulation 2014;129:1914–23.

112. Abman SH, Kinsella JP, Rosenzweig EB, et al. Implications of the U.S. Food and Drug Administration warning against the use of sildenafil for the treatment of pediatric pulmonary hypertension. Am J Respir Crit Care Med 2013;187:572–5.

113. Backes CH, Reagan PB, Smith CV, et al. Sildenafil treatment of infants with bronchopulmonary dysplasia-associated pulmonary hypertension. Hosp Pediatr 2016;6:27–33.

114. Balasubramaniam V, Mervis CF, Maxey AM, et al. Hyperoxia reduces bone marrow, circulating, and lung endothelial progenitor cells in the developing lung: implications for the pathogenesis of bronchopulmonary dysplasia. Am J Physiol Lung Cell Mol Physiol 2007;292:L1073–84.

115. Hansmann G, Fernandez-Gonzalez A, Aslam M, et al. Mesenchymal stem cell-mediated reversal of bronchopulmonary dysplasia and associated pulmonary hypertension. Pulm Circ 2012;2:170–81.
116. Thebaud B. Stem cell-based therapies in neonatology: a new hope. Arch Dis Child Fetal Neonatal Ed 2018;103(6):F583–8.
117. Chang YS, Ahn SY, Yoo HS, et al. Mesenchymal stem cells for bronchopulmonary dysplasia: phase 1 dose-escalation clinical trial. J Pediatr 2014;164:966–72.e6.
118. Ahn SY, Chang YS, Kim JH, et al. Two-Year Follow-up outcomes of premature infants enrolled in the phase I trial of mesenchymal stem cells transplantation for bronchopulmonary dysplasia. J Pediatr 2017;185:49–54.e2.
119. Lim R, Malhotra A, Tan J, et al. First-in-human administration of allogeneic amnion cells in premature infants with bronchopulmonary dysplasia: a safety study. Stem Cells Transl Med 2018;7:628–35.
120. Hellstrom A, Engstrom E, Hard AL, et al. Postnatal serum insulin-like growth factor I deficiency is associated with retinopathy of prematurity and other complications of premature birth. Pediatrics 2003;112:1016–20.
121. Ley D, Hallberg B, Hansen-Pupp I, et al. rhIGF-1/rhIGFBP-3 in preterm infants: a phase 2 randomized controlled trial. J Pediatr 2018. [Epub ahead of print].
122. Challis JR, Lockwood CJ, Myatt L, et al. Inflammation and pregnancy. Reprod Sci 2009;16:206–15.
123. Zakar T, Mesiano S. How does progesterone relax the uterus in pregnancy? N Engl J Med 2011;364:972–3.
124. Pieber D, Allport VC, Hills F, et al. Interactions between progesterone receptor isoforms in myometrial cells in human labour. Mol Hum Reprod 2001;7:875–9.
125. NIH Consensus Panel. Effect of corticosteroids for fetal maturation on perinatal outcomes. NIH Consensus Development Panel on the Effect of Corticosteroids for Fetal Maturation on Perinatal Outcomes. JAMA 1995;273:413–8.
126. Stevens TP, Harrington EW, Blennow M, et al. Early surfactant administration with brief ventilation vs. selective surfactant and continued mechanical ventilation for preterm infants with or at risk for respiratory distress syndrome. Cocharne Database Syst Rev 2007;(4):CD003063.
127. Rigo V, Lefebvre C, Broux I. Surfactant instillation in spontaneously breathing preterm infants: a systematic review and meta-analysis. Eur J Pediatr 2016;175:1933–42.
128. Tyson JE, Wright LL, Oh W, et al. Vitamin A supplementation for extremely-low-birth-weight infants. N Engl J Med 1999;340:1962–8.
129. Brundage KL, Mohsini KG, Froese AB, et al. Bronchodilator response to ipratropium bromide in infants with bronchopulmonary dysplasia. Am Rev Respir Dis 1990;142:1137–42.

Pharmacologic Prevention and Treatment of Neonatal Brain Injury

Check for updates

Melanie A. McNally, MD[a], Janet S. Soul, MDCM, FRCPC[b],*

KEYWORDS

- Neonatal brain injury • Hypoxic-ischemic encephalopathy
- Periventricular leukomalacia • Neuroprotection • Therapeutic hypothermia
- Erythropoietin • Magnesium

KEY POINTS

- Neonatal brain injury is one of the largest contributors to neonatal mortality and long-term neurodevelopmental morbidity worldwide.
- Therapeutic hypothermia is the only approved therapy to decrease term neonatal brain injury. In preterm neonates, prevention of brain injury is currently limited to antenatal steroid administration and other supportive measures.
- Erythropoietin has shown benefit in clinical trials to reduce term and preterm neonatal brain injury, and several other drugs are currently being tested in early phase trials for neonatal hypoxic-ischemic encephalopathy (HIE).
- Clinical trials have demonstrated a role for magnesium in the prevention of preterm neonatal brain injury.

INTRODUCTION

Neonatal brain injury (NBI) remains a common condition despite efforts at prevention, and is most often due to hypoxic-ischemic encephalopathy (HIE) in term neonates, or intraventricular hemorrhage (IVH) and/or periventricular leukomalacia in preterm neonates. With HIE affecting approximately 2 per 1000 live births and prematurity occurring in up to 12% of live births, NBI is one of the largest contributors to neonatal mortality and long-term neurodevelopmental morbidity worldwide.[1–3] Over the last decade, the implementation of therapeutic hypothermia (TH) as standard of care for moderate to severe HIE has been an important first therapy to minimize NBI.[4] However, this intervention is currently limited to term neonates and is only partially

Disclosure Statement: The authors have nothing to disclose.
[a] Department of Neurology, Boston Children's Hospital, 300 Longwood Avenue, Boston, MA 02115, USA; [b] Fetal-Neonatal Neurology Program, Department of Neurology, Boston Children's Hospital, 300 Longwood Avenue, Boston, MA 02115, USA
* Corresponding author.
E-mail address: janet.soul@childrens.harvard.edu

Clin Perinatol 46 (2019) 311–325
https://doi.org/10.1016/j.clp.2019.02.006
0095-5108/19/© 2019 Elsevier Inc. All rights reserved.

perinatology.theclinics.com

effective, with 45% of patients still suffering significant neurodevelopmental disability or death despite treatment. In addition, TH has not been as successfully implemented in low-resource compared with high-resource countries.[5,6] Unfortunately, neuroprotection in the preterm neonate remains limited to general preventive and supportive measures, rather than targeted neuroprotection. Therefore, basic, translational, and clinical research efforts continue to investigate novel and adjuvant neuroprotective strategies for term and preterm brain injury.

When designing therapeutic strategies for NBI, multiple injury mechanisms that often vary with their cause must be considered in the context of a rapidly developing neonatal brain. In addition, pathogenic processes change in the hours to days after insult and injury. The most common post-insult pathways targeted in therapeutic development include oxidative stress, excitotoxicity, apoptotic cell death, and inflammation.[7] To date, treatment strategies that target multiple pathogenic mechanisms (eg, TH) and those that promote cellular repair have shown the most promise clinically. Lastly, because TH is now standard of care for term neonates with moderate-severe HIE, the research community has an ethical obligation to test the effectiveness of any new treatment strategy as an adjuvant to TH.

ERYTHROPOIETIN/DARBEPOETIN

Erythropoietin (Epo) is a glycoprotein cytokine that is a growth factor well known for its role in promoting erythropoiesis in the bone marrow and for the treatment of anemia in neonates. However, receptors for Epo (EpoR) have also been found on oligodendrocytes, astrocytes, microglia, neurons, and endothelial cells throughout the central nervous system, in which Epo plays an important role in normal early brain development.[8,9] Following an episode of hypoxia, levels of EpoR increase without a proportional increase in circulating Epo levels. When these EpoR are left unbound, apoptotic cell death is triggered.[10] Therefore, Epo supplementation is being investigated to increase cell survival after neonatal HIE. In animal models, Epo has proven effective at reducing inflammation, limiting oxidative stress, decreasing apopotosis (in neuronal and oligodendroglial cells), and promoting angiogenesis, neurogenesis, and oligodendrogenesis.[11,12] Notably, there is also interest in darbepoetin (Darbe) as an alternative to Epo. Darbe is an erythropoiesis-stimulating agent that has been biologically modified to be longer acting (eg, once weekly dosing) than Epo, but with similar effectiveness to Epo for treatment of anemia in neonates.[13]

Initial phase I clinical trials of Epo monotherapy (ie, without TH) administered in the first week of life in term newborns with HIE showed feasibility, safety, and some improvement in neurologic outcome. However, the studies were limited by small sample size.[14,15] In a larger randomized, placebo-controlled phase III trial, Epo monotherapy was demonstrated to decrease the combined risk of death or moderate to severe disability at a mean age of 19 months in treatment (40%) compared with placebo groups (70%).[16] However, in the era of TH, clinical trials have shifted to investigating Epo as an adjuvant to TH for neonatal HIE. A phase I, uncontrolled trial of 24 term neonates with HIE who received Epo in addition to TH examined safety and pharmacokinetics.[17] At a mean age of 22 months, only 4.5% of treated neonates had moderate to severe disability, prompting phase II then phase III trials of Epo combined with TH. The phase II trial of TH plus Epo in 50 term neonates with HIE showed that the Epo-treated group had less brain injury on MRI in the first week of life, as well as improved motor function scores at 12 months of life, compared with neonates treated with TH alone.[18] A population pharmacokinetic analysis of the 47 neonates in these 2 trials who received both TH and Epo revealed that birth weight was the only clinical variable that significantly affected Epo pharmacokinetics. An Epo dose of 1000 U/kg every 24 hours for the first 2 days after birth resulted in consistent serum concentrations that had provided neuroprotection in relevant animal models.[19] In light of the growing clinical evidence of safety and therapeutic benefit, a double-blind, placebo-controlled, multicenter phase III trial of high-dose Epo for moderate to severe neonatal HIE is ongoing, with a goal to enroll 500 term neonates.[20]

There have been fewer studies of Darbe than Epo in neonatal HIE. A small randomized, placebo-controlled safety and pharmacokinetic trial evaluated administration of Darbe to term neonates undergoing TH for moderate or severe encephalopathy. The investigators compared a low-dose treatment group (single 2 μg/kg Darbe infusion within 12 hours of birth, n = 10), a high-dose treatment group (a single 10 μg/kg Darbe infusion within 12 hours of birth, n = 10), and a control group (TH alone, n = 10). They found that combining Darbe and TH was safe, and that a 10-μg/kg Darbe infusion was adequate for weekly administration in the neonate. There is an ongoing phase II trial to assess neuroprotection of a single dose of Darbe (10 μg/kg) given to infants of more than 34 weeks gestation with mild encephalopathy who do not qualify for TH (NCT03071861).

Beyond treatment of term neonates with HIE, Epo and Darbe are also being tested as neuroprotective treatments for NBI in preterm neonates. Erythropoietin has well-established safety data in preterm neonates, as it has long been used to treat anemia of prematurity. An early retrospective cohort study examined preterm neonates born at ≤30 weeks gestation who received Epo for anemia. They found that the developmental outcome at a median of 25 months of age was proportional to the cumulative Epo dose received in the neonatal period.[21] In light of increasing evidence in animal models that very high doses of Epo are required for neuroprotection,[22] phase I/II studies were conducted to establish safety and pharmacokinetics of higher doses of Epo in very preterm neonates. In a prospective, dose-escalation trial of 30 preterm neonates, early administration of daily Epo in the first 3 days of life was well tolerated, and doses of 1000 and 2500 U/kg achieved neuroprotective serum levels.[23] Another phase II trial found no increased mortality or adverse effects of daily doses of high-dose Epo (3000 U/kg) administered to 229 preterm neonates in the first 3 days after birth.[24] In light of the promising safety profile, multiple randomized placebo-controlled trials have been completed or initiated to determine a possible neuroprotective effect of Epo with different administration schedules and dosing regimens in preterm neonates. Three trials have been completed; (1) using high-dose Epo and (2) using low-dose Epo. The former included 495 neonates born ≤32 weeks gestation who were randomized to receive 3000 U/kg of Epo in 3 doses over the first 42 hours after birth compared with placebo. At term-equivalent age, the neonates who had received Epo showed lower white and gray matter injury scores on brain MRI than controls.[25] However, there were no differences in 2-year neurodevelopmental outcomes between groups.[26] Although there was no neuroprotective role identified in this large trial, it is possible that a different timing of Epo administration or different doses might be required. In addition, the neurodevelopmental benefit may only be detected at later time points. To this point, a larger trial of 800 preterm neonates born at ≤32 weeks gestation who received lower dosing and longer administration of Epo showed promising results. The treatment group received a single Epo dose of 500 U/kg once in the first 72 hours of life and then every other day for 2 weeks. At 18- to 22-month follow-up assessment, the incidence of mortality and moderate or severe disability was decreased by over 50% in treatment compared with control groups.[27] A similar long-term neurodevelopmental benefit was seen in a much smaller trial of preterm neonates who received 400 U/kg of Epo (n = 27) 3 times a week, Darbe

10 μg/kg once a week (with 2 placebo infusions a week; n = 29), or placebo 3 times a week (n = 24) until they reached 35 weeks corrected gestational age.[28] The study found that both treatment groups (Epo and Darbe) showed significantly better developmental scores and a lower incidence of cerebral palsy at 18 to 20 months,[28] as well as improved behavioral scores at 4 years of age compared with the placebo group.[29] The study was not powered to compare the effectiveness of Darbe versus Epo with regard to neurodevelopmental outcome. Large phase III trials are currently evaluating Epo (NCT02036073 and NCT01378273) and Darbe (NCT03169881) administration in preterm neonates for long-term neuroprotection.

Overall, Epo and Darbe are very promising neuroprotective agents for NBI in term and preterm neonates alike. The several different mechanisms proposed for neuroprotective effects of these agents are likely responsible for their early success in clinical trials. If the ongoing phase III trials demonstrate long-term neurodevelopmental benefit, either Epo or Darbe could be the first neuroprotective agent for preterm NBI outside of standard supportive care. Either drug may provide additional benefit over TH for treatment of HIE in term neonates.

ALLOPURINOL

Allopurinol is a drug traditionally used to treat conditions, such as gout and cancer, by decreasing uric acid levels through inhibition of xanthine oxidase. Allopurinol has additional anti-oxidant properties through chelation of unbound iron and directly scavenging free hydroxyl radicals. Because reactive oxygen species are thought to play an important role in secondary brain injury following reperfusion, allopurinol has been investigated as a therapeutic strategy for NBI.[30] In preclinical studies, allopurinol was shown to decrease brain injury in rodent models of NBI.[31] Multiple clinical studies have been completed, with mixed results. Administration of 40 mg/kg of intravenous allopurinol within 4 hours of birth in neonates with severe HIE was determined to have no toxic effects, to decrease serum-free radical levels, and to improve cerebral blood flow when administered to 11 patients.[32] When examined in a small randomized feasibility study of 32 term neonates with severe HIE (17 received allopurinol and 15 placebo), this same dose did not show improvement in neonatal mortality or short-term neurologic outcome by MRI or electroencephalogram (EEG).[33] However, the study was small and only enrolled neonates with severe encephalopathy (need for resuscitation for at least 5 minutes; cord or first pH <7; multi-organ failure and burst suppression pattern or worse on an amplitude-integrated EEG). Thus the trial was not designed to test drug efficacy. Given the proposed mechanism of action, these authors postulated that administration within 4 hours after birth might have been outside of the therapeutic window and that earlier or antenatal administration should be investigated. In support of this idea, another small randomized control trial tested 40 mg/kg of allopurinol within 2 hours of birth for term neonates with mild, moderate, or severe encephalopathy (this dose was repeated daily for 3 days).[34] Three groups were compared including 30 neonates who received allopurinol (treatment group), 30 neonates who received placebo, and a control group of 20 healthy term neonates. No adverse side effects of allopurinol were found. Serum, but not cerebrospinal fluid levels of nitric oxide (a free radical known to be increased after NBI), were decreased in the treatment group compared with placebo and control groups. In addition, at 12-month follow-up, the treatment group showed better developmental outcome compared with the placebo group. In a follow-up study of the neonates enrolled in these latter 2 randomized trials, neurodevelopmental and cognitive outcomes were assessed at 4 to 8 years of age. There was no difference in mortality or adverse developmental outcome between treatment and control groups. However, a sub-group analysis revealed a significant decrease in the risk of a severe adverse outcome (death or severe disability at long-term follow-up) in neonates with moderate HIE who received allopurinol within 4 hours after birth.[35]

Trials of allopurinol administration to pregnant women have also been conducted to investigate a potential neuroprotective effect of antenatal administration. A small randomized, double-blind feasibility study of 500 mg of intravenous allopurinol given to pregnant women with evidence of fetal hypoxia at greater than 36 weeks gestation showed that antenatal allopurinol was safe and achieved therapeutic levels in arterial cord blood, indicating successful placental crossing.[36] This group also showed that, when levels of allopurinol were therapeutic in arterial cord blood, there was a concurrent decrease in free radical formation (biomarker of hypoxia) and levels of S-100B protein (glial calcium binding protein released with brain injury) in cord blood. Therefore, a larger randomized, placebo-controlled, multicenter trial was conducted. The trial recruited 222 pregnant women at greater than 36 weeks gestation with suspected fetal hypoxia during labor who were randomized to receive antenatal allopurinol (500 mg intravenously) or placebo.[37] Although there were no differences between the groups in immediate clinical outcomes or levels of brain injury markers in cord blood, none of the neonates developed HIE. When post hoc sub-group analyses were completed, there was a decrease in cord blood levels of brain injury markers in female neonates, but not male neonates, when compared with the placebo group. The authors suggested that allopurinol may be effective at preventing hypoxic brain injury in female neonates, but emphasize that this requires further investigation because none of the neonates developed detectable brain injury.

In summary, preliminary clinical trials suggest that postnatal allopurinol administration may provide neuroprotection to neonates with moderate HIE. Antenatal administration may also attenuate hypoxic brain damage in female neonates. However, larger trials will be required to demonstrate the efficacy of allopurinol in preventing brain injury and improving neurologic outcome related to neonatal HIE. In addition, the effect of allopurinol as an adjuvant to TH needs to be tested. There is an ongoing phase III trial in term neonates with moderate or severe HIE receiving TH (NCT03162653, AL-BINO trial). A possible preventive or therapeutic potential of allopurinol for NBI in preterm neonates has not been investigated.

MAGNESIUM

Magnesium is a ubiquitous intracellular cation involved in innumerable enzymatic processes throughout the body. It has been studied as a possible fetal and neonatal neuroprotective agent for decades because of its potential to decrease excitotoxicity by antagonizing postsynaptic N-methyl-D-aspartate receptors and to decrease inflammation through inhibition of the nuclear factor-κB pathway.[38] To date, 6 small randomized placebo-controlled trials have investigated magnesium in term neonates with HIE. One of the studies did include TH, establishing the safety of magnesium administration during cooling. Although no differences in immediate mortality or adverse outcomes were reported, long-term neurodevelopmental data have not been published.[39] Collectively, these trials produced mixed results and were limited by small size (22–60 patients per study) and different dosing and administration regimens. A meta-analysis of these studies suggested that magnesium treatment is protective against short-term adverse outcomes (eg, abnormal neurologic examination, abnormal neuroimaging, or abnormal amplitude-integrated EEG). However, there was no difference between groups in mortality or 18-month neurodevelopmental outcome.[40] Whether or not magnesium could improve long-term neurodevelopmental outcome after term HIE in combination with TH remains unknown.

Magnesium has been more thoroughly investigated as an antenatal neuroprotective strategy for preterm NBI. A Cochrane review of 5 randomized controlled trials examined data from pregnant women who received antenatal magnesium compared with placebo who were at high risk for preterm birth (<37 weeks gestation). A total of 3052 fetuses were exposed to magnesium infusions (treatment group), and 3093 were exposed to saline infusions (placebo group). Primary outcomes included fetal, neonatal, or later mortality, incidence of cerebral palsy, and combined risk of mortality and cerebral palsy. There were no differences between groups in terms of mortality or combined risk, but there was a significant lower incidence of cerebral palsy in survivors (relative risk 0.68). The number needed to treat was 63 women at risk for preterm delivery to prevent 1 case of cerebral palsy.[41] More recently, a meta-analysis of individual participant data from these trials was performed to help develop treatment guidelines. No significant difference in treatment effect was seen related to the risk factors associated with preterm birth, the gestational age at intervention, the total magnesium dose received, or whether magnesium treatment was also administered after birth. The analysis was repeated including 4 of the 5 original trials in which the use of the drug was intended for neuroprotection (4448 fetuses included). With these selected data, there was a significant reduction in the primary outcome of death or cerebral palsy with antenatal magnesium treatment compared with no treatment (relative risk 0.86).[42]

Overall, magnesium shows promise as an antenatal therapeutic strategy for preterm NBI and is considered standard care for mothers at risk for preterm delivery. However, determining what role it might play as an adjuvant treatment with TH for term HIE will require larger clinical trials. The potential benefit of magnesium has also resulted in recommendations for adjusting serum magnesium levels to high normal range in neonates with HIE. Given its low cost and availability, it remains a neuroprotective candidate worthy of further study.

INDOMETHACIN

Indomethacin is a prostaglandin synthetase inhibitor that is commonly used in preterm neonates for closure of a hemodynamically significant patent ductus arteriosus (PDA). Its use is associated with significant decreases in the incidence of symptomatic PDA and need for surgical PDA ligation.[43] As a neuroprotective strategy for preterm brain injury, prophylactic indomethacin has been shown to significantly decrease risk of severe IVH in the first few weeks of life in several randomized controlled trials when compared with placebo or no treatment groups.[43,44] This effect seems to be independent of a neonate's risk of developing IVH.[44] Despite the decreased incidence of severe IVH in the immediate neonatal period, prophylactic indomethacin has not shown clear benefit in decreasing mortality or improving long-term neurodevelopmental outcome when compared with placebo or no treatment groups.[43–45] Interestingly, 1 meta-analysis of 2 recent observational studies suggests that there may be a small reduction in mortality in neonates who received prophylactic indomethacin.[46] However, these authors caution against concluding that this represents a true benefit of the therapy versus chance or confounding given the small effect size and observational nature of the studies.[46] To date, most of the clinical evidence does not support the routine use of indomethacin in improving long-term neurodevelopmental outcome in preterm neonates. However, there may be a benefit in the relatively small number of neonates in whom severe IVH is prevented.

MELATONIN

An endogenous indolamine hormone known for its regulation of the circadian rhythm, melatonin also has potent anti-oxidant and anti-inflammatory effects. Preclinical work in animal models of NBI demonstrates that melatonin confers neuroprotection alone and as an adjuvant therapy with TH.[47–49] Given the observed safety profile in these animal models (even at high doses) and the ease by which it crosses both the placenta and blood-brain barrier, melatonin is a very attractive therapeutic candidate for NBI. In a small prospective randomized trial, 30 term neonates with moderate to severe HIE were randomized to either TH alone or TH with 5 daily enteral doses (10 mg/kg) of melatonin. At 2 weeks of age, an EEG and brain MRI were obtained. Neonates who received adjuvant melatonin were reported to show fewer electrographic seizures by EEG and less white matter injury on brain MRI than the neonates who received TH alone. At 6 months of age, the treatment group showed higher survival without neurodevelopmental abnormalities compared with controls. However, caution should be exercised in extrapolating efficacy from the results of a small early phase trial.[50] An open-label dose escalation phase 1 trial examining combined melatonin and TH treatment of term HIE is actively recruiting (NCT02621944). Although a promising drug with a favorable safety profile, larger, randomized trials with neurodevelopmental outcome measured at a minimum of 18 to 24 months of age are required to establish a definitive therapeutic role for neonatal NBI.

TOPIRAMATE

Topiramate (TPM) is an established anticonvulsant drug with multiple mechanisms of action including inhibiting carbonic anhydrase isoenzymes, decreasing excitatory currents through α-amino-3-hydroxy-5-methyl-4-isoxazoleproprionic acid receptor transmembrane ion channels, and enhancing gamma-aminobutyric acid-mediated inhibitory currents.[51] Preclinical studies have examined the neuroprotective potential of TPM by targeting excitotoxicity during secondary energy failure after HIE. In rodent and piglet models of NBI, TPM alone or in combination with TH attenuates white matter injury and improves long-term cognition and memory.[52,53] Preliminary phase 1 studies in term neonates with HIE established the safety and pharmacokinetics of administering TPM with[54] and without[55] concurrent TH. A dose of 5 mg/kg was shown to produce therapeutic serum levels and no adverse effects were reported in 13 neonates.[55] A recently completed phase II study evaluated the efficacy and safety of TPM in combination with TH.[54] Forty-four term neonates with moderate to severe HIE were randomized to TH alone or TH with adjuvant TPM, administered in 3 daily doses of 10 mg/kg. Serum levels were within reference range during TH, but approximately 50% lower in neonates who were receiving concurrent phenobarbital to treat seizures. No adverse effects were reported. When mortality and severe neurodevelopmental disability were assessed at 18 months, no differences were observed between the control and treatment groups. Interestingly, although the study was not powered to assess this secondary outcome, the authors noted that only 14% of survivors in the treatment group developed epilepsy at follow-up, compared with 30% of survivors receiving TH alone. This trend warrants further clinical study given the potential to decrease the incidence of epilepsy after neonatal HIE. However, larger studies and longer term follow-up are required to determine if TPM can ultimately reduce the incidence of epilepsy later in childhood. Another phase I/II study is underway examining the efficacy of 5 daily TPM doses (5 mg/kg) used in conjunction with

TH for term neonates with moderate to severe HIE (NCT01765218). Results from this trial and larger phase III trials are needed to determine whether TPM confers a neurodevelopmental benefit in neonatal HIE.

XENON

Xenon is an inert inhaled anesthetic with minimal physiologic effects or associated toxicity in patients. It has been investigated as a possible neuroprotective agent in HIE. In preclinical studies, it demonstrates N-methyl-D-aspartate receptor inhibition (decreased excitotoxicity), upregulation of anti-apoptotic proteins and multiple growth factors (decreased neuronal death and enhanced repair), and modulation of inflammatory cytokines (decreased inflammation).[56] In rodent and piglet models of hypoxia-ischemia, xenon enhances neuroprotection when combined with TH.[57,58] Due to the promising preclinical profile, a small, single-arm, dose escalation feasibility study was conducted in neonates with moderate or severe HIE receiving TH. Inhalation of 50% xenon was started in all patients within 11 hours of birth and continued for up to 18 hours during TH. The study found that xenon depressed electrographic seizures, increased sedation, and depressed EEG background without blood pressure reduction in the 14 enrolled neonates. Given the concern for the high cost of xenon, the authors estimated the expense at approximately $15 an hour of xenon delivery arguing that administration is both safe and feasible. At 18- to 20-month follow-up, they also showed that developmental outcomes were no worse than TH alone.[59] Subsequently, a larger feasibility and safety trial was completed which randomized 92 neonates with moderate or severe HIE to TH alone or TH plus inhaled 30% xenon for 24 hours, started by a median of 10 hours after birth. No additive effects were seen in neonatal mortality or early brain injury assessed by neonatal brain MRI in the neonates who received TH plus xenon.[60] Long-term neurodevelopmental follow-up in these patients is still ongoing. Although the primary outcome measures did not show significant benefit, it is possible that neuroprotection from xenon requires higher concentrations and/ or earlier administration. Given the concern that xenon requires specialized tertiary hospital settings for administration, a feasibility study was completed on a portable xenon delivery system. Five neonates received inhaled xenon safely in an ambulance during transport to tertiary centers which could shorten time to initiate xenon therapy.[61] The extent of neuroprotection from inhaled xenon for neonates with HIE, as well as the optimal timing, dosing, and feasibility of broad administration, remain to be determined. The high cost and specialized delivery systems make xenon less likely to be widely adopted for use compared with previously described agents.

SUMMARY

There has been significant expansion of basic science, translational and clinical research studies of NBI in the last 2 decades. With TH becoming standard of care, investigations of other neuroprotective drugs and therapies in term and preterm neonates has significantly increased. The burden of NBI is substantial worldwide and offers enormous potential for therapeutic intervention to lessen life-long neurologic disability. In addition to the approaches described above, other molecular pathways for therapeutic targeting currently being studied in the preclinical realm include stimulation of endogenous stem cell production, modification of epigenetic factors with histone deacetylases, or modification of the immune response to injury. The preclinical pipeline contains many promising agents such as vitamins C and E, desferrioxamine,

Table 1
Neuroprotective agents for neonatal brain injury in clinical trials

Agent	Target	Mechanism of Action	Preclinical Evidence	Clinical Trials
Erythropoetin/ Darbepoetin	Postnatal term and preterm NBI	• Decreases inflammation, oxidative stress, and apoptosis • Increases angiogenesis and neurogenesis	Neuroprotective effects in multiple rodent models and a primate model independently and combined with hypothermia	Term NBI Epo • Completed: I–III (no TH); I and II (+TH) • Enrolling: III (+TH) Term NBI Darbe • Completed: I (+TH); Enrolling: II (no TH) Preterm NBI Epo and Darbe • Completed: I–III; Enrolling: III
Allopurinol	Antenatal and postnatal term NBI	Anti-oxidant	Decreases acute brain edema and sub-acute brain atrophy in a rodent model	Postnatal • Completed: I– III (no TH); Enrolling: III (+TH) Antenatal • Completed: III
Magnesium	Antenatal for preterm NBI. Postnatal for term NBI	Decreases excitotoxicity (NMDA receptor inhibition) and inflammation (NF-κB pathway inhibition)	• Decreases acute histopathologic markers of injury in a sheep model • Inconsistent neuroprotection in rodent models	Postnatal term NBI • Completed: I–III (no TH), I (+TH) Antenatal preterm NBI • Completed: I–III
Melatonin	Postnatal term NBI	Anti-oxidant and anti-inflammatory	• Improves histologic measures of brain injury and behavioral and motor outcomes in a rodent model • Augments neuroprotective protective effects of hypothermia in a piglet model	• Completed: III (+TH) • Enrolling: I (+TH)

(continued on next page)

Table 1
(continued)

Agent	Target	Mechanism of Action	Preclinical Evidence	Clinical Trials
Topiramate	Postnatal term NBI	Decreases excitotoxicity by inhibiting AMPAR and increasing GABA-mediated inhibitory currents	Rodent models: • Lessens histopathological brain injury and improved behavioral outcomes • Lengthens therapeutic window for hypothermia	• Completed: I (no TH); I and II (+TH) • Enrolling: I/II (+TH)
Xenon	Postnatal term NBI	• Decreases excitotoxicity (NMDA receptor inhibition), neuronal death (upregulates anti-apoptotic proteins), and inflammation (modulates cytokines) • Enhances repair (via growth factors)	Augments neuroprotection from hypothermia in rodent and piglet models	• Completed: I and II (+TH)

Abbreviations: AMPAR, α-amino-3-hydroxy-5-methyl-4-isoxazoleproprionic acid receptor; GABA, gamma-aminobutyric acid; NF-κB, nuclear factor-κB; NMDA, N-methyl-ᴅ-aspartate.

N-acetylcysteine, lutein, iminobiotin, resveratrol, omega-3 fatty acids, azithromycin, cannabinoids, and microRNAs. There are also preclinical and clinical studies exploring the benefits of optimization of placental transfusion at birth, enhancing cerebral blood flow and oxygenation after birth, improved seizure control, administration of umbilical cord or bone marrow mesenchymal stem cells, and remote ischemic post-conditioning. Of the pharmacologic agents currently being investigated clinically (summarized in **Table 1**), those that have shown the highest likelihood of success and are closest to clinical implementation include Epo for term and preterm NBI and magnesium for antenatal prevention of preterm NBI. Given the enormous world-wide burden of the sequelae of NBI, more therapies to prevent or treat NBI and optimization of access to neuroprotective strategies for NBI in low resource settings are clearly needed to improve the care and neurologic outcome of preterm and term neonates.

Best practices

What is current practice?

Term neonatal brain injury

- 72 hours of hypothermia (33–34°C) for moderate or severe hypoxic-ischemic encephalopathy
- Supportive care for mild hypoxic-ischemic encephalopathy. Some centers are offering hypothermia to treat mild encephalopathy, but limited data supporting this approach

Preterm neonatal brain injury

- Antenatal steroids, minimizing the use of postnatal dexamethasone
- Some centers administer prophylactic indomethacin to decrease risk of severe IVH
- Supportive care to optimize brain perfusion, oxygenation, and nutrition

What changes in current practice are likely to improve outcomes?

Term neonatal brain injury

- Optimizing delivery of hypothermia
- Erythropoietin with hypothermia being tested in a large multicenter phase III trial

Preterm neonatal brain injury

- Erythropoietin may be beneficial as shown by one published phase III trial and is being tested in another large phase III trial
- Antenatal magnesium to decrease rate of cerebral palsy, currently offered in some centers

Major recommendations

- Therapeutic hypothermia is standard of care in term neonates with moderate or severe hypoxic-ischemic encephalopathy, and can be considered to treat mild encephalopathy
- Prevention and treatment of preterm brain injury through optimization of supportive care and testing of neuroprotective agents, and optimization of access to neuroprotective care for neonatal brain injury in low resource settings

Summary statement

Neuroprotective strategies with strong evidence are currently limited to antenatal steroids and supportive care for preterm neonatal brain injury and therapeutic hypothermia for term hypoxic-ischemic encephalopathy. Pharmacologic agents with the highest likelihood of success and closest to clinical implementation include erythropoietin to minimize term and preterm brain injury and antenatal magnesium to prevent/minimize preterm brain injury

Data from Refs.[4,12,20,38]

REFERENCES

1. Kurinczuk JJ, White-Koning M, Badawi N. Epidemiology of neonatal encephalopathy and hypoxic-ischaemic encephalopathy. Early Hum Dev 2010;86:329–38.
2. Lawn JE, Kinney MV, Black RE, et al. Newborn survival: a multi-country analysis of a decade of change. Health Policy Plan 2012;27:6–28.
3. Black RE, Cousens S, Johnson HL, et al. Global, regional, and national causes of child mortality in 2008: a systematic analysis. Lancet 2010;375:1969–87.
4. Azzopardi DV, Strohm B, Edwards AD, et al. Moderate hypothermia to treat perinatal asphyxial encephalopathy. N Engl J Med 2009;361:1349–58.
5. Montaldo P, Pauliah SS, Lally PJ, et al. Cooling in a low-resource environment: lost in translation. Semin Fetal Neonatal Med 2014;20:1–8.
6. Kali GTJ, Martinez-Biarge M, Van Zyl J, et al. Management of therapeutic hypothermia for neonatal hypoxic ischaemic encephalopathy in a tertiary centre in South Africa. Arch Dis Child Fetal Neonatal Ed 2015;100:F519–23.
7. Johnston MV, Fatemi A, Wilson MA, et al. Treatment advances in neonatal neuroprotection and neurointensive care. Lancet Neurol 2011;10:372–82.
8. Juul SE. Erythropoietin in the neonate. Curr Probl Pediatr 1999;29:133–49.
9. Yu X, Shacka JJ, Eells JB, et al. Erythropoietin receptor signalling is required for normal brain development. Development 2002;129:505–16.
10. Mazur M, Miller RH, Robinson S. Postnatal erythropoietin treatment mitigates neural cell loss after systemic prenatal hypoxic-ischemic injury. J Neurosurg Pediatr 2010;6:206–21.
11. Rangarajan V, Juul SE. Erythropoietin: emerging role of erythropoietin in neonatal neuroprotection. Pediatr Neurol 2014;51:481–8.
12. Juul SE, Pet GC. Erythropoietin and neonatal neuroprotection. Clin Perinatol 2015;42:469–81.
13. Ohls ARK, Christensen RD. A randomized, masked, placebo-controlled study of darbepoetin alfa in preterm infants. Pediatrics 2013;132:e119–27.
14. Zhu C, Kang W, Xu F, et al. Erythropoietin improved neurologic outcomes in newborns with hypoxic-ischemic encephalopathy. Pediatrics 2009;124:e218–26.
15. Elmahdy H, El-Mashad A-R, El-Bahrawy H, et al. Human recombinant erythropoietin in asphyxia neonatorum: pilot trial. Pediatrics 2010;125:e1135–42.
16. Malla RR, Asimi R, Teli MA, et al. Erythropoietin monotherapy in perinatal asphyxia with moderate to severe encephalopathy: a randomized placebo-controlled trial. J Perinatol 2017;37:596–601.
17. Wu YW, Bauer LA, Ballard RA, et al. Erythropoietin for neuroprotection in neonatal encephalopathy: safety and pharmacokinetics. Pediatrics 2012;130:683–91.
18. Wu YW, Mathur AM, Chang T, et al. High-dose erythropoietin and hypothermia for hypoxic-ischemic encephalopathy: a phase II trial. Pediatrics 2016;137:e20160191.
19. Frymoyer A, Juul SE, Massaro AN, et al. High-dose erythropoietin population pharmacokinetics in neonates with hypoxic-ischemic encephalopathy receiving hypothermia. Pediatr Res 2017;81:865–72.
20. Juul SE, Comstock BA, Heagerty PJ, et al. High-dose erythropoietin for asphyxia and encephalopathy (HEAL): a randomized controlled trial – background, aims, and study protocol. Neonatology 2018;113:331–8.
21. Brown MS, Eichorst D, LaLa-Black B, et al. Higher cumulative doses of erythropoietin and developmental outcomes in preterm infants. Pediatrics 2009;124:e681–7.

22. Kellert BA, McPherson RJ, Juul SE. A comparison of high-dose recombinant erythropoietin treatment regimens in brain-injured neonatal rats. Pediatr Res 2007;61:451–5.

23. Juul SE, McPherson RJ, Bauer LA, et al. A phase I/II trial of high-dose erythropoietin in extremely low birth weight infants: pharmacokinetics and safety. Pediatrics 2008;122:383–91.

24. Fauchère JC, Koller BM, Tschopp A, et al. Safety of early high-dose recombinant erythropoietin for neuroprotection in very preterm infants. J Pediatr 2015;167: 52–7.e3.

25. Leuchter RHV, Gui L, Poncet A, et al. Association between early administration of high-dose erythropoietin in preterm infants and brain MRI abnormality at term-equivalent age. JAMA 2014;312:817–24.

26. Natalucci G, Latal B, Koller B, et al. Effect of early prophylactic high-dose recombinant human erythropoietin in very preterm infants on neurodevelopmental outcome at 2 years. JAMA 2016;315:2079–85.

27. Song J, Sun H, Xu F, et al. Recombinant human erythropoietin improves neurological outcomes in very preterm infants. Ann Neurol 2016;80:24–34.

28. Ohls RK, Kamath-Rayne BD, Christensen RD, et al. Cognitive outcomes of preterm infants randomized to darbepoetin, erythropoietin, or placebo. Pediatrics 2014;133:1023–30.

29. Lowe JR, Rieger RE, Moss NC, et al. Impact of erythropoiesis-stimulating agents on behavioral measures in children born preterm. J Pediatr 2017;184:75–80.e1.

30. Arteaga O, Álvarez A, Revuelta M, et al. Role of antioxidants in neonatal hypoxic–ischemic brain injury: new therapeutic approaches. Int J Mol Sci 2017;18. https://doi.org/10.3390/ijms18020265.

31. Palmer C, Towfighi J, Roberts RL, et al. Allopurinol administered after inducing hypoxia-ischemia reduces brain injury in 7-day-old rats. Pediatr Res 1993;33: 405–11.

32. Van Bel F, Shadid M, Moison RM, et al. Effect of allopurinol on postasphyxial free radical formation, cerebral hemodynamics, and electrical brain activity. Pediatrics 1998;101:185–93.

33. Benders MJ, Bos AF, Rademaker CM, et al. Early postnatal allopurinol does not improve short term outcome after severe birth asphyxia. Arch Dis Child Fetal Neonatal Ed 2006;91:F163–5.

34. Gunes T, Ozturk MA, Koklu E, et al. Effect of allopurinol supplementation on nitric oxide levels in asphyxiated newborns. Pediatr Neurol 2007;36:17–24.

35. Kaandorp JJ, Van Bel F, Veen S, et al. Long-term neuroprotective effects of allopurinol after moderate perinatal asphyxia: follow-up of two randomised controlled trials. Arch Dis Child Fetal Neonatal Ed 2012;97. https://doi.org/10.1136/archdischild-2011-300356.

36. Torrance HL, Benders MJ, Derks JB, et al. Maternal allopurinol during fetal hypoxia lowers cord blood levels of the brain injury marker S-100B. Obstet Gynecol Surv 2009;64:705–6.

37. Kaandorp JJ, Benders MJNL, Schuit E, et al. Maternal allopurinol administration during suspected fetal hypoxia: a novel neuroprotective intervention? A multicentre randomised placebo controlled trial. Arch Dis Child Fetal Neonatal Ed 2015;100:F216–23.

38. Lingam I, Robertson NJ. Magnesium as a neuroprotective agent: a review of its use in the fetus, term infant with neonatal encephalopathy, and the adult stroke patient. Dev Neurosci 2018;40:1–12.

39. Rahman S, Siham A, Tuzun H, et al. Multicenter randomized controlled trial of therapeutic hypothermia plus magnesium sulfate versus therapeutic hypothermia plus placebo in the management of term and near-term infants with hypoxic ischemic encephalopathy (The Mag Cool study): a pilot study. J Clin Neonatol 2015;4:158.

40. Tagin M, Shah PS, Lee KS. Magnesium for newborns with hypoxic-ischemic encephalopathy: a systematic review and meta-analysis. J Perinatol 2013;33:663–9.

41. Doyle L, Crowther C, Middleton P, et al. Magnesium sulphate for women at risk of preterm birth for neuroprotection of the fetus. Cochrane Libr 2009;1968:1–96.

42. Crowther CA, Middleton PF, Voysey M, et al. Assessing the neuroprotective benefits for babies of antenatal magnesium sulphate: an individual participant data meta-analysis. PLoS Med 2017;14:1–24.

43. Fowlie P, Davis P, Mcguire W. Prophylactic intravenous indomethacin for preventing mortality and morbidity in preterm infants [review]. Cochrane Database Syst Rev 2010. https://doi.org/10.1002/14651858.CD000174.pub2.

44. Foglia EE, Roberts S, Stoller JZ, et al. Effect of prophylactic indomethacin in extremely low birth weight infants based on the predicted risk of severe intraventricular hemorrhage. Neonatology 2018;113:183–6.

45. Shepherd E, Ra S, Middleton P, et al. Neonatal interventions for preventing cerebral palsy: an overview of Cochrane Systematic Reviews [review]. Cochrane Database Syst Rev 2018. https://doi.org/10.1002/14651858.CD012409.pub2. Available at: www.cochranelibrary.com.

46. Jensen EA, Foglia EE, Schmidt B. Association between prophylactic indomethacin and death or bronchopulmonary dysplasia: a systematic review and meta-analysis of observational studies. Semin Perinatol 2018;42:228–34.

47. Carloni S, Albertini MC, Galluzzi L, et al. Melatonin reduces endoplasmic reticulum stress and preserves sirtuin 1 expression in neuronal cells of newborn rats after hypoxia-ischemia. J Pineal Res 2014;57:192–9.

48. Carloni S, Perrone S, Buonocore G, et al. Melatonin protects from the long-term consequences of a neonatal hypoxic-ischemic brain injury in rats. J Pineal Res 2008;44:157–64.

49. Robertson NJ, Faulkner S, Fleiss B, et al. Melatonin augments hypothermic neuroprotection in a perinatal asphyxia model. Brain 2013;136:90–105.

50. Aly H, Elmahdy H, El-Dib M, et al. Melatonin use for neuroprotection in perinatal asphyxia: a randomized controlled pilot study. J Perinatol 2015;35:186–91.

51. Shank RP, Gardocki JF, Streeter AJ, et al. An overview of the preclinical aspects of topiramate: pharmacology, pharmacokinetics, and mechanism of action. Epilepsia 2000;41:3–9.

52. Liu Y, Barks JD, Xu G, et al. Topiramate extends the therapeutic window for hypothermia-mediated neuroprotection after stroke in neonatal rats. Stroke 2004;35:1460–5.

53. Noh MR, Kim SK, Sun W, et al. Neuroprotective effect of topiramate on hypoxic ischemic brain injury in neonatal rats. Exp Neurol 2006;201:470–8.

54. Filippi L, Fiorini P, Catarzi S, et al. Safety and efficacy of topiramate in neonates with hypoxic ischemic encephalopathy treated with hypothermia (NeoNATI): a feasibility study. J Matern Fetal Neonatal Med 2018;31:973–80.

55. Filippi L, Poggi C, La Marca G, et al. Oral topiramate in neonates with hypoxic ischemic encephalopathy treated with hypothermia: a safety study. J Pediatr 2010;157:361–6.

56. Amer AR, Oorschot DE. Xenon combined with hypothermia in perinatal hypoxic-ischemic encephalopathy: a noble gas, a noble mission. Pediatr Neurol 2018. https://doi.org/10.1016/j.pediatrneurol.2018.02.009.
57. Chakkarapani E, Dingley J, Liu X, et al. Xenon enhances hypothermic neuroprotection in asphyxiated newborn pigs. Ann Neurol 2010;68:330–41.
58. Thoresen M, Hobbs CE, Wood T, et al. Cooling combined with immediate or delayed xenon inhalation provides equivalent long-term neuroprotection after neonatal hypoxia-ischemia. J Cereb Blood Flow Metab 2009;29:707–14.
59. Dingley J, Tooley J, Liu X, et al. Xenon ventilation during therapeutic hypothermia in neonatal encephalopathy: a feasibility study. Pediatrics 2014;133:809–18.
60. Azzopardi D, Robertson NJ, Bainbridge A, et al. Moderate hypothermia within 6 h of birth plus inhaled xenon versus moderate hypothermia alone after birth asphyxia (TOBY-Xe): a proof-of-concept, open-label, randomised controlled trial. Lancet Neurol 2016;15:145–53.
61. Dingley J, Liu X, Gill H, et al. The feasibility of using a portable xenon delivery device to permit earlier xenon ventilation with therapeutic cooling of neonates during ambulance retrieval. Anesth Analg 2015;120:1331–6.

Drugs for the Prevention and Treatment of Sepsis in the Newborn

Sagori Mukhopadhyay, MD, MMSc[a,b,c,d],
Kelly C. Wade, MD, PhD, MSCE[a,b,c,d],
Karen M. Puopolo, MD, PhD[a,b,c,d,*]

KEYWORDS

• Newborn • Sepsis • Antibiotics • Prophylaxis

KEY POINTS

• Early-onset sepsis remains a common clinical concern in neonates with persistently high morbidity and mortality, particularly among preterm infants.
• Antibiotics administered to the mother during the intrapartum period can reduce the risk of some perinatal infections by reducing ascending bacterial colonization and via transplacental antibiotic transfer to the fetus/newborn.
• Ampicillin and gentamicin remain the first-line choice for empiric treatment of early-onset sepsis.
• Understanding antibiotic pharmacology can allow neonatal providers to optimize antibiotic choice and minimize resistance-promoting selection pressures.

INTRODUCTION

Antimicrobial medication use is exceedingly common among neonates. Perinatal antibiotic exposure includes in utero exposure to maternal intrapartum antibiotic prophylaxis (IAP), whether for group B streptococcus (GBS) colonization or concern for maternal intra-amniotic infection (IAI), as well as exposure to empiric antibiotics given directly to the neonate for risk of early-onset sepsis (EOS). These combined indications mean that ~30% to 35% of term neonates in the United States are exposed to antibiotics in the immediate perinatal period. Among extremely preterm neonates

Disclosure Statement: Dr. Mukhopadhyay is supported by funding from the Eunice Kennedy Shriver National Institutes of Child Health and Development through grant K23HD088753.
[a] Section on Newborn Medicine, Pennsylvania Hospital, Philadelphia, PA, USA; [b] Division of Neonatology, Children's Hospital of Philadelphia, Philadelphia, PA, USA; [c] Department of Pediatrics, University of Pennsylvania Perelman School of Medicine, Philadelphia, PA, USA; [d] CHOP Newborn Care, Pennsylvania Hospital, 800 Spruce Street, Philadelphia, PA 19107, USA
* Corresponding author. CHOP Newborn Care, Pennsylvania Hospital, 800 Spruce Street, Philadelphia, PA 19107.
E-mail address: Karen.Puopolo@pennmedicine.upenn.edu

cared for in the neonatal intensive care unit (NICU), antimicrobial exposure is even higher, averaging ~80% for very low-birth-weight (VLBW) neonates.[1] Antibiotics comprise 3 of the 4 most commonly prescribed medications in the NICU.[2] The frequency of antimicrobial administration and the critical, life-saving role these medications play in neonatal care, demand that the neonatal provider have detailed and current knowledge of their mode of action, spectrum of action, and potential toxicities. Over the last 2 decades, reports of highly resistant "superbugs" have called attention to inappropriate prescribing practices and prompted closer monitoring of resistance patterns.[3] Pharmacokinetic (PK) studies in the neonatal population have described dosing regimens that are specific to the unique physiology of neonates and can allow safer and more efficacious dosing. In this review, we will discuss parenteral antibiotics most commonly used in the management of perinatal bacterial infections.

ANTIMICROBIAL PHARMACOLOGY
Pharmacokinetic Considerations of Using Antimicrobials in Neonates

The effect of an antimicrobial medication on the neonate (pharmacodynamic effect) and the effect of the neonate's physiology on drug exposures (PK) depend on multiple factors that are distinct in neonates compared with older children and adults. Dynamic organ development, changing body composition, evolving gene/enzyme expression, and comorbid conditions (eg, prematurity) can all affect drug exposure, efficacy, and toxicity. A paucity of neonatal-specific studies contributes to the significant variation in dose recommendations characteristic of different formulary sources.[4] Standard regimens are often derived from older studies that are limited by lower representation of the extremely preterm neonate, use of intramuscular administration, small sample sizes, and extrapolation from older populations.[5] A study of NICU dosing regimens across 89 NICUs in 21 countries found significant variability across sites, with a tendency to use higher than recommended doses of penicillins and wide variability in vancomycin use.[6] The authors attributed this variability to the scarcity of neonatal studies, discrepancies between standard recommendations and regimens derived from newer PK studies, and difficulties in the dissemination of available information.

Dosing determinations for antimicrobials are based on achieving drug concentrations that are above the minimum inhibitory concentration (MIC) of a pathogen, the level at which an antimicrobial inhibits growth of the organism in vitro. Although a critical determinant of antimicrobial efficacy is attaining and maintaining in vivo drug concentrations above the infecting pathogen's MIC, antimicrobials differ in the exposure metrics associated with pathogen killing. Bacterial killing can depend on: (1) the peak concentration (C_{max}) relative to the MIC (concentration-dependent killing); (2) how long the serum level stays above the MIC (time-dependent killing); or (3) a combination of factors estimated by the total drug exposure, which is represented by the area under the concentration curve for a given dose (AUC-dependent killing). Examples of drugs with each characteristic and its implication for dosing are found in **Table 1**[7]. Initial concentrations depend on the volume of distribution of the drug. Preterm infants may need a higher dose to achieve the same concentration given their higher water content and larger volume of distribution. However, drug elimination is also affected by prematurity.[8] Most antimicrobials used for early infection depend on the kidneys for clearance (with the exception of nafcillin, cleared by the liver). Renal clearance is lower after birth and increases in the first 1 to 2 weeks of life. Neonates less than 32 to 34 weeks gestation often have significantly lower renal clearance than neonates born at older gestation. Because renal clearance increases with postnatal age, it often

Table 1
Pharmacodynamic considerations when dosing antimicrobials

Killing Pattern	Antimicrobial Drug	Goal of Dosing	PK/ Pharmacodynamic Parameter
Concentration-dependent killing	Aminoglycosides	Maximize peak (C_{max}) High dose, long dosing interval	C_{max}/MIC
Time-dependent killing	Penicillins Carbapenams Cephalosporins	Maximize duration of exposure above MIC Short dosing interval and long infusion times	% time > MIC
AUC-dependent killing	Vancomycin Fluconazole	Maximize C_{max} and duration of exposure above MIC. High dose and short interval	AUC_{24}/MIC

Adapted from Table 37-3, Remington and Klein's infectious disease of the fetus and newborn. 8th edition. Philadelphia: Elsevier Saunders; 2016; with permission.

remains lower among premature infants than among their than term counterparts during their NICU stay. Thus, PK studies in neonates often result in altered dosing schedules based on gestational age, postnatal age, and/or postmenstrual age to maintain similar drug exposure across different age groups.

Mechanisms of Antibiotic Action and Resistance

Parenteral antibiotics commonly used in neonates have 3 primary mechanisms of action: (1) disruption of the bacterial cell wall (beta-lactams and vancomycin inhibit peptidoglycan linking in bacterial cell wall); (2) inhibition of protein synthesis (aminoglycosides and macrolides bind to the 30s ribosomal subunit and clindamycin to the 50s ribosomal subunit, inhibiting translation); and (3) inhibition of nucleic acid function (metronidazole disrupts DNA structure and rifampin inhibits RNA formation required for DNA synthesis).[9] Although fluoroquinolones inhibit DNA replication and sulfonamides disrupt bacterial metabolic pathways, these antibiotics are rarely used in neonates.

Bacterial susceptibility to an antibiotic usually results from interference with a pathway essential for the organism's growth and survival. **Intrinsic resistance** occurs when the organism's inherent genotype and/or phenotype renders an antibiotic ineffective. Enterococci are intrinsically resistant to cephalosporins, as penicillin-binding protein these organisms produce does not bind to cephalosporins. Gram-negative organisms are resistant to vancomycin because the large size of the molecule prevents penetration through the outer lipid membrane. Similarly, the thick Gram-positive cell wall confers intrinsic resistance to aminoglycosides by slowing entry into the intracytoplasmic site of action. **Acquired resistance** can occur from nongenetic mechanisms (eg, nondividing bacteria), chromosomal mutation, or horizontal acquisition via mobile genetic elements (eg, transposons, plasmids). Beyond the natural tendency of organisms to acquire resistance, antimicrobial use exerts selection pressures for proliferation of resistant strains.[10] Various medical organizations have all recognized that judicious use of antibiotics is needed to prevent the spread of antimicrobial-resistant organisms.[11,12] Single-center and time-trend studies reveal increasing antimicrobial resistance in neonatal late-onset infections and increasing resistance among GBS and *Escherichia coli* isolates in early-onset infections.[13–17] The known

Table 2
Antibiotics used for intrapartum prophylaxis

Antibiotic	Intrapartum Indication	Placental Kinetics
Penicillin G[18]	Recommended for GBS prophylaxis	Cord blood levels > MIC for GBS <1 h after administration
Ampicillin[19–22]	Recommended for GBS prophylaxis	• Cord blood levels > MIC for GBS with 30 min of maternal administration • Rapid (<1 h after maternal dose) transfer into amniotic fluid • Neonatal serum levels > MIC for GBS at 4 h of age, if dose administered to mother >15 min before delivery
Cefazolin[23–25]	Recommended for GBS prophylaxis in case of mild maternal penicillin allergy (nonanaphylaxis)	• Cord blood levels > MIC GBS within 20 min of maternal administration
Clindamycin[26–28]	Recommended for GBS prophylaxis in case of serious maternal penicillin allergy *and* GBS isolate sensitive to clindamycin	• Cord blood levels ~50% of maternal levels and above MIC for GBS • Poor transfer into amniotic fluid
Vancomycin[29,30]	Recommended for GBS prophylaxis in case of maternal serious penicillin allergy *and* GBS isolate resistant to erythromycin or clindamycin	• Ex vivo placental studies predict cord blood levels <10% of maternal levels. • Study of 13 women demonstrated cord blood levels > MIC for GBS by 30 min after 60–90 min maternal infusion completed
Ampicillin and gentamicin[27,31]	Recommended when there is concern for intrapartum maternal intra-amniotic infection	• Gentamicin reaches lower levels in pregnant compared with nonpregnant women • Cord blood levels ~40% of maternal levels • Poor transfer into amniotic fluid
Cefazolin and gentamicin	Recommended when there is concern for intrapartum maternal intra-amniotic infection, in case of mild maternal penicillin allergy	
Vancomycin and gentamicin	Recommended when there is concern for intrapartum maternal intra-amniotic infection, in case of serious maternal penicillin allergy	

Ampicillin-sulbactam, piperacillin-tazobactam, cefoxitin, cefotetan, and ertapenem are alternative regimens for empiric treatment of maternal intra-amniotic infection.

resistance patterns of common pathogens combined with local antibiograms can inform antibiotic choices of empiric and definitive therapy (**Tables 2** and **3**).

Synergy

Combining beta-lactams with aminoglycosides to increase bactericidal potential occurs frequently in neonates. Synergy is defined as a combination of antimicrobials demonstrating greater activity (greater than 2 log bactericidal activity) against an organism compared with either used alone.[45] Synergy can compensate for some forms of antimicrobial resistance. For example, synergy between cell wall active

Table 3
Microbiology and antibiotic susceptibilities of EOS pathogens

Bacteria in EOS (% of cases)[a]	Ampicillin Susceptibility	Gentamicin Susceptibility	Cephalosporin Susceptibility	General Comments
GBS[32–34] (35.8%)	100% susceptible	Intrinsic resistance but when paired with a beta-lactam, aminoglycosides can act synergistically	100% susceptible	• Drug of choice: penicillin G; ampicillin is alternate • GBS meningitis: higher dose and longer therapy. Some guidelines include gentamicin for synergy (5 d). Complicated or unresponsive cases may require repeat CSF testing to determine therapy duration • Reports of high-level gentamicin-resistant GBS strains in adults with concern for loss of synergy
E coli[13,33,35,36] (24.8%)	~22% susceptible	~90% susceptible Combination therapy with a beta-lactam in meningitis	Case reports of ESBL E coli sepsis in NICUs after maternal travel in high-prevalence areas and in late-onset sepsis	• Drug of choice: based on susceptibility. Commonly cefotaxime • Reports of gentamicin resistance with retained susceptibility to amikacin • ESBL E coli treated with carbapenems • Peripartum transmission of ESBL E coli strains from mother to infant highlight possible role of maternal isolate data to inform antimicrobial choices in infants with poor response to standard empiric therapy

(continued on next page)

Table 3
(continued)

Bacteria in EOS (% of cases)[a]	Ampicillin Susceptibility	Gentamicin Susceptibility	Cephalosporin Susceptibility	General Comments
Viridans streptococci[34,37] (18.9%)	Variable susceptibility; population surveillance susceptibility 67%	Added for synergy in endocarditis in which isolate has intermediate-level resistance to penicillin	Majority susceptible (87% found susceptible to cefepime)	• Drug of choice: penicillin G when penicillin susceptible • Cephalosporin second line for penicillin-resistant strains • Alternate agent: vancomycin
H influenzae[34,38] (4.5%)	Worldwide susceptibility reported ~82%	Susceptible at baseline but not recommended for definitive therapy. Acquired resistance with use has been reported	Worldwide susceptibility high (100% to ceftriaxone)	• Drug of choice: ampicillin in susceptible variants. • Alternate: cephalosporins • Beta-lactamase-negative, ampicillin-resistant variants are difficult to test for susceptibility because the MIC are only slightly elevated from susceptible variants. Such cases may require use of cephalosporins
S aureus[33,39,40] (3.5%)	Most strains resistant due to production of beta lactamases	Susceptible at baseline but not recommended due to better alternates. Variable increase in resistance has been reported worldwide	Variable susceptibility	• Drug of choice for methicillin-sensitive S aureus: oxacillin or nafcillin have better outcomes than vancomycin. • Drug of choice for methicillin-resistant S aureus(MRSA): vancomycin • MRSA in EOS is still rare. In a population study of EOS pathogens S aureus accounted for 0.03 cases/1000 live births in USA and 1/23 cases were MRSA • Maternal history of MRSA colonization/disease can inform antimicrobial choices. • In cases of endocarditis and device-related MRSA infection, addition of gentamicin and rifampin is recommended

Organism				Drug of choice
Enterococcus spp (3.1%)	Enterococcus faecalis mostly sensitive and more frequent cause of EOS. E faecium largely resistant	Intrinsic resistance but has been used synergistically in endocarditis	Intrinsically resistant	• Drug of choice: Penicillin or ampicillin • Alternate: Vancomycin • Rare case reports of neonatal late-onset vancomycin-resistant enterococci treated with linezolid • Gentamicin not recommended if acquired high-level resistance is documented
Group D Streptococcus (1.4%), eg, S bovis	Universally susceptible	May be used for synergy	Susceptible	• Drug of choice: penicillin G
L monocytogenes (1.3%)[41]	Susceptible but bacteriostatic	Intracellular form of Listeria is protected from gentamicin. May be added for synergy	Intrinsically resistant	• Drug of choice: ampicillin with an aminoglycoside • Alternate agent: vancomycin • Reports of ampicillin resistance present in adults and in the food industry
Klebsiella pneumoniae[11,42] (<1%) and other Enterobacteriaceae	Increasingly resistant	Susceptible at baseline. Acquired resistance has been described. Amikacin susceptibility may be retained despite gentamicin resistance	Susceptible. ESBL isolates most cephalosporins including cefepime	• Drug of choice: based on susceptibility with ampicillin or cefotaxime • ESBL pathogen – drug of choice is a carbapenem • K pneumoniae is the most common ESBL Enterobacteriaceae reported in NICU, in late-onset sepsis. Risk factors includes prior antibiotic exposure • Synergistic therapy with gentamicin in meningitis has been recommended
Streptococcus pneumoniae[11] (<1%) and other Gram-positive cocci	Increasing penicillin resistance	Intrinsic resistance	Variable susceptibility	• Drug of choice: based on susceptibility, penicillin or cephalosporin if susceptible and vancomycin with rifampin if penicillin and cephalosporin resistant

[a] Top 10 pathogens associated with invasive EOS occurring 2005–2014 in the United States using absolute frequencies.[33] Resistant patterns are noted in perinatal infection only for GBS and E coli. Remaining susceptible patterns are based on case reports or information on older infants and adults[43,44].

beta-lactams and aminoglycosides can overcome intrinsic resistance by allowing the aminoglycoside to penetrate the cell wall.[46,47] Synergism is used for highly invasive and difficult to sterilize GBS or enterococcal infections, such as endocarditis, meningitis, or infections associated with medical devices. Although both GBS and enterococci can acquire modes of resistance to aminoglycosides, which will render synergy ineffective,[32] some experts recommend treating GBS meningitis with a beta-lactam antibiotic and gentamicin until cerebrospinal fluid (CSF) sterility is achieved,[48] and others recommend using both drugs for the first 5 days of therapy before completing treatment with a beta-lactam alone.[49] However, clinical demonstration of in vitro synergy has been inconsistent and no advantage was found for using a beta-lactam with aminoglycoside versus using beta-lactams alone in a meta-analysis of 69 trials of adult sepsis, with a higher incidence of renal injury with combination therapy.[50]

INTRAPARTUM ANTIMICROBIAL PROPHYLAXIS
Prevention of Perinatal Infection with Group B Streptococcus

Transplacental fetal exposure to intrapartum maternally administered antibiotics is the most common form of perinatal antibiotic treatment. Intrapartum antibiotic prophylaxis to prevent early-onset GBS disease (GBS EOD) is the primary indication for perinatal antibiotic administration. GBS emerged as an important cause of EOS in the United States in the 1970s, and subsequent studies identified maternal gastrointestinal and genitourinary colonization with GBS as the primary risk factor for GBS-specific EOS. The high rate of vertical transmission ($\sim$50%) and subsequent infection ($\sim$1% of infants born to colonized mothers become infected) and the severity of GBS-associated morbidity and mortality prompted the search for public health approaches to disease prevention. Current recommendations focus on universal antenatal screening of pregnant women for GBS colonization using vaginal-rectal cultures obtained at 35 to 37 weeks gestation or in the event of preterm labor or preterm rupture of membranes.[51] Antibiotics used for IAP include penicillin G, ampicillin, cefazolin, clindamycin, and vancomycin (see **Table 2**). Intrapartum antibiotic prophylaxis is hypothesized to prevent neonatal GBS disease in 3 ways: (1) by temporarily decreasing maternal colonization burden; (2) by preventing surface and mucus membrane colonization of the fetus/neonate; and (3) by reaching the MIC of the antibiotic for killing GBS.[19,20]

Penicillin G and Ampicillin

Penicillin G and ampicillin are beta-lactam antibiotics that differ in structure by a single amino group. These antibiotics inhibit bacterial cell synthesis and are bactericidal. Although penicillin G is metabolized in the liver, it is largely excreted unchanged in urine. Group B streptococcus remains susceptible to beta-lactam antibiotics with ampicillin and penicillin G best studied for their role as GBS IAP. Maternally administered penicillin G readily crosses the placenta, reaches cord blood peak levels by 1 hour, and rapidly declines by 4 hours reflecting elimination of the antibiotic by the fetal kidney into amniotic fluid.[18] Both peak and nadir cord blood levels are above the GBS MIC when administered to the mother every 4 hours. Ampicillin has been detected in cord blood within 30 minutes and in amniotic fluid within 45 minutes of maternal administration.[19] One study measured ampicillin levels in 115 newborns after maternal IAP and detected levels above the GBS MIC at 4 hours of age when maternal dosing occurred at least 15 minutes before delivery.[21] Ampicillin IAP has been shown to decrease maternal vaginal colonization within 2 hours of administration and to prevent neonatal surface colonization in 97% to 100% of cases if IAP was given at least 4 hours before delivery.[20,22]

Cefazolin

Cefazolin is a first-generation cephalosporin. Like ampicillin and penicillin, cefazolin inhibits cell wall synthesis and is bactericidal. The drug is recommended for GBS IAP for women with nonanaphylaxis penicillin allergy. Cefazolin rapidly crosses the placenta and is detected in cord blood at levels above the GBS MIC within 20 minutes after maternal administration.[23,24] One study included 25 women administered cefazolin 20 minutes to 7 hours before planned Cesarean section delivery. Cord blood and amniotic fluid levels of cefazolin above the GBS MIC were detected in virtually all cases regardless of the timing relative to delivery.[25]

Clindamycin

Clindamycin is a synthetic lincosamide antibiotic derivative recommended for IAP among women with serious (anaphylaxis) penicillin allergy if the colonizing GBS isolate is sensitive. Clindamycin inhibits bacterial protein synthesis and is considered bacteriostatic. Few data inform the potential effectiveness of clindamycin as GBS IAP. One study of GBS-positive women found that vaginal cultures had no viable GBS if clindamycin was administered 4 hours before delivery.[26] In another study, peak cord blood levels of clindamycin occurred ~20 minutes after the maternal dose was given, but levels were only ~50% of simultaneous maternal levels.[27] Clindamycin was not detected in amniotic fluid in 9 specimens obtained 30 to 90 minutes after maternal dose. Clindamycin is metabolized by the liver; 1 study of oral maternally administered clindamycin found the drug concentrates in fetal liver but accumulates in amniotic fluid only after multiple maternal doses.[28]

Group B streptococcus are increasingly resistant to clindamycin as well as to macrolide antibiotics such as erythromycin. The same genetic elements responsible for clindamycin resistance also cause erythromycin resistance.[52] Antibiotic sensitivity testing for GBS should include erythromycin and clindamycin; strains identified as erythromycin resistant but clindamycin sensitive should also be assessed by D-test to identify inducible clindamycin resistance. Clindamycin resistance was identified in 12.7% of ~3500 tested GBS isolates collected in 4 states from 1998 to 2003, with an increasing trend over time.[53] Erythromycin resistance was also identified in one-third of all GBS isolates and is no longer recommended for GBS IAP. One report from Canada in 2010 to 2011 found 26.6% of 158 GBS isolates resistant,[54] whereas another study in upstate New York found resistance in 38.4% of 688 GBS isolates.[55] The bacteriostatic mechanism of antimicrobial action, incomplete placental transfer and unclear fetal/neonatal PK suggest that clindamycin may not provide the same level of protection from GBS infection as provided by beta-lactam antibiotic IAP, even with susceptible isolates.

Vancomycin

Group B streptococci are universally sensitive to vancomycin, a bactericidal glycopeptide antibiotic that inhibits cell wall synthesis of Gram-positive bacteria. Vancomycin is recommended for GBS IAP in women with serious (anaphylaxis) penicillin allergy if colonized with clindamycin-resistant GBS. Ex vivo studies with placental lobules suggest that vancomycin crosses the placental poorly, with fetal-side blood levels only ~10% of maternal levels.[29] In contrast, a study of 13 women undergoing elective Cesarean section delivery found that cord blood levels of vancomycin above the GBS MIC could be achieved within 30 minutes of maternal drug administration.[30] No data were reported in this study concerning amniotic fluid or newborn blood levels of vancomycin after birth. As with clindamycin, there is insufficient evidence to inform the efficacy of vancomycin for prevention of neonatal GBS disease.

Prevention of All-Bacterial Cause Early-Onset Sepsis

The American College of Obstetricians and Gynecologists (ACOG) recommends the use of IAP for the prevention of neonatal EOS when there is concern for suspected or confirmed maternal IAI. ACOG guidance defines a *confirmed* diagnosis of IAI as that made by amniotic fluid Gram stain and/or culture or by placental histopathology. *Suspected* IAI is defined by maternal intrapartum fever (either a single maternal intrapartum temperature $\geq 39.0°C$ or persistent temperature of $38.0°C–38.9°C$) in combination with maternal leukocytosis, purulent cervical drainage, and/or fetal tachycardia. In addition, current ACOG guidance is for the administration of IAP when otherwise unexplained maternal fever occurs in isolation. Recommended intrapartum antibiotic regimens for treatment of confirmed or suspected IAI or isolated fever include ampicillin, cefazolin, clindamycin, or vancomycin, each in combination with gentamicin.[31]

ANTIMICROBIAL THERAPY FOR NEONATAL EARLY-ONSET SEPSIS
Early-Onset Sepsis

Neonatal EOS is defined as blood or CSF culture-confirmed infection that occurs 0 to 6 days after birth.[51] This is the primary indication for antibiotic use in the immediate neonatal period. Antibacterial choice for empiric therapy is based on the population epidemiology of EOS, whereas definitive therapy is tailored to the specific organism cultured and to the reported antimicrobial susceptibilities. The 2 most frequent EOS pathogens in United States are GBS (0.22 cases per 1000 live births) and *E coli* (0.18 cases per 1000 live births).[33] The proportionate contribution of *E coli* to EOS has increased with decreasing incidence of early-onset GBS disease, such that it is the most common pathogen in some areas[17,33] and in the VLBW population.[56] Fungal species (most commonly *Candida albicans* and *Candida parapsilosis*) account for less than 1% of EOS cases and occur primarily among VLBW infants[57]; therapy for fungal EOS will not be addressed in this review. Early-onset sepsis remains a significant cause of neonatal morbidity; mortality is unusual (<2%) among infected term infants, but is as high as 30% to 50% among neonates born less than 29 weeks gestation.[58,59]

Choice of Empiric Therapy for Early-Onset Sepsis

The most frequent choice for empiric EOS therapy is a beta-lactam such as ampicillin plus gentamicin.[1,3] This combination provides adequate coverage for most common Gram-positive pathogens including GBS, viridans streptococci, *Enterococcus* sp and *Listeria monocytogenes*, as well as *E coli* and other Gram-negative bacteria. However, the evolving resistance patterns in *E coli* have led to concerns about the adequacy of current empiric choices.[17] In a multistate surveillance report of EOS cases, 78% of the *E coli* isolates were resistant to ampicillin and 10% resistant to gentamicin.[33] In addition, 24/25 cases of gentamicin-resistant strains were also resistant to ampicillin. A single center report from Spain similarly found that, among 65 *E coli* isolates over 21 years, 75% were resistant to ampicillin and 12% to gentamicin.[17]

Few randomized trials have compared neonatal empiric regimens, and a 2004 Cochrane review found insufficient studies to determine an optimal regimen.[60] An open-label, cluster-randomized trial among 283 neonates with suspected EOS compared regimens of gentamicin combined with either ampicillin or penicillin and found no difference in treatment failure. A trend to increased all-cause mortality was observed among infants born less than 26 weeks gestation treated with penicillin, unexplained by early mortality or later colonization.[61,62] Most other studies have been observational in design. The NeonIN prospective surveillance study across multiple units in the United Kingdom over a period of 10 years found that the combination of penicillin or aminopenicillin and an aminoglycoside provided 93% to 96% coverage, with better performance of ampicillin (versus penicillin) in the preterm population.[3] In a cohort of 258 neonates with E coli bacteremia, 123 (48%) cases had ampicillin-resistant isolates. Neonates with ampicillin-resistant E coli were more likely to be born to mothers treated with antenatal antibiotics but were otherwise similar. There were no overall difference in mortality and no effect of the composition of the empiric antibiotic regimen on 30-day mortality or duration of bacteremia.[63]

Although third-generation cephalosporin susceptibility remains high in E coli, multiple factors argue against use of cephalosporins as initial empiric therapy. A study investigating the odds of neonatal mortality in 24,111 episodes of empiric ampicillin/cefotaxime use with 104,803 episodes of empiric ampicillin/gentamicin use in the first 21 days of life, found a significant increased odds of mortality with cefotaxime when controlling for multiple patient-level characteristics.[64] Other studies have associated cephalosporin use with increased risk of subsequent fungal infection[65] and selection of highly resistant organisms.[10] Cefotaxime lacks intrinsic activity against other common early pathogens such as Listeria and Enterococcus. In addition, although ~80% of VLBW infants are started on empiric therapy,[1] only ~5% will have an E coli infection.[66] Most of these isolates will be sensitive to gentamicin. Thus, ampicillin and gentamicin remains the optimal empiric choice, with broader spectrum use limited to high-risk infants with poor response or when preliminary microbiologic results identify Gram-negative organisms.

Antibiotics Used in Management of Early-Onset Sepsis

In the following sections we describe the common antimicrobials used for EOS in the NICU and factors that determine use (**Table 3**). Specific dose recommendations can be found in available formularies and the AAP Red Book.

Ampicillin

As noted above, ampicillin is a semisynthetic formulation derived from penicillin in which the extra amino groups increase its penetration in the Gram-negative cell membrane, broadening its antimicrobial activity. It is indicated for treatment of EOS with L monocytogenes, susceptible Haemophilus influenzae, Streptococcus spp, Enterococcus spp, and Gram-negative organisms when susceptibility has been documented.

Ampicillin mediates time-dependent bacterial killing, and frequent dosing allows the drug concentration to remain above the MIC for prolonged periods, which is thought to improve efficacy. Because ampicillin undergoes renal clearance, neonates (both premature and term) with relatively immature renal function will maintain required levels with less frequent dosing. Although this is also the case for infants with acute renal dysfunction, ampicillin doses are rarely adjusted for renal insufficiency owing to lack of neonatal PK data and relatively low drug toxicity. An open-label PK study of 28 infants born at less than 34 weeks gestation and 45 infants born at greater than 34 weeks gestation demonstrated a significant increase in clearance with increasing gestation and postnatal age.[67] This supports gestation-specific dosing regimens to achieve the required drug exposure above MIC for GBS and E coli. Ampicillin-associated adverse effects in older children, such as diarrhea, rash, and increased bleeding tendency are rarely reported in neonates. Increased colonization with *Klebsiella pneumonia* has been noted with empiric early use compared with penicillin use.[61] Increased risk of seizures have been shown with high doses in simulated models,[68] which emphasize the need for PK and toxicity studies in neonates.

Gentamicin

Aminoglycosides irreversibly bind to the 30s subunit of the bacterial ribosome, inhibiting protein synthesis and ultimately killing the organism. Gentamicin, tobramycin, and amikacin are the most frequently used aminoglycosides in neonates.[2] Tobramycin provides superior coverage for most strains of *Pseudomonas*, and amikacin may be chosen for treatment of gentamicin-resistant organisms.[17] But, in the absence of drug shortage, gentamicin remains the most appropriate choice for empiric therapy for EOS. Although many Gram-negative organisms are susceptible to aminoglycosides, concern for cumulative toxicity with prolonged therapy and poor outcomes in adult patients with Gram-negative sepsis managed with aminoglycoside monotherapy[69] has led to gentamicin being used mainly in combination therapy.

Extended-interval, high-dose regimens in neonatal EOS are designed to achieve peak concentrations over MIC of 8 to 10, while still achieving trough concentrations of less than 2 mg/L.[70] Aminoglycoside peak concentrations above MIC are related to bacterial killing. Higher doses are needed in preterm neonates to achieve a similar peak concentration due their greater volume of distribution. Because gentamicin is eliminated through the kidneys, neonates with renal immaturity or injury clear the drug less efficiently. As a result, longer dosing intervals are recommended in premature neonates, neonates with kidney injury, and neonates in the first few days of life when renal clearance is lower. Retrospective analysis of clinically obtained gentamicin levels in 994 preterm and 455 term infants found a significant effect of gestational age and postnatal age on drug clearance.[71] This study validated the need for higher doses (5 mg/kg/dose) in extremely preterm neonates along with extended frequency of dosing (every 48 hours) to reach required therapeutic targets. Longer interval dosing of every 36 hours has also been recommended for neonates with hypoxic injury undergoing therapeutic hypothermia to obtain required trough levels.[72] The prevalence of renal and ototoxicity is difficult to establish in neonates due to multiple competing factors. Prolonged therapy and therapy in neonates with significant renal compromise should be managed by following serum drug levels to ensure appropriate trough levels.

Cefotaxime

Cefotaxime is the most common systemic cephalosporin used in neonates.[2] A broad-spectrum, low-toxicity antibiotic with excellent CSF penetration,[73] cefotaxime targets specific penicillin-binding proteins, which results in an extended spectrum compared with ampicillin. Cefotaxime is most frequently added to empiric regimens to broaden coverage against Gram-negative bacilli (particularly when ampicillin-resistant *E coli* is a concern) or provide coverage in suspected meningitis. Cefepime and ceftazidime may be used when cefotaxime is unavailable, but the very broad-spectrum coverage provided by these antibiotics (eg, for *Pseudomonas* and other extended spectrum beta-lactamase [ESBL] organisms) is not currently indicated for empiric treatment of neonatal EOS. Ceftriaxone is rarely used in newborns due to its high avidity for serum albumin and increased risk of hyperbilirubinemia, as well as its incompatibility with calcium-containing fluids.

Similar to ampicillin and other renally cleared drugs with time-dependent killing, low-dose, frequent-interval regimens maximize the time cefotaxime levels remains above

MIC. A study using scavenged blood specimens from 100 neonates born at 23 to 42 weeks gestation found that failure to shorten the dosing interval after the first week among neonates born greater than 32 weeks gestation was associated with subtherapeutic cefotaxime levels. This study recommended interval adjustments by gestational age at birth as well as by postnatal age.[74] Adverse drug reactions with cephalosporins (including allergy, diarrhea, bleeding, seizures, bone marrow suppression) have been primarily reported in adults. As noted above, neonatal cephalosporin use is associated with increased fungal colonization, infection, and increased mortality.[10,64]

Penicillin

Penicillin G is a water-soluble intravenous formulation with a narrow spectrum and a long therapeutic history of use in neonates. Other formulations used include benzathine and procaine penicillin that allow for slow release from deep intramuscular injections and are indicated for management of congenital syphilis. Penicillin and an aminoglycoside are used in combination as empiric therapy in some neonates,[3] but not commonly in the United States. Penicillin remains the recommended definitive therapy for GBS, groups C and G streptococci, *Treponema pallidum*, and susceptible strains of viridans streptococci and enterococci.[34]

Pathogen killing by penicillin is determined by the time for which unbound drug in the serum remains above the MIC. It is recommended that levels be above the MIC for ~50% of the dosing interval. Like other beta-lactam antibiotics, penicillin is cleared by the kidney and interval adjustments should be made for preterm neonates and term neonates in the first days after birth.[75] A study of 18 infants born less than 28 weeks gestation found that a common penicillin dose recommendation (50,000 units/kg/dose every 12 h) resulted in peak and trough concentrations in these infants that exceeded the MIC_{90} value for GBS (MIC value that inhibits 90% of isolates) by 1000- and 100-fold, respectively. Current recommendations involve much higher doses for treatment of GBS meningitis[34] (250,000–450, 000 units/kg/d in 3 divided doses). The authors of that study noted that, even with reduced penicillin penetration of the blood brain barrier (CSF: serum concentration ratio of ~5%–10%),[76] current regimens would consistently exceed MIC for GBS in the CSF, an observation that has been made by others.[7] Such studies highlight the difficulties of optimizing dosing recommendations among high-risk very preterm neonates with serious infections.

Piperacillin-Tazobactum

A semisynthetic beta-lactam, piperacillin is a broad-spectrum antibiotic with activity against *Staphylococcus aureus*, most *Streptococcus* sp, *H influenzae*, *Neisseria meningitidis*, *L monocytogenes*, multiple Gram-negative rods, and many anaerobes. The tazobactum component acts to protect the piperacillin component from beta-lactamase degradation. This antibiotic is infrequently indicated in the immediate neonatal period and more commonly used for late-onset sepsis and necrotizing enterocolitis. Piperacillin-tazobactam use showed the highest absolute increase from 2005 to 2010 among antimicrobials used in 305 NICUs in the United States.[2] Its wide spectrum includes anaerobes, and its safety profile makes it a useful choice in polymicrobial infection and in cases of intra-abdominal pathology. Whereas some ESBL-producing Enterobacteriaceae demonstrate in vitro sensitivity to piperacillin-tazobactam, carbepenems remain the recommended drug of choice,[34] with superior results demonstrated in adults.[77]

As with most penicillins, piperacillin-tazobactam mediates time-dependent killing, with renal clearance that increases with gestational and postnatal age. A PK study in 71 neonates born 26 to 41 weeks gestation found that birth weight and postmenstrual age significantly affected the dosing regimen.[78] Another study of 32 neonates born at 23 to 40 weeks gestation found that postmenstrual age alone was adequate to determine dosing regimen and that prolonged infusions were not necessary to achieve therapeutic targets.[79] Adverse effects are rarely noted in neonates.[80]

Meropenem

Meropenem is a carbapenem beta-lactam antibiotic with a broad spectrum against *Pseudomonas* and ESBL-producing bacteria. Unlike imipenem, it is labeled for use in premature neonates by the US Food and Drug Administration. Methicillin-resistant staphylococci and most enterococci are resistant to meropenem. Meropenem is the drug of choice when an ESBL bacteria is isolated, or when there is known maternal ESBL colonization in a neonate with suspicion of EOS.

Meropenem also mediates time-dependent killing with renal clearance and requires interval adjustments with increases in gestational and postnatal age. A significant impact of postmenstrual age and serum creatinine levels was reported in a prospective PK study of 188 neonates born at 23 to 40 weeks gestation with suspected intra-abdominal infection.[81] Although CSF levels measured in 9 neonates were variable, they were consistently above the therapeutic target. Meropenem is considered safer than imipenem for decreasing the seizure threshold by binding with GABA receptors in the brain.[7] In a review of adverse events associated with meropenem administration in 200 neonates, only 2 cases were considered drug related, including 1 case of fungal infection.[82] In a randomized control trial of 102 infants with late-onset, Gram-negative sepsis, continuous infusion of meropenem compared with intermittent bolus dosing was associated with less renal dysfunction.[83]

Vancomycin

This glycopeptide acts by inhibiting peptidoglycan cell wall formation and is infrequently indicated shortly after birth. Vancomycin is primarily used for beta-lactam-resistant organisms such as enterococci, staphylococci, and *Streptococcus pneumoniae*.[34]

Vancomycin is excreted unchanged by the kidneys and demonstrates time-dependent killing that is best reflected in 24-hour area under the curve (AUC_{24}) for serum concentration divided by MIC. Neonatal vancomycin dosing regimens remain subject to debate.[6,84] In adults, efficacy is associated with doses that achieve an exposure target of AUC/MIC greater than 400 or serum steady-state trough levels of 15 to 20 mg/L. The latter has been determined to be a useful surrogate measure of AUC/MIC 400 when the MIC is ≤ 1 mg/L.[85] However, in neonates, a trough level of 7 to 11 mg/L resulted in ~90% of cases attaining AUC_{24} greater than 400.[86] This AUC/MIC efficacy exposure target is difficult to achieve for organisms with an MIC greater than 1 mg/L.[84] Nephrotoxicity and ototoxicity along with rash, red man syndrome, and altered colonization have been reported in adults with vancomycin use, but the incidence among neonates is unclear.[84] Overall, the unexplained variability of drug exposure in PK studies supports the use of trough drug levels to tailor prolonged management.[87]

Oxacillin/Nafcillin

These semisynthetic derivatives of penicillins are not affected by penicillinases produced by staphylococci. In adults with methicillin-sensitive *S aureus* infection, the use of beta-lactam antibiotics is associated with improved survival compared with vancomycin.[39] Oxacillin/nafcillin are the drugs of choice for methicillin-sensitive *S aureus*, which is isolated in neonatal EOS in less than 5% of cases.[33] Nafcillin is cleared by the liver and oxacillin by the kidney. Few recent studies have informed neonatal PK dosing.[5,88] Both drugs have a similar safety profile to other penicillins and demonstrate time-dependent killing.

SUMMARY

Monitoring the incidence and microbiology of perinatal infections is critical to informing the choice of antibiotic for infection prophylaxis and therapy. Changes in antimicrobial susceptibilities of common pathogens and increasing survival of extremely preterm neonates highlight the inadequacies of available drug information for the neonate. The goals of antibiotic therapy should be to attain the desired effect with minimal toxicity for the individual while reducing selection pressures for the unit and the community. Placental antibiotic kinetics and neonatal-specific PK studies are needed to better define optimal prophylactic and therapeutic dosing regimens for perinatal infection prevention and treatment.

Best Practices

What is the current practice for choosing drugs for the prevention and treatment of sepsis in the newborn?

Best practices and guidelines

- Guidelines for use of maternal intrapartum antibiotic prophylaxis to prevent neonatal early-onset sepsis caused by group B *Streptococcus* and other perinatal pathogens are provided by the Centers for Disease Control and Prevention, the American College of Obstetrics and Gynecology, the American Academy of Pediatrics

- Guidance on the administration of empiric antibiotics owing to concern for neonatal early-onset sepsis is informed by national epidemiologic data and provided by the American Academy of Pediatrics

- Optimal antibiotic choice for the administration of empiric antibiotics owing to concern for neonatal early-onset sepsis can also be informed by local data on the antibiotic sensitivity profiles of local infecting organisms

Major recommendations

- Review and use national guidance on intrapartum and neonatal antibiotic choice for prevention and empiric treatment of neonatal early-onset sepsis

- Collaborate with infection control personnel to obtain local data on the antibiotic sensitivity profiles of infecting organisms to optimize empiric antibiotic choice

- Minimize prolonged use of antibiotics when cultures are sterile

- Use the narrowest-spectrum effective antibiotic when antibiotic sensitivity data are obtained for infecting organisms

- Account for the gestational age, postnatal age, and renal and liver function of the individual infant when choosing drug dose and dosing interval

Summary statement

Optimal drug choices for neonatal sepsis prevention and treatment are informed by microbiologic data, use the narrowest-spectrum effective antibiotic, and account for gestational age, postnatal age, and organ function to optimize antibiotic effectiveness, minimize drug toxicities, and avoid resistance-promoting selection pressures.

Data from Refs.[31,33,51,89–91]

REFERENCES

1. Flannery DD, Ross RK, Mukhopadhyay S, et al. Temporal trends and center variation in early antibiotic use among premature infants. JAMA Netw Open 2018; 1(1):e180164.
2. Hsieh EM, Hornik CP, Clark RH, et al. Medication use in the neonatal intensive care unit. Am J Perinatol 2014;31(9):811–21.
3. Cailes B, Kortsalioudaki C, Buttery J, et al. Antimicrobial resistance in UK neonatal units: NeonIN infection surveillance network. Arch Dis Child Fetal Neonatal Ed 2018;103(5):F474–8.
4. Dallefeld S, Hornik CD, Zimmerman K, et al. Antibiotic dosing considerations for term and preterm infants. In: Bentiz WE, Smith PB, editors. Neonatology questions and controversies: infectious disease and pharmacology. 1st edition. Philadelphia: Elsevier; 2018. p. 167.
5. Pacifici GM. Clinical pharmacokinetics of penicillins, cephalosporins and aminoglycosides in the neonate: a review. Pharmaceuticals (Basel) 2010;3(8):2568–91.
6. Metsvaht T, Nellis G, Varendi H, et al. High variability in the dosing of commonly used antibiotics revealed by a Europe-wide point prevalence study: implications for research and dissemination. BMC Pediatr 2015;15:41.
7. Wade KC, Benjamin DK. Chapter 37: clinical pharmacology of anti-infective drugs. In: Wilson CB, Nizet V, Maldonado YA, et al, editors. Remington and Klein's Infectious Diseases of the Fetus and Newborn Infant. 8th edition. Philadelphia: Elsevier Saunders; 2016. p. 1160–211.
8. Bueva A, Guignard J. Renal function in preterm neonates. Pediatr Res 1994; 36(5):572.
9. Neu HC, Gootz TD. Antimicrobial chemotherapy. In: Baron S, editor. Medical Microbiology. 4th edition. Galveston (TX): University of Texas Medical Branch at Galveston; 1996. Chapter 11. Available at: https://www.ncbi.nlm.nih.gov/books/NBK7986/. Accessed August 22, 2018.
10. Le J, Nguyen T, Okamoto M, et al. Impact of empiric antibiotic use on development of infections caused by extended-spectrum beta-lactamase bacteria in a neonatal intensive care unit. Pediatr Infect Dis J 2008;27(4):314–8.
11. Centers of disease control and prevention. Threat report 2013 2013. Available at: http://www.cdc.gov/drugresistance/threat-report-2013/. Accessed August 22, 2018.
12. Society for Healthcare Epidemiology of America, Infectious Diseases Society of America, Pediatric Infectious Diseases Society. Policy statement on antimicrobial stewardship by the society for healthcare epidemiology of America (SHEA), the infectious diseases society of America (IDSA), and the pediatric infectious diseases society (PIDS). Infect Control Hosp Epidemiol 2012;33(4):322–7.
13. Oteo J, Cercenado E, Fernandez-Romero S, et al. Extended-spectrum-beta-lactamase-producing Escherichia coli as a cause of pediatric infections: report of a neonatal intensive care unit outbreak due to a CTX-M-14-producing strain. Antimicrob Agents Chemother 2012;56(1):54–8.
14. Cantey JB, Sreeramoju P, Jaleel M, et al. Prompt control of an outbreak caused by extended-spectrum beta-lactamase-producing Klebsiella pneumoniae in a neonatal intensive care unit. J Pediatr 2013;163(3):672–9.e1-3.
15. Carr D, Barnes EH, Gordon A, et al. Effect of antibiotic use on antimicrobial antibiotic resistance and late-onset neonatal infections over 25 years in an Australian tertiary neonatal unit. Arch Dis Child Fetal Neonatal Ed 2017;102(3):F244–50.

16. Schrag SJ, Zell ER, Lynfield R, et al. A population-based comparison of strategies to prevent early-onset group B streptococcal disease in neonates. N Engl J Med 2002;347(4):233–9.

17. Mendoza-Palomar N, Balasch-Carulla M, Gonzalez-Di Lauro S, et al. *Escherichia coli* early-onset sepsis: trends over two decades. Eur J Pediatr 2017;176(9): 1227–34.

18. Barber EL, Zhao G, Buhimschi IA, et al. Duration of intrapartum prophylaxis and concentration of penicillin G in fetal serum at delivery. Obstet Gynecol 2008;112(2 Pt 1):265–70.

19. Yow MD, Mason EO, Leeds LJ, et al. Ampicillin prevents intrapartum transmission of group B streptococcus. JAMA 1979;241(12):1245–7.

20. Boyer KM, Gadzala CA, Kelly PD, et al. Selective intrapartum chemoprophylaxis of neonatal group B streptococcal early-onset disease. III. interruption of mother-to-infant transmission. J Infect Dis 1983;148(5):810–6.

21. Berardi A, Rossi C, Creti R, et al. Group B streptococcal colonization in 160 mother-baby pairs: a prospective cohort study. J Pediatr 2013;163(4):1099–10104.e1.

22. de Cueto M, Sanchez MJ, Sampedro A, et al. Timing of intrapartum ampicillin and prevention of vertical transmission of group B streptococcus. Obstet Gynecol 1998;91(1):112–4.

23. Brown CE, Christmas JT, Bawdon RE. Placental transfer of cefazolin and piperacillin in pregnancies remote from term complicated by Rh isoimmunization. Am J Obstet Gynecol 1990;163(3):938–43.

24. Groff SM, Fallatah W, Yang S, et al. Effect of maternal obesity on maternal-fetal transfer of preoperative cefazolin at cesarean section. J Pediatr Pharmacol Ther 2017;22(3):227–32.

25. Fiore Mitchell T, Pearlman MD, Chapman RL, et al. Maternal and transplacental pharmacokinetics of cefazolin. Obstet Gynecol 2001;98(6):1075–9.

26. Knight KM, Thornburg LL, McNanley AR, et al. The effect of intrapartum clindamycin on vaginal group B streptococcus colony counts. J Matern Fetal Neonatal Med 2012;25(6):747–9.

27. Weinstein AJ, Gibbs RS, Gallagher M. Placental transfer of clindamycin and gentamicin in term pregnancy. Am J Obstet Gynecol 1976;124(7):688–91.

28. Philipson A, Sabath LD, Charles D. Transplacental passage of erythromycin and clindamycin. N Engl J Med 1973;288(23):1219–21.

29. Nanovskaya T, Patrikeeva S, Zhan Y, et al. Transplacental transfer of vancomycin and telavancin. Am J Obstet Gynecol 2012;207(4):331.e1–6.

30. Laiprasert J, Klein K, Mueller BA, et al. Transplacental passage of vancomycin in noninfected term pregnant women. Obstet Gynecol 2007;109(5):1105–10.

31. Heine RP, Puopolo KM, Beigi R, et al. Committee on obstetric practice. committee opinion no. 712: intrapartum management of intraamniotic infection. Obstet Gynecol 2017;130(2):e95.

32. Sendi P, Furitsch M, Mauerer S, et al. Chromosomally and extrachromosomally mediated high-level gentamicin resistance in streptococcus agalactiae. Antimicrob Agents Chemother 2016;60(3):1702–7.

33. Schrag SJ, Farley MM, Petit S, et al. Epidemiology of invasive early-onset neonatal sepsis, 2005 to 2014. Pediatrics 2016;138(6). https://doi.org/10.1542/peds.2016-2013.

34. American Academy of Pediatrics. In: Kimberlin DW, Brady MT, Jackson MA, Long SS, editors. Red Book: 2018 Report of the Committee on Infectious Diseases. Itasca, IL: American Academy of Pediatrics; 2018.

35. Hayat S, Berry N, Lewis A, et al. An outbreak of ESBL-producing *E. coli* in a NICU.

36. Peretz A, Skuratovsky A, Khabra E, et al. Peripartum maternal transmission of extended-spectrum beta-lactamase organism to newborn infants. Diagn Microbiol Infect Dis 2017;87(2):168–71.

37. Diekema DJ, Beach ML, Pfaller MA, et al, SENTRY Participants Group. Antimicrobial resistance in viridans group streptococci among patients with and without the diagnosis of cancer in the USA, Canada and Latin America. Clin Microbiol Infect 2001;7(3):152–7.

38. Tristram S, Jacobs MR, Appelbaum PC. Antimicrobial resistance in *Haemophilus influenzae*. Clin Microbiol Rev 2007;20(2):368–89.

39. McDanel JS, Perencevich EN, Diekema DJ, et al. Comparative effectiveness of beta-lactams versus vancomycin for treatment of methicillin-susceptible *Staphylococcus aureus* bloodstream infections among 122 hospitals. Clin Infect Dis 2015;61(3):361–7.

40. Schmitz FJ, Fluit AC, Gondolf M, et al. The prevalence of aminoglycoside resistance and corresponding resistance genes in clinical isolates of staphylococci from 19 European hospitals. J Antimicrob Chemother 1999;43(2):253–9.

41. Wilson CB, Nizet V, Maldonado YA, et al. Remington and Klein's infectious diseases of the fetus and newborn infant. Philadelphia: Elseiver; 2016.

42. Li X, Xu X, Yang X, et al. Risk factors for infection and/or colonisation with extended-spectrum beta-lactamase-producing bacteria in the neonatal intensive care unit: a meta-analysis. Int J Antimicrob Agents 2017;50(5):622–8.

43. Pfaller MA, Jones RN, Doern GV, et al. Bacterial pathogens isolated from patients with bloodstream infection: frequencies of occurrence and antimicrobial susceptibility patterns from the SENTRY antimicrobial surveillance program (United States and Canada, 1997). Antimicrob Agents Chemother 1998;42(7):1762–70.

44. Diekema DJ, Pfaller MA, Jones RN, SENTRY Participants Group. Age-related trends in pathogen frequency and antimicrobial susceptibility of bloodstream isolates in north America: SENTRY antimicrobial surveillance program, 1997-2000. Int J Antimicrob Agents 2002;20(6):412–8.

45. Tamma PD, Cosgrove SE, Maragakis LL. Combination therapy for treatment of infections with gram-negative bacteria. Clin Microbiol Rev 2012;25(3):450–70.

46. Swingle HM, Bucciarelli RL, Ayoub EM. Synergy between penicillins and low concentrations of gentamicin in the killing of group B streptococci. J Infect Dis 1985;152(3):515–20.

47. Eliopoulos GM, Moellering RC Jr. Antibiotic synergism and antimicrobial combinations in clinical infections. Rev Infect Dis 1982;4(2):282–93.

48. Edwards MS, Nizet V, Baker CJ. Chapter 12: group B streptococcal infections, p 411–56. In: Wilson CB, Nizet V, Maldonado YA, et al, editors. Remington and Klein's Infectious Diseases of the Fetus and Newborn Infant. 8th edition. Philadelphia: Elsevier-Saunders; 2016. p. 411–56.

49. Neonatal infection (early onset): antibiotics for prevention and treatment (CG149). Available at: https://www.nice.org.uk/guidance/cg149. Accessed August 22, 2018.

50. Paul M, Lador A, Grozinsky-Glasberg S, et al. Beta lactam antibiotic monotherapy versus beta lactam-aminoglycoside antibiotic combination therapy for sepsis. Cochrane Database Syst Rev 2014;(1):CD003344.

51. Verani JR, McGee L, Schrag SJ, Division of Bacterial Diseases, National Center for Immunization and Respiratory Diseases, Centers for Disease Control and Prevention (CDC). Prevention of perinatal group B streptococcal disease–revised guidelines from CDC, 2010. MMWR Recomm Rep 2010;59(RR-10):1–36.

52. Hawkins PA, Law CS, Metcalf BJ, et al. Cross-resistance to lincosamides, strep-togramins A and pleuromutilins in *Streptococcus agalactiae* isolates from the USA. J Antimicrob Chemother 2017;72(7):1886–92.

53. Castor ML, Whitney CG, Como-Sabetti K, et al. Antibiotic resistance patterns in inva-sive group B streptococcal isolates. Infect Dis Obstet Gynecol 2008;2008:727505.

54. Back EE, O'Grady EJ, Back JD. High rates of perinatal group B streptococcus clindamycin and erythromycin resistance in an upstate New York hospital. Antimi-crob Agents Chemother 2012;56(2):739–42.

55. Sherman K, Whitehead S, Blondel-Hill E, et al. Penicillin susceptibility and macrolide-lincosamide-streptogramin B resistance in group B streptococcus iso-lates from a Canadian hospital. Can J Infect Dis Med Microbiol 2012;23(4):196–8.

56. Puopolo KM, Mukhopadhyay S, Hansen NI, et al. Identification of extremely pre-mature infants at low risk for early-onset sepsis. Pediatrics 2017;140(5). https://doi.org/10.1542/peds.2017-0925.

57. Barton M, O'Brien K, Robinson JL, et al. Invasive candidiasis in low birth weight preterm infants: risk factors, clinical course and outcome in a prospective multi-center study of cases and their matched controls. BMC Infect Dis 2014;14:327.

58. Weston EJ, Pondo T, Lewis MM, et al. The burden of invasive early-onset neonatal sepsis in the United States, 2005-2008. Pediatr Infect Dis J 2011;30(11):937–41.

59. Stoll BJ, Hansen NI, Bell EF, et al. Trends in care practices, morbidity, and mor-tality of extremely preterm neonates, 1993-2012. JAMA 2015;314(10):1039–51.

60. Mtitimila EI, Cooke RW. Antibiotic regimens for suspected early neonatal sepsis. Cochrane Database Syst Rev 2004;(4).CD004495.

61. Metsvaht T, Ilmoja ML, Parm U, et al. Ampicillin versus penicillin in the empiric therapy of extremely low-birthweight neonates at risk of early onset sepsis. Pe-diatr Int 2011;53(6):873–80.

62. Metsvaht T, Ilmoja ML, Parm U, et al. Comparison of ampicillin plus gentamicin vs. penicillin plus gentamicin in empiric treatment of neonates at risk of early onset sepsis. Acta Paediatr 2010;99(5):665–72.

63. Bergin SP, Thaden JT, Ericson JE, et al. Neonatal *Escherichia coli* bloodstream infections: clinical outcomes and impact of initial antibiotic therapy. Pediatr Infect Dis J 2015;34(9):933–6.

64. Clark RH, Bloom BT, Spitzer AR, et al. Empiric use of ampicillin and cefotaxime, compared with ampicillin and gentamicin, for neonates at risk for sepsis is asso-ciated with an increased risk of neonatal death. Pediatrics 2006;117(1):67–74.

65. Benjamin DK Jr, Stoll BJ, Gantz MG, et al. Neonatal candidiasis: epidemiology, risk factors, and clinical judgment. Pediatrics 2010;126(4):e865–73.

66. Stoll BJ, Hansen NI, Sanchez PJ, et al. Early onset neonatal sepsis: the burden of group B streptococcal and *E. coli* disease continues. Pediatrics 2011;127(5):817–26.

67. Tremoulet A, Le J, Poindexter B, et al. Characterization of the population pharma-cokinetics of ampicillin in neonates using an opportunistic study design. Antimi-crob Agents Chemother 2014;58(6):3013–20.

68. Hornik CP, Benjamin DK Jr, Smith PB, et al. Electronic health records and phar-macokinetic modeling to assess the relationship between ampicillin exposure and seizure risk in neonates. J Pediatr 2016;178:125–9.e1.

69. Leibovici L, Paul M, Poznanski O, et al. Monotherapy versus beta-lactam-aminoglycoside combination treatment for gram-negative bacteremia: a prospec-tive, observational study. Antimicrob Agents Chemother 1997;41(5):1127–33.

70. Eliopoulos GM, Drusano GL, Ambrose PG, et al. Back to the future: using amino-glycosides again and how to dose them optimally. Clin Infect Dis 2007;45(6): 753–60.
71. Fuchs A, Guidi M, Giannoni E, et al. Population pharmacokinetic study of genta-micin in a large cohort of premature and term neonates. Br J Clin Pharmacol 2014;78(5):1090–101.
72. Frymoyer A, Meng L, Bonifacio SL, et al. Gentamicin pharmacokinetics and dosing in neonates with hypoxic ischemic encephalopathy receiving hypother-mia. Pharmacotherapy 2013;33(7):718–26.
73. Pacifici GM. Pharmacokinetics of cephalosporins in the neonate: a review. Clinics (Sao Paulo) 2011;66(7):1267–74.
74. Leroux S, Roue JM, Gouyon JB, et al. A population and developmental pharma-cokinetic analysis to evaluate and optimize cefotaxime dosing regimen in neo-nates and young infants. Antimicrob Agents Chemother 2016;60(11):6626–34.
75. Muller AE, DeJongh J, Bult Y, et al. Pharmacokinetics of penicillin G in infants with a gestational age of less than 32 weeks. Antimicrob Agents Chemother 2007; 51(10):3720–5.
76. Lutsar I, McCracken GH Jr, Friedland IR. Antibiotic pharmacodynamics in cere-brospinal fluid. Clin Infect Dis 1998;27(5):1117–27.
77. Harris PNA, Tambyah PA, Lye DC, et al. Effect of piperacillin-tazobactam vs mer-openem on 30-day mortality for patients with *E coli* or *Klebsiella pneumoniae* bloodstream infection and ceftriaxone resistance: a randomized clinical trial. JAMA 2018;320(10):984–94.
78. Li Z, Chen Y, Li Q, et al. Population pharmacokinetics of piperacillin/tazobactam in neonates and young infants. Eur J Clin Pharmacol 2013;69(6):1223–33.
79. Cohen-Wolkowiez M, Watt KM, Zhou C, et al. Developmental pharmacokinetics of piperacillin and tazobactam using plasma and dried blood spots from infants. Antimicrob Agents Chemother 2014;58(5):2856–65.
80. Berger A, Kretzer V, Apfalter P, et al. Safety evaluation of piperacillin/tazobactam in very low birth weight infants. J Chemother 2004;16(2):166–71.
81. Smith PB, Cohen-Wolkowiez M, Castro LM, et al. Population pharmacokinetics of meropenem in plasma and cerebrospinal fluid of infants with suspected or complicated intra-abdominal infections. Pediatr Infect Dis J 2011;30(10):844–9.
82. Cohen-Wolkowiez M, Poindexter B, Bidegain M, et al. Safety and effectiveness of meropenem in infants with suspected or complicated intra-abdominal infections. Clin Infect Dis 2012;55(11):1495–502.
83. Shabaan AE, Nour I, Elsayed Eldegla H, et al. Conventional versus prolonged infusion of meropenem in neonates with Gram-negative late-onset sepsis: a ran-domized controlled trial. Pediatr Infect Dis J 2017;36(4):358–63.
84. Jacqz-Aigrain E, Zhao W, Sharland M, et al. Use of antibacterial agents in the neonate: 50 years of experience with vancomycin administration. Semin Fetal Neonatal Med 2013;18(1):28–34.
85. Alvarez R, Lopez Cortes LE, Molina J, et al. Optimizing the clinical use of vanco-mycin. Antimicrob Agents Chemother 2016;60(5):2601–9.
86. Frymoyer A, Hersh AL, El-Komy MH, et al. Association between vancomycin trough concentration and area under the concentration-time curve in neonates. Antimicrob Agents Chemother 2014;58(11):6454–61.
87. Pacifici GM, Allegaert K. Clinical pharmacokinetics of vancomycin in the neonate: a review. Clinics (Sao Paulo) 2012;67(7):831–7.
88. Banner W Jr, Gooch WM 3rd, Burckart G, et al. Pharmacokinetics of nafcillin in infants with low birth weights. Antimicrob Agents Chemother 1980;17(4):691–4.

89. Nanduri SA, Petit S, Smelser C, et al. Epidemiology of invasive early-onset and late-onset group B streptococcal disease in the United States, 2006 to 2015: multistate laboratory and population-based surveillance. JAMA Pediatr 2019. https://doi.org/10.1001/jamapediatrics.2018.4826.
90. Puopolo KM, Benitz WE, Zaoutis TE. Committee on fetus and newborn; committee on infectious diseases. Management of neonates born at ≤34 6/7 weeks' gestation with suspected or proven early-onset bacterial sepsis. Pediatrics 2018;142(6) [pii:e20182896].
91. Puopolo KM, Benitz WE, Zaoutis TE. Committee on fetus and newborn; committee on infectious diseases. Management of neonates born at ≥35 0/7 weeks' gestation with suspected or proven early-onset bacterial sepsis. Pediatrics 2018;142(6) [pii:e20182894].

Analgesia, Opioids, and Other Drug Use During Pregnancy and Neonatal Abstinence Syndrome

Hendrée E. Jones, PhD[a,b,c,*], Walter K. Kraft, MD[d]

KEYWORDS

- Neonatal abstinence syndrome • NAS • Neonatal opioid withdrawal • NOWS
- Neonatal • Addiction • Opioid use disorder • Prenatal

KEY POINTS

- A life course perspective helps patients stop substance use. Pregnancy is a critical time for behavior change. Healing opioid use disorder requires an individualized multifactorial approach.
- Buprenorphine formulations (alone and those with naloxone) and methadone show relative safety and efficacy for the fetus, mother, and child. Medications works best with comprehensive physical, psychological, and case management.
- Infants with significant in utero opioid exposure need observation for neonatal abstinence syndrome (NAS). At least half of infants with NAS can be managed solely with nonpharmacologic approaches.
- Future genetic factor research may yield (1) infant risk stratification to minimize NAS intensity and duration and (2) optimizing NAS treatments based on drug disposition and effect differences.

Disclosure Statement: H.E. Jones has no relationship with a commercial company that has a direct financial interest in subject matter or materials discussed in article or with a company making a competing product. W.K. Kraft has received research funding from Chiesi.

[a] Department of Obstetrics and Gynecology, University of North Carolina at Chapel Hill, UNC Horizons, 410 North Greensboro Street, Chapel Hill, NC, USA; [b] Department of Psychiatry and Behavioral Sciences, School of Medicine, Johns Hopkins University, Baltimore, MD, USA; [c] Department of Obstetrics and Gynecology, School of Medicine, Johns Hopkins University, Baltimore, MD, USA; [d] Clinical Research Unit, Department of Pharmacology and Experimental Therapeutics, Thomas Jefferson University, 1170 Main Building, 132 South 10th Street, Philadelphia, PA 19107-5244, USA
* Corresponding author. Department of Obstetrics and Gynecology, UNC Horizons, University of North Carolina at Chapel Hill, 410 North Greensboro Street, Chapel Hill, NC 27510.
E-mail address: Hendree_Jones@med.unc.edu

Clin Perinatol 46 (2019) 349–366
https://doi.org/10.1016/j.clp.2019.02.013
0095-5108/19/© 2019 Elsevier Inc. All rights reserved.

OPIOID USE CONTINUES TO RISE AMONG THE GENERAL POPULATION: PREGNANT WOMAN ARE NOT SPARED

The opioid crisis was a recognized threat to public health in the United States since 2009 when annual deaths due to opioid overdose surpassed motor vehicle accidents.[1] Nationally,630,000 people died from a drug overdose between 1999 and 2016 with opioid deaths 5 times higher in 2016 compared with 1999.[2] Although more men than women report illicit (eg, heroin) and nonmedical (eg, prescription opioids) opioid use, it is a concerning problem for women.[3] For heroin, women tend to use smaller amounts, for less time, and are less likely to inject it compared with men.[4–7] For prescription opioids, women report using them (eg, oxycodone, hydrocodone, fentanyl) to relieve pain (physical and psychological), reduce weight, reduce stress, and reduce exhaustion.[8] Although fewer women than men died from opioid overdoses in 2016 (ie, 7109 women and 9978 men), from 1999 to 2016, prescription opioid overdose deaths rose more rapidly for women (sevenfold) than for men (fourfold). Thus, gender-responsive interventions need development to reduce overdose deaths.

OPIOID USE OCCURS ON A CONTINUUM: IDENTIFICATION AND TREATMENT IS NEEDED FOR OPIOID USE DISORDERS DURING PREGNANCY

All substance use, including opioids, occurs on a continuum that encompasses no, occasional, and regular use. Substance use occurring despite adverse consequences leads to a diagnosis of opioid use disorder (OUD) that is graded as mild, moderate, or severe. For women who continue to use opioids after pregnancy awareness, the Diagnostic and Statistical Manual, Fifth Edition (DSM-5) criteria indicates that they have at least a mild OUD that merits intervention. Consistent with the general population, the prevalence of OUD during pregnancy, measured at delivery, has greatly increased from 1999 to 2014 (from 1.5 per 1000 to 6.5 per 1000 delivery hospitalizations; $P<.05$).[9] Likewise, the diagnosis of neonatal abstinence syndrome (NAS) (see the section "Defining neonatal abstinence syndrome" for definition) has increased from 1.2 per 1000 hospital births in 2000 to 8.0 per 1000 in 2014.[10] This almost sevenfold increase in NAS nationally suggests that approximately every 15 minutes an infant is born with a NAS diagnosis.[11,12]

Before women can be treated for OUD during pregnancy, they must be identified. Opioid and/or other substance use is most commonly initiated before pregnancy. Thus, all women of childbearing age deserve regular screening for substance use problems to prevent and respond to substance-exposed pregnancies. The American College of Obstetrics and Gynecology (ACOG) recommends repeated substance use disorder screening across prenatal visits.[13] Of note, substance use screening (via instrument/questionnaire) differs from drug testing (via *confirmed* biologic samples, such as urine via gas chromatography–mass spectrometry). A positive urine drug screen is not a diagnosis of a substance use disorder; such results indicate only the presence or absence of the parent drug and/or its metabolites indicating recent substance use.[14] Universal *voluntary* screening using a validated instrument must be conducted with a nonpunitive, supportive treatment approach.

A life course perspective is needed to help patients stop harmful substance use. For women, the pregnancy life event can be a critical time for behavior change. Ending substance use, including opioids, requires an individualized multifactorial approach. Factors associated with the risk of substance use disorders are genetic (eg, ~50% of substance use disorder vulnerability),[15] as well as environmental issues specific to women (eg, 40%–70% of women in treatment have been the victim of physical or sexual abuse).[16,17] Thus, treatment first requires access to appropriate care and a personalized approach. Access to the appropriate level of care is the first step of treatment initiation, engagement, and retention. For women with OUD who become pregnant, prenatal care and OUD treatment ideally require integration or at least co-ordination of providers.[18] Appropriate perinatal care also includes identifying and responding to multiple life domain needs such as physical health, concurrent sub-stance use (eg, tobacco, alcohol, and marijuana), dental health, psychological health, interpersonal, economic, housing, parenting, and family. Such comprehensive treat-ment must be continued based on the patient's needs, often encompassing at least a year after pregnancy ends.

BUPRENORPHINE AND METHADONE: PART OF A COMPLETE TREATMENT APPROACH

An important, but not only, part of care of women with OUD includes the use of opioid agonist medication (buprenorphine or methadone). Recommendations to use metha-done pharmacotherapy over medically assisted withdrawal (also known commonly as detoxification) resulted from reports of medically assisted withdrawal leading to maternal opioid relapse and fetal demise.[19,20] Although data to date do not support an association between medically assisted withdrawal and fetal demise, they also do not support either equivalence or benefit of such an approach relative to maternal opioid agonist pharmacotherapy.[20,21] In fact, medically assisted withdrawal can increase the risk of maternal relapse (up to 100%), reduce treatment engagement (treatment completion rates as low as 9%),[21] and fail to prevent NAS. Given these issues, medically assisted withdrawal is not considered a first-line approach and needs more systematic investigation to determine its role, if any, as a treatment approach to OUD during the perinatal period. In contrast to medically assisted withdrawal, medication treatment us-ing either buprenorphine or methadone is endorsed by the ACOG,[22] American Society for Addiction Medicine,[23] United Nations,[24] World Health Organization,[25] and other government agencies[26] as the optimal approach for treating OUD during pregnancy.

Buprenorphine or methadone, if taken in adequate doses, can stabilize the OUD of the pregnant woman and prevent relapse.[27,28] Methadone treatment, compared with untreated use of heroin, improves maternal medical outcomes (eg, less human immu-nodeficiency virus [HIV] infection due to reduced drug risk, decreased preeclampsia risk, and more obstetric visits completed).[29] For the fetus, methadone versus untreated OUD has been associated with less fetal death, less fetal exposure to cycles of heroin-induced intoxication and withdrawal,[30] and improved fetal growth.[27] Buprenorphine is approved by the Food and Drug Administration (FDA) to treat OUD and has been inves-tigated in pregnant patients.[31] The MOTHER study[32] assessed buprenorphine compared with methadone in a randomized trial that focused on pregnant women with OUD throughout pregnancy and their neonates. Both buprenorphine and metha-done had similar maternal and delivery outcomes. Relative to methadone, among pa-tients retained in the study, in utero buprenorphine-exposed neonates required 89% less morphine to treat NAS, spent 58% less time in the hospital being medicated for NAS, and spent 43% less time in the hospital. A systematic review of research regarding buprenorphine to treat OUD during pregnancy concludes the following: (1) buprenor-phine and methadone have comparable maternal outcomes; (2) buprenorphine pro-duces less fetal heart rate and movement suppression; (3) buprenorphine produces less severe NAS; (4) both drugs are compatible with breastfeeding; and (5) deleterious effects of buprenorphine on subsequent infant development are not apparent.[33]

The FDA approved products containing both buprenorphine and naloxone (an opioid antagonist added to deter buprenorphine product injecting the medication) to treat adult OUD. All labels include pregnancy, neonatal, and lactation information and note the accepted use of the medication during the perinatal period if the benefits outweigh the risks. Although the product insert contains updated information, national and international guidance documents are slow to catch up with science to support the use of combination products. Buprenorphine + naloxone during pregnancy shows no obvious adverse maternal or neonatal outcomes, a reduced incidence of NAS, lower peak NAS scores, and shorter overall mean length of hospitalization than neonates with in utero methadone exposure.[34–36] Prospective large-sample results would benefit future practice.

Every national and international guideline on the treatment of OUD endorses buprenorphine and methadone as the first-line approach for pregnant women. In addition, federal regulations require priority access to opioid treatment programs for pregnant women (eg, no need to fully meet DSM-5 criteria for OUD to initiate medication). However, only a third of pregnant women who qualify actually receive opioid agonist pharmacotherapy in the United States.[37] Thus, although treatment programs have increased capacity to treat more pregnant women with OUD, focusing on certain risk groups and increasing utilization of opioid medication should be emphasized (eg, young, unemployed, uninsured have less access).[38] Further, increasing the numbers of active medical buprenorphine prescribers is needed to expand access for all pregnant patients.

WOMEN RECEIVING BUPRENORPHINE OR METHADONE DURING PREGNANCY: PAIN MANAGEMENT: LABOR, DELIVERY, AND POSTPARTUM

Delivery universally produces acute pain with a clearly defined onset and resolution.[39] Women with OUD require assessment for appropriate analgesia and anesthesia options, with adequate pain management provided at delivery. Regardless of treatment status, women with OUD may by hyperanalgesic, have opioid tolerance, and need greater amounts of opioid for relief of pain compared with patients without OUD.[40] Pain medication must be provided regardless of current or past OUD. For women treated with buprenorphine or methadone, the medication should not be withheld or altered in terms of quantity or frequency of dosing during labor and delivery or the immediate postpartum period. Women treated with buprenorphine or methadone for OUD can experience adequate pain control postpartum with the use of other opioids in combination with acetaminophen and a nonsteroidal anti-inflammatory drugs.[41] Women receiving methadone during pregnancy were found to have similar analgesic requirements and response during labor but required more opioid analgesic after cesarean delivery when compared with women not on methadone maintenance.[39] Of great importance, women who use heroin or prescription opioids and/or are prescribed chronic opioids (including methadone or buprenorphine) should *not* receive opioid agonist/antagonist pain medications (eg, butorphanol, nalbuphine, and pentazocine) for acute pain because these medications may cause an acute opioid withdrawal syndrome.[42]

BREASTFEEDING IS COMPATIBLE AND ENCOURAGED: BUPRENORPHINE OR METHADONE

Breastfeeding helps to build a strong mother-infant bond and provides optimal nutrition and passive immunization for the child. Women with OUD may struggle with using their breasts for food (eg, due to sexual abuse and trauma). They may also struggle with the responsibilities of motherhood (eg, no parenting role models due to being raised in foster care, loss of custody of other children, their own adverse childhood experiences). Successful establishment of breastfeeding can be quite empowering for some women. Women should not be forced to breastfeed. Women receiving buprenorphine or methadone should be encouraged to breastfeed if they are HIV negative.[43] Women with hepatitis B or C may also breastfeed as long as the nipple and surrounding areola are not cracked and/or bleeding to avoid direct contact with maternal blood.[44] If this does occur, women should be encouraged to pump and discard breast milk and to resume nursing when the skin has healed. Because negligible amounts of methadone are excreted in human milk across the dose range, there is no contraindication to nursing while prescribed methadone.[45] Although little buprenorphine or methadone is transferred in breast milk, the act of breastfeeding may ease neonatal withdrawal from opioids.[46] Similarly, little buprenorphine is excreted in breast milk, and its low oral bioavailability is not thought to impact NAS or infant behavior.[47] Given that some women use other substances while taking buprenorphine or methadone, such substances deserve discussion. Neonatal exposure to nicotine may cause irritability, poor feeding, and sleep disruption.[48] Infants can have irritability, gastrointestinal disruptions, and sleep issues with cocaine exposure.[49] Breastfeeding during maternal use of benzodiazepines should be discouraged. ACOG discourages any use of cannabis during preconception, pregnancy, and lactation.[50] Finally, alcohol use and breastfeeding are not compatible.

The need for treatment continues postpartum. A review of methadone discontinuation in pregnant and postpartum women concluded that methadone discontinuation at or up to 6 months postpartum was 56%.[51] Although the discontinuation reasons are elusive, program policies that withdraw medication from women after delivery and loss of Medicaid coverage may be contributing issues. Opioid-related overdoses contribute to pregnancy-associated deaths in many states (11%–20% of cases).[52,53] At 12 months postpartum, treatment retention negatively correlated with illicit drug use during the third trimester.[54] Expanding coverage of OUD treatment for pregnant and postpartum women is critical to maternal and neonatal health.[55]

DEFINING NEONATAL ABSTINENCE SYNDROME

In utero transfer of opioids is associated with a withdrawal syndrome in the neonate after the umbilical cord is cut. The pathobiology of opioid withdrawal prompts a similar set of physical signs in the neonate as in the adult, although the manifestations and medical implications differ. As in adults, the neonate with significant symptoms will have difficulty with gastrointestinal function with loose stools and vomiting, autonomic dysfunction with temperature dysregulation and sneezing, and neurologic signs of irritability and tremors. Unlike the adult, the neonate differs in a developmental arc of growth and development. Severe withdrawal impairs the ability of the neonate to feed properly, which can lead to poor weight gain and development. Irritability also impairs maternal-infant bonding. The mechanistic basis for the clinical presentation is not fully defined; however, tolerance to opioids is primarily medicated by receptor downregulation coupled with upregulation in the cyclic adenosine monophosphate pathway.[56] Although NAS is a nonspecific term, it has traditionally referred to signs due to primarily opioid withdrawal and its defining manifestations are those associated with opioid withdrawal. To more clearly link the etiology of the discrete syndrome to an in utero exposure, federal agencies have suggested the more specific term neonatal opioid withdrawal syndrome (NOWS).[57]

Although not causing a withdrawal syndrome severe enough requiring individualized treatment on their own, many medications and exposures along with in utero opioid exposure can worsen the severity of neonatal withdrawal symptoms (eg, tobacco or medications such as antidepressants, benzodiazepines, and gabapentin).[58–63] Other factors that impact the need for pharmacologic treatment include concurrent use of alcohol, tobacco, and other drugs.[63] Maternal methadone dose as a potential modifiable covariate of NAS severity has been extensively investigated, with varied methodological quality of studies. Although meta-analysis did not identify a statistically significant difference in outcomes between high-dose and low-dose methadone, there is a trend suggestive of a modest maternal dose–NAS severity relationship.[64] This dose relationship, if it exists, is at best loosely tied to the severity of withdrawal signs and not relevant in terms of choosing a maternal dose or differential NAS treatment approaches. Lower maternal methadone doses have been associated with higher rates of illicit drug use. ACOG and others suggest that maternal doses of methadone should not be reduced solely to reduce NAS severity.[52]

NEONATAL ABSTINENCE SYNDROME TREATMENT APPROACHES

Infants with documented or suspected in utero opioid exposure need monitoring with a standard assessment instrument. Although a number of scoring systems have been developed,[65–68] the Finnegan[69] remains the de facto standard for clinical care. A score of greater than 8 is highly correlated with in utero opioid exposure, even in the absence of declared use during pregnancy.[70] When informed by at least moderate pretest probability, performance in defining a high degree of symptoms is excellent. Elements that make up the score have drifted over time, with individual sites modifying the instrument over the years. These changes reflect practice changes (eg, removal of seizures only seen in the early NAS practice history). Thus, the terms "Finnegan" or "modified Finnegan" generally describe scoring systems that vary in minor ways across sites. Regardless of the NAS scoring instrument used, key elements are ensuring uniformity in scoring through a process of continuous training and quality assessment of nursing staff. In-service sessions paired with observed assessment by a site-level gold standard assessor comprises quality NAS assessment.

Attempts to simplify NAS assessment approaches (Jones and colleagues,[71,72] Isemann and colleagues[73]) include quick screening instruments with a goal of predicting those infants most likely to need pharmacologic treatment. Others have focused on shortening the Finnegan while retaining the instrument's discrimination for both identifying the neonates who need pharmacologic treatment and informing treatment decisions following medication initiation. Maguire and colleagues[74] and Gomez-Pomar and colleagues[75] used quantitative methods comparing Finnegan as the gold standard with the explicit goal to remove less informative scoring elements to reduce nursing burden. Most recently, the scoring elements have focused on the infant's ability to eat, sleep, and be consoled (sometimes identified by the acronym ESC). This approach was 1 of 8 elements comprising a quality improvement project.[76,77] The ESC approach has not been compared with the Finnegan and the test characteristics of sensitivity, specificity, and receiver operator curves have not been published. Comprehensive approaches to NAS treatment that include ESC as one of many elements have demonstrated decreased resource utilization. However, which specific interventions are responsible for less resource utilization is unknown. The benefits in reduction of nursing time with the use of ESC score have not been quantitated. In addition, NAS is a condition with heterogeneous expression of symptoms covering multiple organ systems. Systematic evaluation of ESC compared with the Finnegan scoring systems would be welcomed to assess if simplification of the score to 3 domains results in missing signs of concern in certain neonates, or if it provides a similar result to current standard assessment tools.

NONPHARMACOLOGIC TREATMENT OF NEONATAL ABSTINENCE SYNDROME

All neonates, regardless of initial manifestations, should first be treated with nonpharmacologic approaches. Nonpharmacologic approaches should not be considered an alternative to medication therapy, but instead the baseline for all patients. Nonpharmacologic approaches are effective in reducing the number of infants treated with pharmacologic treatments.[76,78] No standard set of interventions constitute a definitive "nonpharmacologic treatment bundle." Some sites have embarked on large-scale changes to NAS care. These approaches often yield an impressive reduction in length of stay. Such interventions involve many changes at once and it is difficult to identify which specific intervention is associated with the greatest impact. Interventions, such a use of small, frequent formula feedings for those not breastfeeding, have not been (and likely will never be) individually examined but are considered safe and widely practiced. A few key interventions have been examined more closely. Those with the most evidence to support are breastfeeding, rooming in, swaddling, and skin-to-skin contact.[79] Breastfeeding is associated with clear improvements in NAS outcomes of need for treatment, duration of hospitalization, and length of pharmacologic treatment.[80,81] In retrospective studies, rooming in has been associated with significant improvement in outcomes.[82–84] These interventions select out a very specific group of mothers who are able to be integrated into the neonatal care plan. In addition to these specific interventions, parallel attention to trust building with mothers is a key element in fostering the health of infants with NAS. Above all, successful outcomes are more likely when the parents trust the caregiver's and clinician's approach interactions with an understanding of the stages of addiction recovery and a lack of preconceived notions of how an individual parent Is anticipated to act. Ideally, the flow of information from the newborn nursery to the mother occurs before the baby is born. This includes a discussion of scoring, treatment approaches, and empowering mothers to aid in activities that have been shown to reduce the need for pharmacologic treatment.

PHARMACOLOGIC TREATMENT OF NEONATAL ABSTINENCE SYNDROME

Pharmacologic treatment is used in neonates with severe NAS (**Fig. 1**). End points in clinical trials of pharmacologic therapy are length of treatment and duration of hospitalization. However, these measures assume that the other goals of treatment (relief of

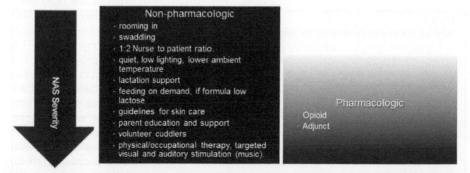

Fig. 1. Approach to infants with in utero opioid exposure. All infants should be provided a base of nonpharmacologic therapies. Specific measures will vary with the ability of the local site to provide. Some potential approaches are listed. Pharmacologic therapy is added only in those for whom symptoms are not controlled with nonpharmacologic means.

discomfort, appropriate growth and development, and maximizing parental bonding) are being met. Some of these goals are less easily quantified. It is possible for example, that low doses of control medications and aggressive weaning schedules could reduce length of stay but at the cost of accepting a higher degree of infant discomfort. Weight and some measure of symptom scores could capture this difference, but mother-infant bonding is more difficult to assess. Thus, despite the primacy of length of treatment in clinical trials, secondary measures of neonatal well-being should be considered when judging various treatments.

The foundation of pharmacologic treatment for opioid NAS is replacement with an opioid. Compared with other classes of agents, the opioids are consistently superior in clinical trials and retrospective examinations. This is consistent with observations in the treatment of adult opioid withdrawal.[85,86] Continued elevated symptom scores and clinical signs of severe NAS trigger the use of pharmacologic treatment. Doses are titrated up until signs/symptoms are controlled, or a second medication is added. After a period of clinical stability, doses are gradually weaned to a target dose and then discontinued. Regardless of the specific drugs or regimens used, standardization of treatment is a key element in optimizing therapy. Published examples in which improvement programs stressing uniform use of institutional treatment protocol have resulted in 15% to 50% reduction in length of treatment and duration of hospitalization.[87–91]

There are significant differences in treatment regimens between institutions. Eighty percent of US sites use morphine as the primary opioid, with the remainder using methadone.[91] A small but growing number of sites are using buprenorphine as the primary opioid. In the inpatient setting, all 3 opioids have excellent safety records. Comparing morphine and methadone efficacy, the randomized controlled data suggest an advantage of methadone (**Table 1**). The largest multicenter study of 117 neonates with mixed in utero exposure (~60% methadone and 30% buprenorphine) demonstrated a 14% shorter mean length of treatment with methadone than morphine.[92] Real-world data from the Pediatrix Clinical Data Warehouse of 7667 infants showed a 22% reduction in length of hospitalization for neonates treated with methadone compared with morphine.[93] Sublingual buprenorphine was compared with oral morphine in the BBORN, a blinded controlled study in 63 neonates almost all who were exposed to methadone in utero.[94] Buprenorphine had a 42% shorter length of stay compared with a weight-based morphine comparison. Hall and colleagues[95,96] reported retrospective cohort data from southern Ohio

Table 1
Methadone versus morphine: median length of treatment

Author	Design	n	Morphine (Number of Days)	Methadone (Number of Days)	P
Lainwala et al,[112] 2005	Retrospective	46	36	40	NS
Hall et al,[88] 2014	Retrospective	383	16[a]	16[a]	NS
Young et al,[113] 2015	Retrospective	26	7[a]	38[a]	.001
Brown et al,[114] 2015	Blinded RCT	31	21	14	.008
Davis et al,[92] 2018	Blinded RCT	183	15	11.5	.02
Tolia et al,[93] 2018	Retrospective	7667	23[b]	18[b]	<.001

Abbreviations: NS, not significant; RCT, randomized controlled trial.
[a] Mean.
[b] Length of stay.

of 212 neonates treated with buprenorphine compared with 349 treated with morphine and morphine as a comparison cohort. Buprenorphine use was associated with a 29% reduction in length of treatment. Compared with the BBORN controlled trial, the buprenorphine and morphine treatment regimens differed, and the Ohio cohort had more heterogeneous exposures in utero. The similarity of effect size using different study designs, populations, and drug regimens suggests an advantage for buprenorphine. The preparation used in all published reports contains 30% ethanol. The safety profile of ethanol in infants has not been established, but serum concentrations after buprenorphine administration generally fall within regulatory guidelines.[97]

Ultimately, the answer to "what is the best opioid for NAS?" is not straightforward. We have the results of randomized controlled trials, but the better question is "what is the best opioid treatment regimen for which neonate?" A treatment protocol identifies not only the specific opioid, but defines starting dose, rate of up-titration, maximum dose, weaning rate, and a cessation dose. Other differences are the severity score cut points used to initiate and intensify pharmacologic treatment, as well as the choice and dose of other pharmacologic adjunct therapy. Up to this point, the endpoint used to gauge success of a regimen has been the drug dose, and not the drug concentration within the neonate. Pharmacometric modeling is a quantitative approach that has particular value in the neonatal population. The strengths include an ability to (1) use a small number of blood draws per patient, (2) define the variability in pharmacokinetics between individuals, (3) identify covariates associated with the variation, (4) incorporate developmental changes with maturation of hepatic and renal function, and (5) establish a relationship between drug exposure and pharmacodynamic response. A number of investigators have begun to use pharmacometrics to describe drug behavior in NAS[98–101] and to generate dosing regiments.[102]

NONOPIOID ADJUNCT THERAPY

Phenobarbital and clonidine are nonopioid drugs that can be used in conjunction with an opioid. These adjunctive therapies aim to synergize treatment. Several small studies compared an adjunct medication with an opioid to treat NAS. Commonly, an adjunct is given only when symptoms are not controlled and then weaned before cessation of the opioid. Other centers will wean the opioid first and discontinue the adjunct later as an inpatient or outpatient. This approach is much more common for phenobarbital than clonidine. The third approach is that of parallel opioid and clonidine therapy, with a goal of reducing opioid exposure, as well as length of treatment. Neither the optimal adjunctive drug nor treatment regimen have been clearly defined for specific populations.

TREATMENT LOCATION

NAS treatment has increasingly moved out of the intensive care unit to areas of the hospital with less stimulation. Alternatively, specialized areas have been designated that are optimized not only in environment control, but also in staff support. There are treatment protocols in which pharmacologic treatment is transitioned to the outpatient management with methadone. Another approach is to discharge with phenobarbital as the primary pharmacologic therapy after inpatient opioid weaning. Inpatient pharmacologic treatment is consistently reported as being associated with longer lengths of hospitalization compared with outpatient weaning, but shorter total duration of treatment.[103] The best documented experience is a population-based retrospective cohort study of 532 neonates primarily treated with phenobarbital.[104]

Consistent with prior studies, the median (interquartile range) length of pharmacologic therapy was significantly shorter in inpatients compared with outpatients. However, neonates treated as outpatients had an increased number of emergency room visits within 6 months of discharge when compared with those treated as inpatients alone. Although not statistically significant, the point estimate odds ratio for an emergency visit at 6 weeks, or any hospitalization at 6 or 24 weeks was approximately 1.5 for outpatient compared with inpatient treatment. This suggests that caution is indicated when transitioning a neonate to outpatient treatment, which should be considered only when there is a comprehensive support structure in place and pediatricians are familiar and comfortable with weaning a neonate as an outpatient.

GENETICS

OUD heritability in adults, derived from an examination of twins, is high and accounts for approximately 50% of the risk being genetic.[15] Similar data are lacking for neonates, but a small investigation of in utero opioid exposure revealed high concordance of NAS scores and need for treatment in 5 of 7 mostly dizygotic twin sets.[105] Primarily single-nucleotide polymorphism (SNP) approaches in adults have identified variants in the mu-opioid receptor (OPRM1), delta-opioid receptor (OPRD1), the dopamine D2 receptor (DRD2), and brain-derived neurotrophic factor.[106] Initial studies in neonates with in utero opioid exposure suggested OPRRM1 118A > G AG/GG and COMT 158A > G AG/GG genotype were associated with improved outcomes in NAS.[107] A microarray replication identified pointwise, but not experiment-wise significance of these 2 SNPs as well as OPRK1 rs702764 C allele and PNOC rs732636 A allele.[108] Genes in the inflammatory pathway have also been implicated,[109] as well as epigenetic factors.[110,111] In aggregate, early signals suggest that with larger sample sizes, more definitive causal relationships can be established and may lead to a better understanding of NAS biology. Several factors should be noted in comparing adult and neonatal genetic investigations of opioid withdrawal. First, the phenotypic endpoints in neonates are small and generally well established. However, there is drift in standard of care with a greater emphasis on nonpharmacologic care, so a metric such as the need for pharmacologic therapy may differ between older and more recent cohorts. Endpoints of length of stay will vary between institutions, depending on a specific pharmacologic regimen used. The use of morphine equivalents between different opioids widely used in adults and lacks validation in neonates, so comparisons between institutions with different drug regimens are problematic. Alternatively, there is increasing standardization of regimens. All neonates are at least initially treated in the hospital, and the electronic health record provides the ability to generate accurate data with more ease than in adults. The pathology is somewhat simpler in that NAS is withdrawal and not addiction. Future directions will generate larger and more comprehensive data sets with standard data elements. The long-term goal would be to have more solidly associated genetic factors that would allow for the generation of a risk score that would allow for (1) risk stratification of neonates to optimize intensity and duration of monitoring of symptoms and (2) optimizing pharmacologic treatments based on differences in drug disposition and effect. Personalized models will not be based on a single SNP, but polygenic and include nongenetic covariates associated with severity, such as gestational age and other maternal substance use. Such models are aspirational and genetics remains a research tool at the current time.

Best Practices

What is the current practice for

The treatment of women who have substance use disorders, including OUD during the pregnancy period and how their infants cared for.

Best Practice/Guidelines/Care Path Objective

What changes in current practice are likely to improve outcomes?

- All maternal and child health care providers need to be trained to engage all women in a short conversation (universal screening), to provide nonjudgmental feedback/advice about substance use, as needed, and have the knowledge to refer patients to appropriate treatment options. Such actions can improve maternal and infant outcomes.
- For pregnant and postpartum women with an OUD, national and international guidelines recommend the use of methadone and buprenorphine as medications over medically supervised withdrawal given that withdrawal yields high relapse rates and untreated addiction can lead to worse outcomes. However, only a third of pregnant women who qualify, actually receive opioid agonist pharmacotherapy in the United States. Thus, increasing the numbers of active medical buprenorphine prescribers is needed to expand access for all perinatal patients.
- Although national and international guidance recommends encouraging breastfeeding in women receiving methadone or buprenorphine who are not using illicit drugs, and who have no other contraindications (eg, HIV infection), not all providers follow this practice. Thus, more providers need education and support to help women.
- Women who have an opioid use during pregnancy are at high risk of postpartum mortality, and need access to adequate postpartum psychosocial support services, including substance use disorder treatment, relapse prevention programs, case management, and parenting support.
- Approaching NAS treatment from a dyad perspective may improve outcomes. NAS treatment has increasingly moved out of the Intensive care unit to areas of the hospital with less stimulation. Alternatively, specialized areas have been designated that are optimized not only in environment control, but also in staff support When the mother or other caregiver is part of the NAS care approach, fewer resources may be needed.

Major Recommendations

- Taking a life course perspective and dyadic approach to the care and treatment of mothers for substance use disorders (including OUD) and their prenatally substance-exposed child will promote healthy outcomes.

- Treatment access to methadone and buprenorphine for pregnant and postpartum women is needed.

- Treatment cannot end at the postpartum period, the mother-child dyad continues to need support and resources are needed to provide adequate comprehensive care to them.

- Newer NAS approaches need to be evaluated in a rigorously scientific manner.

Summary Statement

Healing women who have substance use disorders, including OUD, requires an individualized multifactorial approach. Methadone and buprenorphine are important parts of treatment and work best with comprehensive physical, psychological, and case management. Infants with significant in utero opioid exposure need observation for NAS. At least half of infants with NAS can be managed solely with nonpharmacologic approaches. A dyadic approach to care is an important key to improving outcomes for the mother and child.

Data from The American College of Obstetricians and Gynecologists. Opioid use and opioid use disorder in pregnancy. Committee Opinion No. 711. American College of Obstetricians and Gynecologists. Obstet Gynecol 2017;130:e81–94; and Substance Abuse and Mental Health Services Administration. Clinical guidance for treating pregnant and parenting women with opioid use disorder and their infants. 2018 SMA18-5054. Available at: https://store.samhsa.gov/product/Clinical-Guidance-for-Treating-Pregnant-and-Parenting-Women-With-Opioid-Use-Disorder-and-Their-Infants/SMA18-5054. Accessed March 13, 2019.

REFERENCES

1. Waite T. American security today. DEA: fentanyl-related overdose deaths rising at an alarming rate 2016. Available at: https://americansecuritytoday.com/dea-fentanyl-related-overdose-deaths-rising-alarming-rate/. Accessed September 15, 2018.
2. Centers for disease control and prevention (CDC). Drug overdose death data 2017. Available at: https://www.cdc.gov/drugoverdose/index.html. Accessed September 15, 2018.
3. Center for behavioral health statistics and quality. Results from the 2016 national survey on drug use and health: detailed tables. Rockville (MD): Substance Abuse and Mental Health Services Administration; 2017. Available at: https://www.samhsa.gov/data/sites/default/files/NSDUH-DetTabs-2016/NSDUH-DetTabs-2016.pdf. Accessed September 15, 2018.
4. Powis B, Griffiths P, Gossop M, et al. The differences between male and female drug users: community samples of heroin and cocaine users compared. Subst Use Misuse 1996;31(5):529–43.
5. Bryant J, Brener L, Hull P, et al. Needle sharing in regular sexual relationships: an examination of serodiscordance, drug using practices, and the gendered character of injecting. Drug Alcohol Depend 2010;107(2–3):182–7.
6. Lum PJ, Sears C, Guydish J. Injection risk behavior among women syringe exchangers in San Francisco. Subst Use Misuse 2005;40(11):1681–96.
7. Dwyer R, Richardson D, Ross MW, et al. A comparison of HIV risk between women and men who inject drugs. AIDS Educ Prev 1994;6(5):379–89.
8. McHugh RK, Devito EE, Dodd D, et al. Gender differences in a clinical trial for prescription opioid dependence. J Subst Abuse Treat 2013;45(1):38–43.
9. Haight SC, Ko JY, Tong VT, et al. Opioid use disorder documented at delivery hospitalization - United States, 1999-2014. MMWR Morb Mortal Wkly Rep 2018;67(31):845–9.
10. Winkelman TNA, Villapiano N, Kozhimannil KB, et al. Incidence and costs of neonatal abstinence syndrome among infants with Medicaid: 2004-2014. Pediatrics 2018;141(4). https://doi.org/10.1542/peds.2017-3520.
11. Patrick SW, Schumacher RE, Benneyworth BD, et al. Neonatal abstinence syndrome and associated health care expenditures: United States, 2000-2009. JAMA 2012;307(18):1934–40.
12. Ko JY, Patrick SW, Tong VT, et al. Incidence of neonatal abstinence syndrome - 28 states, 1999-2013. MMWR Morb Mortal Wkly Rep 2016;65(31):799–802.
13. American College of Obstetricians and Gynecologists, Committee on Health Care for Undeserved Women. ACOG committee opinion no. 343: psychosocial risk factors: perinatal screening and intervention. Obstet Gynecol 2006;108(2):469–77.
14. Terplan M, Minkoff H. Neonatal abstinence syndrome and ethical approaches to the identification of pregnant women who use drugs. Obstet Gynecol 2017;129(1):164–7.
15. Berrettini W. A brief review of the genetics and pharmacogenetics of opioid use disorders. Dialogues Clin Neurosci 2017;19(3):229–36.
16. Martin SL, English KT, Clark KA, et al. Violence and substance use among North Carolina pregnant women. Am J Public Health 1996;86(7):991–8.
17. Okuda M, Olfson M, Hasin D, et al. Mental health of victims of intimate partner violence: results from a national epidemiologic survey. Psychiatr Serv 2011;62(8):959–62.

18. Murphy J, Goodman D, Johnson MC, et al. The comprehensive addiction and recovery act: opioid use disorder and midwifery practice. Obstet Gynecol 2018;131(3):542–4.

19. Center for Substance Abuse Treatment. 1993. Available at: http://adaiclearinghouse.org/downloads/TIP-2-Pregnant-Substance-Using-Women-83.pdf. Accessed March 18, 2019.

20. Jones HE, Terplan M, Meyer M. Medically assisted withdrawal (detoxification): considering the mother-infant dyad. J Addict Med 2017;11(2):90–2.

21. Terplan M, Laird HJ, Hand DJ, et al. Opioid detoxification during pregnancy: a systematic review. Obstet Gynecol 2018;131(5):803–14.

22. ACOG Committee on Health Care for Underserved Women, American Society of Addiction Medicine. ACOG committee opinion no. 524: opioid abuse, dependence, and addiction in pregnancy. Obstet Gynecol 2012;119(5):1070–6.

23. Kampman K, Jarvis M. American Society of Addiction Medicine (ASAM) national practice guideline for the use of medications in the treatment of addiction involving opioid use. J Addict Med 2015;9(5):358–67.

24. United Nations. International standards for the treatment of drug use disorders. Vienna (Austria): United Nations; 2016. Commission on Narcotic Drugs Fifty-Ninth Session.

25. World Health Organization. Guidelines for the identification and management of substance use and substance use disorders in pregnancy. Geneva (Switzerland): World Health Organization; 2014.

26. Substance Abuse and Mental Health Services Administration. Federal guidelines for opioid treatment programs. HS publication no. (SMA)PEP 15-FEDGUIDEOTP. Rockville (MD): Substance Abuse and Mental Health Services Administration; 2015.

27. Kaltenbach K, Berghella V, Finnegan L. Opioid dependence during pregnancy. Effects and management. Obstet Gynecol Clin North Am 1998;25(1):139–51.

28. Center for substance abuse treatment. Medication-assisted treatment for opioid addiction in opioid treatment programs inservice training. HHS publication no. (SMA) 09-4341. Rockville (MD): Substance Abuse and Mental Health Services Administration; 2008. Available at: https://Store.samhsa.gov/shin/content/SMA09-4341/SMA09-4341.pdf.

29. Jones HE. Specialty treatment for women. In: Strain EC, Stitzer ML, editors. Methadone treatment for opioid dependence. Baltimore (MD): Johns Hopkins University Press; 2006. p. 455–84.

30. Kandall SR, Albin S, Gartner LM, et al. The narcotic-dependent mother: fetal and neonatal consequences. Early Hum Dev 1977;1(2):159–69.

31. Jones HE, Heil SH, Baewert A, et al. Buprenorphine treatment of opioid-dependent pregnant women: a comprehensive review. Addiction 2012; 107(Suppl 1):5–27.

32. Jones HE, Kaltenbach K, Heil SH, et al. Neonatal abstinence syndrome after methadone or buprenorphine exposure. N Engl J Med 2010;363(24):2320–31.

33. Zedler BK, Mann AL, Kim MM, et al. Buprenorphine compared with methadone to treat pregnant women with opioid use disorder: a systematic review and meta-analysis of safety in the mother, fetus and child. Addiction 2016;111(12):2115–28.

34. Debelak K, Morrone WR, O'Grady KE, et al. Buprenorphine + naloxone in the treatment of opioid dependence during pregnancy-initial patient care and outcome data. Am J Addict 2013;22(3):252–4.

35. Lund IO, Fischer G, Welle-Strand GK, et al. A comparison of buprenorphine + naloxone to buprenorphine and methadone in the treatment of opioid dependence during pregnancy: maternal and neonatal outcomes. Subst Abuse 2013;7:61–74.

36. Jumah NA, Edwards C, Balfour-Boehm J, et al. Observational study of the safety of buprenorphine+naloxone in pregnancy in a rural and remote population. BMJ Open 2016;6(10):e011774.

37. Martin CE, Longinaker N, Terplan M. Recent trends in treatment admissions for prescription opioid abuse during pregnancy. J Subst Abuse Treat 2015;48(1): 37–42.

38. Krans EE, Bogen D, Richardson G, et al. Factors associated with buprenorphine versus methadone use in pregnancy. Subst Abus 2016;37(4):550–7.

39. Meyer M, Wagner K, Benvenuto A, et al. Intrapartum and postpartum analgesia for women maintained on methadone during pregnancy. Obstet Gynecol 2007; 110(2 Pt 1):261–6.

40. Weaver M, Schnoll S. Abuse liability in opioid therapy for pain treatment in patients with an addiction history. Clin J Pain 2002;18(4 Suppl):S61–9.

41. Jones HE, O'Grady K, Dahne J, et al. Management of acute postpartum pain in patients maintained on methadone or buprenorphine during pregnancy. Am J Drug Alcohol Abuse 2009;35(3):151–6.

42. Strain EC, Preston KL, Liebson IA, et al. Precipitated withdrawal by pentazocine in methadone-maintained volunteers. J Pharmacol Exp Ther 1993;267(2): 624–34.

43. McCarthy JJ, Posey BL. Methadone levels in human milk. J Hum Lact 2000; 16(2):115–20.

44. Section on Breastfeeding. Breastfeeding and the use of human milk. Pediatrics 2012;129(3):e827–41.

45. Jansson LM, Velez M, Harrow C. Methadone maintenance and lactation: a review of the literature and current management guidelines. J Hum Lact 2004; 20(1):62–71.

46. Abdel-Latif ME, Pinner J, Clews S, et al. Effects of breast milk on the severity and outcome of neonatal abstinence syndrome among infants of drug-dependent mothers. Pediatrics 2006;117(6):e1163–9.

47. Marquet P, Chevrel J, Lavignasse P, et al. Buprenorphine withdrawal syndrome in a newborn. Clin Pharmacol Ther 1997;62(5):569–71.

48. Pichini S, Puig C, Zuccaro P, et al. Assessment of exposure to opiates and cocaine during pregnancy in a Mediterranean city: preliminary results of the "meconium project.". Forensic Sci Int 2005;153(1):59–65.

49. Jones W. Cocaine use and the breastfeeding mother. Pract Midwife 2015;18(1): 19–22.

50. American College of Obstetricians and Gynecologists Committee on Obstetric Practice. Committee opinion no. 637: marijuana use during pregnancy and lactation. Obstet Gynecol 2015;126(1):234–8.

51. Wilder C, Lewis D, Winhusen T. Medication assisted treatment discontinuation in pregnant and postpartum women with opioid use disorder. Drug Alcohol Depend 2015;149:225–31.

52. Committee on Obstetric Practice. Committee opinion no. 711: opioid use and opioid use disorder in pregnancy. Obstet Gynecol 2017;130(2):e81–94.

53. Metz TD, Rovner P, Hoffman MC, et al. Maternal deaths from suicide and overdose in Colorado, 2004-2012. Obstet Gynecol 2016;128(6):1233–40.

54. O'Connor AB, Uhler B, O'Brien LM, et al. Predictors of treatment retention in postpartum women prescribed buprenorphine during pregnancy. J Subst Abuse Treat 2018;86:26–9.
55. Schiff DM, Patrick SW, Terplan M. Maternal health in the United States. N Engl J Med 2018;378(6):587.
56. Anand KJ, Willson DF, Berger J, et al. Tolerance and withdrawal from prolonged opioid use in critically ill children. Pediatrics 2010;125(5):e1208–25.
57. FDA. Neonatal Opioid withdrawal syndrome and medication-assisted treatment with methadone and buprenorphine 2016. Available at: https://www.fda.gov/Drugs/DrugSafety/ucm503630.htm. Accessed August 8, 2017.
58. Law KL, Stroud LR, LaGasse LL, et al. Smoking during pregnancy and newborn neurobehavior. Pediatrics 2003;111(6 Pt 1):1318–23.
59. Food and Drug Administration. FDA drug safety communication: antipsychotic drug labels updated on use during pregnancy and risk of abnormal muscle movements and withdrawal symptoms in newborns. Silver Spring, MD: U.S. Food and Drug Administration Location; 2011.
60. Koren G, Matsui D, Einarson A, et al. Is maternal use of selective serotonin re-uptake inhibitors in the third trimester of pregnancy harmful to neonates? CMAJ 2005;172(11):1457–9.
61. Huybrechts KF, Bateman BT, Desai RJ, et al. Risk of neonatal drug withdrawal after intrauterine co-exposure to opioids and psychotropic medications: cohort study. BMJ 2017;358:j3326.
62. Jones HE, Heil SH, Tuten M, et al. Cigarette smoking in opioid-dependent pregnant women: neonatal and maternal outcomes. Drug Alcohol Depend 2013; 131(3):271–7.
63. Desai RJ, Huybrechts KF, Hernandez-Diaz S, et al. Exposure to prescription opioid analgesics in utero and risk of neonatal abstinence syndrome: population based cohort study. BMJ 2015;350:h2102.
64. Cleary BJ, Donnelly J, Strawbridge J, et al. Methadone dose and neonatal abstinence syndrome-systematic review and meta-analysis. Addiction 2010;105(12): 2071–84.
65. Zahorodny W, Rom C, Whitney W, et al. The neonatal withdrawal inventory: a simplified score of newborn withdrawal. J Dev Behav Pediatr 1998;19(2):89–93.
66. Lipsitz PJ. A proposed narcotic withdrawal score for use with newborn infants. A pragmatic evaluation of its efficacy. Clin Pediatr (phila) 1975;14(6):592–4.
67. Ostrea E. Infants of drug-dependent mothers. In: Burg F, Ingelfinger J, Wald R, editors. Current pediatric therapy. 14th edition. Philadelphia: WB Saunders; 1993. p. 800–1.
68. Green M, Suffet F. The neonatal narcotic withdrawal index: a device for the improvement of care in the abstinence syndrome. Am J Drug Alcohol Abuse 1981;8(2):203–13.
69. Finnegan LP, Connaughton JF Jr, Kron RE, et al. Neonatal abstinence syndrome: assessment and management. Addict Dis 1975;2(1–2):141–58.
70. Zimmermann-Baer U, Notzli U, Rentsch K, et al. Finnegan neonatal abstinence scoring system: normal values for first 3 days and weeks 5-6 in non-addicted infants. Addiction 2010;105(3):524–8.
71. Jones HE, Harrow C, O'Grady KE, et al. Neonatal abstinence scores in opioid-exposed and nonexposed neonates: a blinded comparison. J Opioid Manag 2010;6(6):409–13.
72. Jones HE, Seashore C, Johnson E, et al. Measurement of neonatal abstinence syndrome: evaluation of short forms. J Opioid Manag 2016;12(1):19–23.

73. Isemann BT, Stoeckle EC, Taleghani AA, et al. Early prediction tool to identify the need for pharmacotherapy in infants at risk of neonatal abstinence syndrome. Pharmacotherapy 2017;37(7):840–8.

74. Maguire D, Cline GJ, Parnell L, et al. Validation of the Finnegan neonatal abstinence syndrome tool-short form. Adv Neonatal Care 2013;13(6):430–7.

75. Gomez Pomar E, Finnegan LP, Devlin L, et al. Simplification of the Finnegan neonatal abstinence scoring system: retrospective study of two institutions in the USA. BMJ Open 2017;7(9):e016176.

76. Wachman EM, Grossman M, Schiff DM, et al. Quality improvement initiative to improve inpatient outcomes for neonatal abstinence syndrome. J Perinatol 2018;38(8):1114–22.

77. Grossman MR, Berkwitt AK, Osborn RR, et al. An initiative to improve the quality of care of infants with neonatal abstinence syndrome. Pediatrics 2017;139(6). https://doi.org/10.1542/peds.2016-3360.

78. Holmes AV, Atwood EC, Whalen B, et al. Rooming-in to treat neonatal abstinence syndrome: improved family-centered care at lower cost. Pediatrics 2016;137(6). https://doi.org/10.1542/peds.2015-2929.

79. Ryan G, Dooley J, Gerber Finn L, et al. Nonpharmacological management of neonatal abstinence syndrome: a review of the literature. J Matern Fetal Neonatal Med 2019;32(10):1735–40.

80. Tsai LC, Doan TJ. Breastfeeding among mothers on opioid maintenance treatment: a literature review. J Hum Lact 2016;32(3):521–9.

81. Short VL, Gannon M, Abatemarco DJ. The association between breastfeeding and length of hospital stay among infants diagnosed with neonatal abstinence syndrome: a population-based study of in-hospital births. Breastfeed Med 2016;11:343–9.

82. Newman A, Davies GA, Dow K, et al. Rooming-in care for infants of opioid-dependent mothers: implementation and evaluation at a tertiary care hospital. Can Fam Physician 2015;61(12):e555–61.

83. Abrahams RR, Kelly SA, Payne S, et al. Rooming-in compared with standard care for newborns of mothers using methadone or heroin. Can Fam Physician 2007;53(10):1722–30.

84. McKnight S, Coo H, Davies G, et al. Rooming-in for infants at risk of neonatal abstinence syndrome. Am J Perinatol 2016;33(5):495–501.

85. Gowing L, Ali R, White JM, et al. Buprenorphine for managing opioid withdrawal. Cochrane Database Syst Rev 2017;(2):CD002025.

86. Gowing L, Farrell M, Ali R, et al. Alpha(2)-adrenergic agonists for the management of opioid withdrawal. Cochrane Database Syst Rev 2016;(5):CD002024.

87. Burnette T, Chernicky L, Towers CV. The effect of standardizing treatment when managing neonatal abstinence syndrome. J Matern Fetal Neonatal Med 2018;1–5. https://doi.org/10.1080/14767058.2018.1465038.

88. Hall ES, Wexelblatt SL, Crowley M, et al. A multicenter cohort study of treatments and hospital outcomes in neonatal abstinence syndrome. Pediatrics 2014;134(2):e527–34.

89. Hall ES, Wexelblatt SL, Crowley M, et al. Implementation of a neonatal abstinence syndrome weaning protocol: a multicenter cohort study. Pediatrics 2015;136(4):e803–10.

90. Asti L, Magers JS, Keels E, et al. A quality improvement project to reduce length of stay for neonatal abstinence syndrome. Pediatrics 2015;135(6):e1494–500.

91. Patrick SW, Schumacher RE, Horbar JD, et al. Improving care for neonatal abstinence syndrome. Pediatrics 2016;137(5). https://doi.org/10.1542/peds.2015-3835.

92. Davis JM, Shenberger J, Terrin N, et al. Comparison of safety and efficacy of methadone vs morphine for treatment of neonatal abstinence syndrome: a randomized clinical trial. JAMA Pediatr 2018;172(8):741–8.

93. Tolia VN, Murthy K, Bennett MM, et al. Morphine vs methadone treatment for infants with neonatal abstinence syndrome. J Pediatr 2018;203:185–9.

94. Kraft WK, Adeniyi-Jones SC, Chervoneva I, et al. Buprenorphine for the treatment of the neonatal abstinence syndrome. N Engl J Med 2017;376(24):2341–8.

95. Hall ES, Isemann BT, Wexelblatt SL, et al. A cohort comparison of buprenorphine versus methadone treatment for neonatal abstinence syndrome. J Pediatr 2016;170:39–44.e1.

96. Hall ES, Rice WR, Folger AT, et al. Comparison of neonatal abstinence syndrome treatment with sublingual buprenorphine versus conventional opioids. Am J Perinatol 2018;35(4):405–12.

97. Kraft WK, Adeniyi-Jones SC, Ehrlich ME. Buprenorphine for the neonatal abstinence syndrome. N Engl J Med 2017;377(10):997–8.

98. Liu T, Lewis T, Gauda E, et al. Mechanistic population pharmacokinetics of morphine in neonates with abstinence syndrome after oral administration of diluted tincture of opium. J Clin Pharmacol 2016;56(8):1009–18.

99. Moore JN, Healy JR, Thoma BN, et al. A population pharmacokinetic model for vancomycin in adult patients receiving extracorporeal membrane oxygenation therapy. CPT Pharmacometrics Syst Pharmacol 2016;5(9):495–502. Available at: http://www.ncbi.nlm.nih.gov/pmc/articles/PMC5036424/.

100. Wiles JR, Isemann B, Mizuno T, et al. Pharmacokinetics of oral methadone in the treatment of neonatal abstinence syndrome: a pilot study. J Pediatr 2015;167(6):1214–20.e3.

101. Xie HG, Cao YJ, Gauda EB, et al. Clonidine clearance matures rapidly during the early postnatal period: a population pharmacokinetic analysis in newborns with neonatal abstinence syndrome. J Clin Pharmacol 2011;51(4):502–11.

102. Hall ES, Meinzen-Derr J, Wexelblatt SL. Cohort analysis of a pharmacokinetic-modeled methadone weaning optimization for neonatal abstinence syndrome. J Pediatr 2015;167(6):1221–5.e1.

103. Murphy-Oikonen J, McQueen K. Outpatient pharmacologic weaning for neonatal abstinence syndrome: a systematic review. Prim Health Care Res Dev 2018;1–9. https://doi.org/10.1017/S1463423618000270.

104. Maalouf FI, Cooper WO, Slaughter JC, et al. Outpatient pharmacotherapy for neonatal abstinence syndrome. J Pediatr 2018;199:151–7.e1.

105. Pandey R, Pandey Sapkota N, Kumar D. Neonatal abstinence syndrome: twins case series. Front Pediatr 2017;5:242.

106. Crist RC, Reiner BC, Berrettini WH. A review of opioid addiction genetics. Curr Opin Psychol 2018;27:31–5.

107. Wachman EM, Hayes MJ, Brown MS, et al. Association of OPRM1 and COMT single-nucleotide polymorphisms with hospital length of stay and treatment of neonatal abstinence syndrome. JAMA 2013;309(17):1821–7.

108. Wachman EM, Hayes MJ, Sherva R, et al. Variations in opioid receptor genes in neonatal abstinence syndrome. Drug Alcohol Depend 2015;155:253–9.

109. Fielder A, Coller J, Hutchinson M, et al. Neonatal abstinence syndrome in methadone exposed infants: role of genetic variability. Drug Alcohol Depend 2015;146:e202–84.

110. Wachman EM, Hayes MJ, Shrestha H, et al. Epigenetic variation in OPRM1 gene in opioid-exposed mother-infant dyads. Genes Brain Behav 2018;17(7):e12476.
111. Wachman EM, Hayes MJ, Lester BM, et al. Epigenetic variation in the mu-opioid receptor gene in infants with neonatal abstinence syndrome. J Pediatr 2014; 165(3):472–8.
112. Lainwala S, Brown ER, Weinschenk NP, et al. A retrospective study of length of hospital stay in infants treated for neonatal abstinence syndrome with methadone versus oral morphine preparations. Adv Neonatal Care 2005;5(5):265–72.
113. Young ME, Hager SJ, Spurlock D Jr. Retrospective chart review comparing morphine and methadone in neonates treated for neonatal abstinence syndrome. Am J Health Syst Pharm 2015;72(23 Suppl 3):S162–7.
114. Brown MS, Hayes MJ, Thornton LM. Methadone versus morphine for treatment of neonatal abstinence syndrome: a prospective randomized clinical trial. J Perinatol 2015;35(4):278–83.

Balancing the Use of Medications While Maintaining Breastfeeding

Palika Datta, PhD[a], Teresa Baker, MD[b], Thomas W. Hale, PhD[a],*

KEYWORDS

- Medications • Breastfeeding • Pharmacokinetics • Drug transfer
- Relative infant dose

KEY POINTS

- Use of medications during lactation is common.
- It is essential to understand the physiochemical properties that facilitate the transfer of drugs and the pharmacokinetics of individual drugs in human breast milk.
- Studies of the effect of drugs in breast milk on infant wellbeing and subsequent development are limited.
- Most drugs can safely be used in breastfeeding mothers, but a risk versus benefit assessment is always required before use for each drug.

INTRODUCTION

Human milk is the best source of an infant's nutrition. Benefits include stimulating growth, immunity, and neurobehavioral development, as well as protection against infection. It is perfectly suited for the infant's gastrointestinal tract and has numerous factors that promote growth and maturation of a relatively permeable neonatal gastrointestinal tract. Breastfeeding also provides benefit to the mother including a significant reduction in breast cancer risk.[1,2] The American Academy of Pediatrics and the World Health Organization both recommend exclusive breast milk feeding for at least 6 months, followed by continued complementary feeding until a minimum of 12 months has passed. Although recent studies suggest that the number of women who choose to exclusively breast milk feed is increasing (approximately 72% initiate breastfeeding), those who discontinue breastfeeding on the advice from their health care providers remains high. One of the primary reasons given by providers for

Disclosure Statement: The authors declare no conflict of interest.
[a] Department of Pediatrics, Texas Tech University Health Sciences Center, 1400 Wallace Boulevard, Amarillo, TX 79106, USA; [b] Department of Obstetrics and Gynecology, Texas Tech University Health Sciences Center, 1400 Coulter Street, Amarillo, TX 79106, USA
* Corresponding author.
E-mail address: thomas.hale@ttuhsc.edu

patients to discontinue breastfeeding is to restart medications. Many women receive medication or some other therapeutic agent while breastfeeding.[3]

Since so many women take medications in the weeks and months after delivery, one of the most common questions encountered in pediatrics and obstetrics concerns the use of drugs in breastfeeding mothers. Information on the extent of drug excretion in human milk is not available for many drugs, and data from animals may not correlate with that observed in humans. In the absence of data, health care professionals often advise mothers to discontinue breastfeeding when taking a medication to maximize safety. In the past 20 years, our understanding of the kinetics of drug entry into human milk has improved significantly. Most of the physicochemical properties that facilitate the transfer of drugs into breast milk (such as molecular weight, pharmacokinetics, and lipophilic properties) have now been studied in detail and are well known for many medications. This article provides a better understanding of the physiology and pharmacology of breastfeeding and the general principles of medication transfer to the breastfed infant.

PHYSIOLOGY OF LACTATION

A basic understanding of the physiology of breast milk production is important to make decisions regarding medications for the breastfeeding mother.[4] Lactogenesis is defined as the process by which the mammary glands produce and secrete milk, and occurs in 4 stages. The alveolar cell is the principal site for milk production. Neville[5] describes 5 steps for milk synthesis and secretion by the mammary alveolus, including 4 major transcellular and 1 paracellular pathway. They are (1) exocytosis (merocrine secretion) of milk protein and lactose in Golgi-derived secretory vesicles, (2) milk fat secretion via milk fat globules (apocrine secretion), (3) secretion of ions and water across the apical membrane, (4) pinocytosis-exocytosis (eg, of immunoglobulins), and (5) paracellular pathways for plasma components and leukocytes. During lactation, few of the constituents of breast milk are transferred directly from maternal blood.

Stage 1 of lactogenesis begins during mid-pregnancy and is characterized by full alveolar development and maturation of the glandular tissues of the breast so that it is competent to secrete milk (colostrum). During gestation, high levels of circulating progesterone inhibit the production of milk. Stage 2 of lactogenesis occurs during the first 2 to 4 days postpartum. An incremental increase in colostrum secretion occurs in concert with the decrease in levels of progesterone. Colostrum is a thick yellow liquid comprised mostly of protein, especially secretory immunoglobulins, as well as lactose and low levels of fat compared with mature milk. Pharmacologic doses of progesterone or estrogen administered early in the postnatal period may disrupt the orderly progression of stage 2 lactogenesis.

During stage 2 of lactogenesis, the intercellular gaps within the mammary tissue widens, which allows large molecules and interstitial fluids (such as maternal IgG or large drug moieties up to 800 Da) to pass more easily into the colostrum. With the decrease in circulating progesterone and high prolactin levels induced by frequent nursing, the alveolar cells enlarge and seal off the intercellular gaps thereby inhibiting the passage of moieties greater than 200 to 300 Da. During postpartum days 2 to 5, there is a dramatic increase in mammary blood flow and oxygen and glucose uptake by the breast.

After 2 to 7 days postpartum, lactation enters an indefinite period of milk production that was formerly called galactopoiesis, but is now referred to as stage 3 lactogenesis. Prolactin is the single most important galactopoietic hormone, and selective inhibition of prolactin secretion by bromocriptine or ergot derivatives will disrupt lactogenesis altogether. Stimulation of the nipple and areola or even behavioral cues cause the release of oxytocin from the mother's posterior pituitary and subsequent reflex contraction of the alveolar complex leading to ejection of milk from the breast. During this 1- to 2-day period, the transfer of drugs into milk may be significant, but the volume transferred (30–60 mL/d) and hence the dose to the infant is minimal.

The final stage of lactation, stage 4 lactogenesis, involves involution and cessation of breastfeeding. As milk production is reduced and finally ceases, large intercellular gaps may again arise between alveolar cells. Such gaps allow larger molecules to pass easily into the breast milk. Although the drug exposure may increase slightly during this period, the markedly decreased volume of breast milk will deliver a significantly reduced total dose to the infant. Moreover, metabolically, the older child is better able to metabolize and excrete drugs.

FACTORS DETERMINING TRANSFER OF DRUGS INTO BREAST MILK

It is essential to understand the mechanisms associated with the passage of drugs, proteins, and lipids across the apical membrane of the alveolar cell. The state of the alveolar cells, and the physiochemistry of the medication itself, are 2 important factors that control the transport of drugs. The following physiochemical factors affect the transfer of drugs into breast milk:

Drug Concentration

The strongest determinant of drug transfer into breast milk is the maternal plasma (non-protein bound) concentration of the drug. Whereas most drugs transfer into milk largely as a function of equilibrium forces between the plasma and milk compartment, there are a few drugs for which the milk/plasma ratio is significantly elevated, more than would be expected by passive diffusion alone. Such drugs are likely excreted into breast milk by active transport processes, giving a milk/plasma (M/P) ratio greater than 1. Examples of such drugs include nitrofurantoin (M/P = 6),[6] cimetidine (M/P = 5.5),[7] acyclovir (M/P = 4.1),[8] ranitidine (M/P = 6.7–23.8),[9] and iodine (M/P = 23).[10,11] Iodine is so readily transported to the infant via breast milk, that almost 27% of the maternal dose is ingested by the infant, which can lead to clinically hazardous levels.[10]

Molecular Weight of the Drug

The passive diffusion of a medication across a lipid bilayer is largely determined by the molecular weight of the compound. Drugs with a low molecular weight (<500 Da) are more likely to transfer across the membrane.[12] High-molecular-weight products, such as heparin (12–15,000 Da) and most monoclonal antibodies (molecular weight >150,000 Da), are largely excluded from breast milk owing to their size alone. Small amounts may diffuse between cells, but this is usually clinically insignificant. Many of the new monoclonal IgG preparations (eg, infliximab, certolizumab, etanercept) are effectively excluded from the milk compartment because of size alone.

Lipid Content

The lipid content of milk is high, ranging from 2.3% in foremilk to as high as 8% in hindmilk. The higher the lipophilic nature of a drug, the better it is able to penetrate through lipid bilayers (including those of lactocytes) and concentrate in the milk compartment. The pK_a of a drug is a unique physicochemical property that controls its ionization state when in solution. Because the pH of milk (pH 7.2) is less than that of plasma (pH 7.4), some drugs with a high pK_a can become trapped in the milk compartment.[13,14] While interesting, this is a rare occurrence.

In summary, drugs with high maternal plasma levels, low molecular weights, poor ionization, high lipophilic nature, limited volume of distribution, and low protein binding capacity often produce higher levels in breast milk.

ESTIMATION OF DRUG EXPOSURE

Another measure of the ability of a drug to transfer into human milk is the M/P ratio. Drugs with a high M/P ratio are often lipid soluble and small in molecular weight. A high M/P ratio may lead one to assume that the dose of the drug transferred is high, which may not necessarily be the case. Ultimately, the maternal plasma concentration of a drug is the most important factor that determines the dose transferred to the infant. Drugs that are highly protein bound and produce low "free plasma" levels of drug will ultimately result in lower levels in milk.

Another clinically useful estimate of the amount of drug transferred to the breastfeeding infant is the relative infant dose (RID). This value is typically expressed as a percentage of the maternal dose that is received by the infant. The RID formula (below) is standardized by the weight of the mother and the daily intake of milk by an infant, assumed to be 150 mL/kg/d. In general, whereas an RID less than 10% is considered acceptable in a healthy postnatal infant, a value greater than 25% may have a therapeutic effect on the infant if absorbed through the gastrointestinal tract. Most drugs have an RID less than 1%, and only around 3% of drugs have an RID greater than 25%.

$$RID(\%) = \frac{Absolute\ Infant\ Dose(mg/kg/day)}{Maternal\ Dose(mg/kg/day)}$$

PHARMACOKINETICS AND BIOAVAILABILITY OF DRUGS

The metabolic capacity of infants changes as they age and is almost that of an adult at 12 months of age. However, little is known about the oral absorption and bioavailability of medications in infants.[15] In newborn infants, gastric emptying time is delayed and intestinal absorption is irregular. Slower intestinal absorption tends to be advantageous, as this would tend to keep plasma concentrations of medications lower in the infant.[16] Premature infants, who have more vulnerable renal and hepatic systems, are at greater risk than term infants. The absorption of medications by the infant is affected by many different factors, including the dose administered to the mother, the bioavailability of the drug in the mother, the amount of drug transferred into her breast milk, and ultimately the bioavailability of the drug in the infant. Most medications must be absorbed into the infant's plasma compartment to produce untoward effects. Drugs administered orally are absorbed through the intestines into the portal circulation, and then pass through the liver before their delivery to the rest of the body. Often, the liver sequesters and metabolizes drugs, thus eliminating their systemic effect. This is particularly true of opiates (eg, morphine) and cannabis products, which are largely eliminated from the circulation during their first pass through the liver. Fortunately, many medications with poor oral bioavailability in adults are also poorly absorbed in infants, thus limiting drug exposure. Morphine is a classic example, for which 75% of the drug is sequestered in the liver following the first pass.

SELECTED DRUG CLASSES
Analgesics

Pain experienced during the early postpartum period is common in breastfeeding mothers. Ibuprofen and acetaminophen are perhaps the 2 most widely used analgesics in this setting. Fortunately, a moderate amount of data exists on these drugs and their use in breastfeeding mothers (**Table 1**).[17]

Acetaminophen is a good choice for the treatment of pain or fever in lactating mothers because adverse effects are rare in breastfed infants. Levels of acetaminophen depend largely on the maternal dose, but are generally low at less than 6.4% of the maternal dose. Following a 1 g intravenous (IV) maternal dose of acetaminophen, the peak plasma concentration was 28 mg/L 15 minutes after administration. According to one report, following a 2 g IV dose of acetaminophen in postpartum mothers, maternal plasma levels decreased from 22.5 to 3.9 mg/L within 6 hours.[18] Following a single IV dose, a maternal peak plasma concentration of 28 mg/L suggests that a breastfed infant would receive a dose of 19.6 to 28 mg/d (M/P = 1) or about 4 to 6 mg/kg/d. This is far lower than the clinical doses currently recommended for infants (10–15 mg/kg/dose).

Ibuprofen is also a good analgesic for breastfeeding mothers because less than 0.7% of the maternal dose is transferred in breast milk to the infant.[19] Ketorolac is another popular non-steroidal anti-inflammatory agent, but is more controversial. It can produce bleeding problems and reduce renal function in some postpartum women; however, documented levels in breast milk are insignificant. In a study of 10 lactating women who received 10 mg ketorolac orally 4 times daily, the RID was estimated at 0.2% of the maternal dose.[20] Studies of the COX2 inhibitor, celecoxib, suggest that it is also a safe analgesic for breastfeeding mothers. Knoppert and colleagues[21] estimated that an infant receives a dose of approximately 20 μg/kg/d. When studied in the author's laboratory, the absolute infant dose averaged 9.8 μg/kg/d and the mean RID was only 0.30% in women receiving a 200 mg daily dose.[22] Aspirin (acetylsalicylic acid) is a commonly used drug and its levels in milk range from low to undetectable. Used intermittently and in low dose, aspirin probably poses little to no risk to a breastfed infant. Unfortunately, the risk of Reye's syndrome remains largely unknown. Most cases of Reye's syndrome in the past occurred among adolescents using therapeutic doses of aspirin (650 mg or more) to treat viral fevers. Aspirin has an unusual pharmacokinetic profile in that it binds to platelets in the portal circulation and then is removed almost completely during the first pass through the liver. In the liver, aspirin is almost completely metabolized to salicylic acid within 2 hours of administration. A recent study reported an RID of salicylic acid at 0.4% in 7 breastfeeding women who were consuming 81 mg doses of aspirin. This study suggests that, following the use of acetylsalicylic acid, only its metabolite salicylic acid was found in human milk and in very low concentrations.[23]

Opiate analgesics such as morphine, codeine, hydrocodone, fentanyl, and meperidine have been well studied in breastfeeding women. Although morphine, hydrocodone, and fentanyl are generally preferred to control pain in the postnatal period, there have been recent efforts to avoid opiates because of their rapid metabolism and potential for addiction. Breast milk levels are reported to be low and the oral bioavailability of morphine is low in exposed infants. Hydrocodone and codeine have been used in large populations of breastfeeding mothers for many years with only occasional somnolence noted in term infants. However, new data concerning the rapid metabolism that occurs in some patients urges caution in the use of these opioids. The American College of Obstetrics and Gynecology still recommends these opioids when necessary to control severe pain.[24] Narcotic agents such as oxycodone, pentazocine, propoxyphene, and meperidine are not recommended for use in the lactating mother. Relatively high amounts of oxycodone are transferred into human milk, and central nervous system depression has been reported in up to 20% of infants exposed during breastfeeding.[25] Hydromorphone levels in milk are low, averaging

Table 1
Commonly used medications during lactation

Medications	Relative Infant Dose (%) Range	Recommendations
Analgesics		
Acetaminophen	6.4–24.2	Should be safe. No adverse effects observed
Celecoxib	0.3–0.7	Considered safe
Aspirin	2.5–10.8	Safe at low doses, caution at higher doses
Ibuprofen	0.12–0.66	Safe to use
Naproxen	3.3	Compatible, but only with short courses. Excessive bleeding reported
Indomethacin	1.2	Compatible, but only short courses
Ketorolac	0.14–0.2	Safe to use
Hydrocodone	2.2–3.7	Safe, but use with caution. Sedation observed
Morphine	9–35	Compatible in normal doses. Caution in high doses
Codeine	0.6–0.8	Safe, but use with caution, especially in premature infants
Fentanyl	2.9–5	Concerns, infant to be monitored
Hydromorphone	0.7	Safe, but concerns expressed
Antibiotics		
Amoxicillin	0.95	Compatible. Observe infant for diarrhea or changes in gut flora
Cephalexin	0.39–1.47	Compatible. Observe infant
Dicloxacillin	0.6–1.4	Compatible. Observe infant for diarrhea
Azithromycin	5.9	Safe, infant to be observed
Erythromycin	1.4–1.7	Safe, observe infant for diarrhea
Doxycycline	4.2–13.3	Compatible for short-term use (<3 wk). Avoid chronic dosing
Tetracycline	0.6	Compatible for short-term use. Oral absorption low
Clindamycin	0.9–1.8	Compatible. One case of pseudomembranous colitis reported. Observe infant for diarrhea
Metronidazole	12.6–13.5	Moderate transfer. No adverse effects reported in exposed infants
Vancomycin	6.5–6.6	Compatible. Poor oral bioavailability. Dose via milk subclinical
Antidepressants		
Amitriptyline	1.0–2.8	Safe. Observe infant for sedation
Bupropion	0.1–1.9	Compatible. Do not use in patients subject to seizures
Citalopram, escitalopram	3.56–5.37	Caution, somnolence reported
Desipramine	0.3–0.9	Compatible. Observe for sedation
Doxepin	0.3	Metabolite accumulation in milk. Respiratory arrest and sedation reported
Fluoxetine	1.6–14.6	Probably safe. Avoid high maternal dose in early postpartum period
Paroxetine	1.2–2.8	Compatible
Sertraline	0.4–2.2	Compatible, and the preferred selective serotonin reuptake inhibitors
Venlafaxine	6.8–8.1	Probably safe, relatively high RID

about 0.67% of the maternal dose.[26] However, a recent case report suggested that repeated use of high-dose hydromorphone (4 mg every 4 hours) led to respiratory difficulties in a full-term infant at 6 days of life.[27] After a dose of naloxone, the infant recovered rapidly.

Antibiotics

Antibiotics are commonly used in breastfeeding mothers. Numerous studies have been published reviewing the transfer of antibiotics into human milk.[28,29] Virtually all penicillins and cephalosporins have been studied and are known to produce only trace levels in milk. The use of these drugs is generally considered safe.[30–36] Amoxicillin reaches very low concentrations in human milk after maternal administration of 1 g. Some change in infant intestinal flora could be expected. The transfer of tetracycline antibiotics (such as doxycycline and tetracycline) into human breast milk is very low. The bioavailability of these products in the infant is poor, as they tend to precipitate out of solution in the presence of calcium in milk. Doxycycline absorption is delayed but not blocked, and its absorption may be significant over time. Short-term use of tetracyclines for up to 3 to 5 weeks is permissible and may be preferred in certain circumstances. The use of fluoroquinolones during lactation is controversial. Although the dose the infant receives via breast milk is low, a case of pseudomembranous colitis has been reported (although this can occur with any antibiotic).[37] In one group of infants exposed to fluoroquinolones for up to 20 days, a greenish discoloration of the infants' teeth was noted at 12 to 23 months of age.[38] Calcium salts are believed to compromise the bioavailability of ciprofloxacin; hence, high levels of calcium found in human milk may suppress the oral bioavailability in an infant. In one study of 10 women who received 750 mg of ciprofloxacin every 12 hours, breast milk levels ranged from 3.79 mg/L at 2 hours post-dose to 0.02 mg/L at 24 hours.[39] Ciprofloxacin ophthalmic products are poorly absorbed and blood levels are low.

The use of the antiprotozoal agent metronidazole in breastfeeding women is controversial. Discovered in 1960s, metronidazole is reputedly mutagenic. Whereas claims of mutagenicity are still evident in rodent studies, no such effect has been found in humans. Topical and vaginal preparations of metronidazole are of little concern to a breastfeeding mother because of limited systemic absorption via these routes of administration. Following oral doses of 1200 mg/d, the maximum concentration in breast milk was 15.5 mg/L.[40] Although the RID of metronidazole is moderate (approximating 13% of the maternal dose), no adverse effects have been reported in infants. Although most antibiotics are considered suitable during breastfeeding, the pK_a profile of each drug must be evaluated to ensure safety in the breastfeeding infant.[41]

Sulfonamides

Sulfamethoxazole is still commonly used in combination with trimethoprim (sulfamethoxazole/trimethoprim) for various infections, now including methicillin-resistant *Staphylococcus aureus*. The RID of sulfamethoxazole and trimethoprim is 2.32% to 2.95% and 3.9% to 9.0%, respectively.[42] These doses are still far lower than typical doses used to treat infants in a clinical setting. However, mothers of infants with hyperbilirubinemia or with glucose-6-phosphate dehydrogenase deficiency should use sulfonamides with caution, particularly during the first 6 weeks postpartum.

Antifungal Medications

Antifungal medications used during breastfeeding are prescribed mainly for yeast infections. Nystatin is virtually unabsorbed when given orally, thus its transfer into breast milk is minimal. Fluconazole transfers into human breast milk with an RID of 16%,[43,44] which is far less than the clinical doses commonly prescribed in infants. As such, it is regarded as safe for breastfeeding mothers. Candida infections of the nipple are actually extremely rare and these products should no longer be used topically on the mother's nipples or orally for this indication as is sometimes done with fluconazole.[45]

Antihypertensive Medications

The use of antihypertensive medications in breastfeeding mothers, particularly those whose infants were born preterm, requires a high degree of vigilance. Diuretics and beta-blockers are commonly used for this indication. They are safe for use in breastfeeding women, with some precautions. The level of transfer into breast milk differs markedly. They are all weak bases, but differ in lipid solubility and protein binding. Several beta-blockers, such as atenolol and acebutolol,[46] have been associated with cyanosis, bradycardia, and hypotension in breastfed infants, although these cases are rare.[46,47] Preferred beta-blockers include metoprolol and propranolol, both of which produce minimal levels in breast milk. No significant side effects have yet been reported in breastfeeding infants. Studies in breastfeeding mothers using hydralazine and methyldopa suggest that levels in breast milk are low. Calcium channel blockers, particularly verapamil and nifedipine, have been studied extensively, produce low levels in breast milk, and have not been associated with adverse events in exposed infants. Nifedipine levels in breast milk are particularly low at less than 0.01 mg/kg/d.[48]

Angiotensin converting enzyme inhibitors have been extensively studied in breastfeeding mothers. Captopril and enalapril (but not nadolol) are preferred because breast milk levels for these 2 agents are low.[49–51] Since angiotensin converting enzyme inhibitors can cause severe nephrotoxicity in the offspring, especially when used in the last trimester of pregnancy, they should be used with caution. This is especially true in premature infants.

Diuretics including hydrochlorothiazide and furosemide have been studied in breastfeeding mothers. In one study of a mother receiving a 50 mg dose of hydrochlorothiazide each morning, milk levels were almost 25% of maternal plasma levels. However, serum levels of hydrochlorothiazide in the infant were undetectable (<20 ng/mL).[52] Most thiazide diuretics are considered compatible with breastfeeding if doses are kept low. Although the oral bioavailability of furosemide in newborn infants is low, it is frequently used in neonates to treat fluid overload.

Antidepressants

Maternal depression is known to have detrimental effects on parenting and child development.[53] Almost all of the tricyclic antidepressants have been studied in breastfeeding mothers and suggest that levels of these agents have little to no effect on breastfed infants. Patient compliance is poor with the tricyclic antidepressants due to anticholinergic symptoms such as xerostomia, blurred vision, and sedation. The RID of amitriptyline is less than 1.5% of the maternal dose.[54] Studies thus far have been unable to detect the drug in the plasma of breastfed infants. Doxepin should best be avoided because of reported cases of hypotonia, poor suckling, vomiting, and jaundice in newborn infants.[55] Desipramine levels in breast milk are minimal; one study of desipramine suggests an RID of 1% following a dose of 30 mg/d.[56]

The selective serotonin reuptake inhibitors are presently the mainstay of treatment of depression, primarily because they are effective and have minimal toxicity. Clinical studies of breastfeeding mothers taking sertraline, fluvoxamine, or paroxetine indicate that the transfer of these medications into human milk is minimal. Consistent information has been recently published, suggesting little or no effect on breastfed infants exposed to these antidepressants.[57] Sertraline seems to be the most commonly used agent, and studies including more than 50 exposed infants suggest that levels in breast milk and infant plasma range from low to undetectable. Fluoxetine has been studied in at least 29 breastfeeding infants. Fluoxetine transfers into human milk in higher concentrations, ranging as high as 9% of the maternal dose.[58] Because of its long half-life, active metabolites, and potential for accumulation in breast milk, it is advisable to avoid its use in breastfeeding women. In several cases, severe side effects such as colic, excessive sedation, seizures, or coma have been reported.[59-62] Therefore, fluoxetine is less preferred unless lower doses are used during pregnancy and in the early postpartum period. Citalopram and its newer congener, escitalopram, transfer into milk in moderate concentrations. In a study of 7 women receiving an average of 0.41 mg/kg/d of citalopram, the average breast milk level was 97 μg/L for citalopram and 36 μg/L for its metabolite (RID = 3.7%).[63] Low concentrations of citalopram were noted in the infants' plasma (2.0–2.3 μg/L). At this time, citalopram should be used with caution in mothers who are breastfeeding premature infants, because of the risk of apnea. In a recent study of 8 breastfeeding women taking an average of 10 mg/d of escitalopram, the total RID of escitalopram and its metabolite was reported to be 5.3%.[64] The drug and its metabolite were undetectable in most of the infants tested and no adverse events were reported. Neonatal withdrawal symptoms have been commonly reported in infants exposed to selective serotonin reuptake inhibitors in utero, including fluoxetine, sertraline, and orparoxetine. These symptoms consist of poor adaptation, irritability, jitteriness, and poor gaze control.[65-67]

Antipsychotics

The incidence of psychotic disorders during the postpartum period is higher than at any other time during a woman's life. This time period also coincides with breastfeeding. As a result, safety data on use of antipsychotics during breastfeeding are critical. First-generation antipsychotic agents, phenothiazines, seem to be safe, as demonstrated by lactation studies that have consistently reported M/P ratios of less than 1. Ten reports including a total of 28 infants exposed to antipsychotic agents through nursing reported no adverse events in most cases.[68] Haloperidol is commonly used to treat schizophrenia and Tourette syndrome. Its transfer into breast milk is reportedly minimal (RID ≤0.2%–11.2%).[69-71] Several new reports suggest that the newer atypical antipsychotics may be a better choice for breastfeeding mothers, but little information is currently available on these agents. Aripiprazole, for example, is transferred into breast milk in low concentrations, with levels reported to peak around 3 hours and plateaus around 12 hours after maternal administration.[72] However, recent evidence suggests aripiprazole may suppress prolactin levels and reduce milk production.[73] Risperidone levels are also reportedly to be quite low with an estimated RID of 0.6% to 6.5% and without any reported sedation in breastfed infants.[74,75] In several studies of olanzapine, the RID ranged from 0.9% to 1.12%.[76-78] In contrast, clozapine achieves relatively high concentrations in breast milk and infant serum. Because agranulocytosis and somnolence have been reported in breastfed infants,[79] clozapine is generally considered contraindicated during breastfeeding.

Cytotoxic/Chemotherapy Drugs

The diagnosis of cancer can occur in breastfeeding mothers. Most chemotherapeutic drugs are highly cytotoxic and are typically regarded as contraindicated during lactation because of the possibility of significant adverse effects in the infant (**Table 2**). Although cisplatin is transferred into breast milk, studies investigating its concentration remain conflicting; some studies report minimal concentrations and others report doses as high as 9%.[80] Given these observations, breastfeeding is best avoided in patients receiving cisplatin treatment. Carboplatin and paclitaxel have also been detected in breast milk. Although carboplatin concentrations have been found to be lower, paclitaxel can still be detected 13 days after a single dose.[81] Methotrexate transfer was determined for 12 consecutive days in one patient being treated for choriocarcinoma. Peak breast milk level was measured at 2.3 µg/L 10 hours after administration of 22.5 mg/d.[82] In a more recent case study of a mother being treated with a dose of 92 mg intramuscularly for placenta accreta, levels in milk were low, with an RID of only 0.11% and 0.02% for methotrexate and 7-OH-methtrexate, respectively.[83]

Fluorouracil is an anticancer medication that is rapidly converted into inactive metabolites and has a short half-life. As such, it is unlikely to be transferred into breast milk.[80] Cyclophosphamide is a pro-drug that is converted to its active form by hepatic enzymes. Its active metabolites have a short half-life, but are known to be highly cytotoxic. In one patient who received daily infusions of 2.8 g, the average RID over a period of 4 days varied from 4.7% on day 1 to 0.9% on day 4.[84] Ipilimumab, a monoclonal antibody used for the treatment of metastatic melanoma, was found in moderately high concentrations in breast milk even 5 days after infusion.[85] Thus far, there is only one case report of a woman given ipilimumab 3 mg/kg IV every 3 weeks for 4 doses postpartum. Breast milk levels increased 5 days after the infusion and continued to increase with subsequent doses. The average level of ipilimumab in breast milk was 75.36 ng/mL, which corresponded to an average infant dose of 53,481 ng/d. The authors further quantified the amount of drug an infant would receive over an 84-day course of maternal therapy as 4.5 mg. In this case, the woman was asked not to breastfeed until 3 weeks after her last infusion. The safety of this medication in lactation remains unknown. Because most chemotherapy drugs are highly

Table 2
Cytotoxic and drugs of abuse

Medications	Relative Infant Dose (%) Range	Recommendations
Cytotoxic drugs		
Cyclophosphamide	0.9–4.7	High caution. Possible immune suppression
Cyclosporine	0.05–3	High caution
Doxorubicin	2.44	High caution
Methotrexate	0.11–0.95	Use with caution
Paclitaxel	13.9–22.9	High caution
Carboplatin	1.8	High caution
Drugs of abuse		
Cocaine	Not known	Withdrawal symptoms observed
Heroin	Not known	Tremors, restlessness, vomiting, poor feeding observed
Marijuana (100 mg)	2.5	Long half-life for some compounds
Phencyclidine	Not known	Potent hallucinogen
Methadone	1.9–6.5	Use with caution. Withdrawal symptoms observed

toxic, extreme caution should be exercised before using such medications in a lactating mother.

Illicit Substances and Recreational Drugs

A large proportion of women consume illicit substances or alcohol during pregnancy and lactation. Whether or not to recommend breastfeeding in this population is controversial. It is important to recognize that breastfeeding provides enormous benefit to the infant and these may supersede the risk of certain illicit drugs. Drinking alcohol while breastfeeding is not recommended. That said, alcohol is rapidly metabolized in an adult and discarding any breast milk for 2 to 2.5 hours after the consumption of each 4 oz of alcohol will remove virtually all alcohol from the mother's plasma and milk compartment. The risk of harmful effects to infants from exposure to recreational drugs such as cocaine, heroin, and phencyclidine hydrochloride is significant, not only from direct exposure of the infant to the drug, but also from accompanying behavioral and environmental influences. The transfer of cocaine in breast milk is likely high because of its high lipid solubility, low molecular weight, and pK_a of 8.6. Infants exposed to cocaine through breast milk can display agitation, irritability, seizures, hypertension, and tachycardia.[78] Heroin is metabolized to morphine, which can transfer into milk relatively easily because of its lipid solubility and low protein binding. However, numerous clinical studies have shown that, given its large first-pass removal from the plasma, morphine is actually one of the safer opiates to use in breastfeeding mothers. In heroin addicts, however, the dose commonly used is supra-therapeutic and the risk to the infant from high doses of IV heroin is significant. Heroin addicts should not breastfeed, not only because of the drug's effect on the infant, but also because of the drug's effect on the mother.

Methadone has been extensively studied and does transfer into breast milk with an RID of 1.9% to 6.5%.[86] Infants may become dependent after prolonged exposure and withdrawal of methadone or breastfeeding may induce withdrawal effects in the breastfed infant. Nevertheless, methadone therapy in breastfeeding women is considered safe.

Cannabis is one of the most widely used phytocannabinoid drugs. Studies on long-term neurobehavioral effects have largely been limited to observational and animal data. Legalization of recreational cannabis has raised concerns in pregnant and breastfeeding women because effects on the developing brain are still unclear. Inhaled delta-9-tetrahydrocannabinol (THC), the most psychoactive compound, rapidly enters the plasma compartment and then redistributes primarily to the liver, brain, and adipose tissues (because it is highly lipid soluble). The result is high immediate plasma concentrations (within minutes) and longer central nervous system levels (2 hours). The secretion of small to moderate amounts of THC into breast milk has been reported in some older studies. A more recent pilot pharmacokinetic study examined the transfer of THC and its metabolite into human breast milk.[80] In this study, 8 women who were exclusively breastfeeding their 2- to 5-month-old infants were instructed to abstain from cannabis use for 24 hours before collecting their baseline sample, after which they smoked a pre-weighed strain containing 23.2% THC (inhaled in 3–4 hits over a period of 20 minutes) and then collected timed milk samples. The average concentration of THC in breast milk was 53.5 ng/mL and peaked at 1 hour after inhalation. The estimated RID was 2.5% (range 0.4%–8.7%) and the average infant dose was estimated to be 8 μg/kg/d. It is important to remember that absorption of THC is poor following oral ingestion, with only about 1% to 5% bioavailability. Most THC is cleared during the first pass by the liver. Other studies suggest that, in chronic users, plasma levels are detectable over a longer period of time (several weeks). With this chronic use, levels of THC are exponentially higher and are maintained for longer periods. Further studies of chronic THC administration and the impact on breastfed infants are currently underway.

SUMMARY

Infants have little to gain from exposure to medication via breast milk, but they do have much to gain from continued breastfeeding. Several strategies are available to allow mothers to continue breastfeeding while taking certain medications. These include: (1) avoiding breastfeeding for 4 to 6 hours after ingestion of a drug to avoid peak levels (ie, pump and discarding), (2) the combined use of formula and breast milk in cases in which the risk or dose of the drug is exceptionally high, and/or (3) pumping and discarding milk during therapy and returning to breastfeeding after discontinuing the drug. Whereas some drugs produce high levels in milk, others produce much lower levels. Another strategy is to switch to an alternative medication that has a better safety profile. Each case must be individually assessed, taking into account the importance of the treatment, the timing of therapy, the choice of medications, the mode of action, the ability of the infant to tolerate the medication, the overall toxicity of the drug itself, and the importance of maintaining breastfeeding.

Best practices

What is the current practice?

Use of medications during breastfeeding.

What changes in current practice are likely to improve outcomes?

Current data using innovative and sensitive techniques are providing better estimates of drug exposure during the postnatal period, especially during lactation. These data provide information for health professionals to advise lactating women.

Major recommendations

To minimize drug exposure and toxicity in infants, it is important to determine a relative risk-benefit analysis for each individual drug and infant. The prevalent use of drugs during nursing indicates a real need to increase studies of drugs used in this population.

REFERENCES

1. Shantakumar S, Terry MB, Teitelbaum SL, et al. Reproductive factors and breast cancer risk among older women. Breast Cancer Res Treat 2007;102(3):365–74.
2. Kim Y, Choi JY, Lee KM, et al. Dose-dependent protective effect of breast-feeding against breast cancer among ever-lactated women in Korea. Eur J Cancer Prev 2007;16(2):124–9.
3. Bennett P. 2nd edition. Drugs and human lactation, vol. 1. New York: Elsevier; 1996.
4. Newton ER. Lactation and breastfeeding. In: Gabbe SG, Niebyl JR, Simpson JL, et al, editors. Obstetrics: normal and problem pregnancies. 7th ed. Philadelphia: Elsevier; 2017. p. 517–48.
5. Neville MC. Physiology of lactation. Clin Perinatol 1999;26(2):251–79.
6. Gerk PM, Kuhn RJ, Desai NS, et al. Active transport of nitrofurantoin into human milk. Pharmacotherapy 2001;21(6):669–75.
7. Oo CY, Kuhn RJ, Desai N, et al. Active transport of cimetidine into human milk. Clin Pharmacol Ther 1995;58(5):548–55.

8. Lau RJ, Emery MG, Galinsky RE. Unexpected accumulation of acyclovir in breast milk with estimation of infant exposure. Obstet Gynecol 1987;69(3 Pt 2):468–71.

9. Kearns GL, McConnell RF Jr, Trang JM, et al. Appearance of ranitidine in breast milk following multiple dosing. Clin Pharm 1985;4(3):322–4.

10. Delange F, Chanoine JP, Abrassart C, et al. Topical iodine, breastfeeding, and neonatal hypothyroidism. Arch Dis Child 1988;63(1):106–7.

11. Postellon DC, Aronow R. Iodine in mother's milk. JAMA 1982;247(4):463.

12. Auerbach KG. Breastfeeding and maternal medication use. J Obstet Gynecol Neonatal Nurs 1999;28(5):554–63.

13. Howard CR, Lawrence RA. Drugs and breastfeeding. Clin Perinatol 1999;26: 447–78.

14. Begg EJ, Duffull SB, Hackett LP, et al. Studying drugs in human milk: time to unify the approach. J Hum Lact 2002;18(4):323–32.

15. Alcorn J, McNamara PJ. Pharmacokinetics in the newborn. Adv Drug Deliv Rev 2003;55(5):667–86.

16. Besunder JB, Reed MD, Blumer JL. Principles of drug biodisposition in the neonate. A critical evaluation of the pharmacokinetic-pharmacodynamic interface (part I). Clin Pharmacokinet 1988;14(4):189–216.

17. Hale TW. Medications & mothers' milk. New York: Springer; 2019.

18. Kulo A, van de Velde M, de Hoon J, et al. Pharmacokinetics of a loading dose of intravenous paracetamol post caesarean delivery. Int J Obstet Anesth 2012; 21(2):125–8.

19. Weibert RT, Townsend RJ, Kaiser DG, et al. Lack of ibuprofen secretion into human milk. Clin Pharm 1982;1(5):457–8.

20. Wischnik A, Manth SM, Lloyd J, et al. The excretion of ketorolac tromethamine into breast milk after multiple oral dosing. Eur J Clin Pharmacol 1989;36(5):521–4.

21. Knoppert DC, Stempak D, Baruchel S, et al. Celecoxib in human milk: a case report. Pharmacotherapy 2003;23(1):97–100.

22. Hale TW, McDonald R, Boger J. Transfer of celecoxib into human milk. J Hum Lact 2004;20(4):397–403.

23. Datta P, Rewers-Felkins K, Kallem RR, et al. Transfer of low dose aspirin into human milk. J Hum Lact 2017;33(2):296–9.

24. ACOG Committee Opinion No. 742 summary: postpartum pain management. Obstet Gynecol 2018;132(1):252–3.

25. Lam J, Kelly L, Ciszkowski C, et al. Central nervous system depression of neonates breastfed by mothers receiving oxycodone for postpartum analgesia. J Pediatr 2012;160(1):33–7.e2.

26. Edwards JE, Rudy AC, Wermeling DP, et al. Hydromorphone transfer into breast milk after intranasal administration. Pharmacotherapy 2003;23(2):153–8.

27. Schultz ML, Kostic M, Kharasch S. A case of toxic breast-feeding? Pediatr Emerg Care 2019;35(1):e9–10.

28. Nahum GG, Uhl K, Kennedy DL. Antibiotic use in pregnancy and lactation: what is and is not known about teratogenic and toxic risks. Obstet Gynecol 2006; 107(5):1120–38.

29. Ben-Ari J, Samra Z, Nahum E, et al. Oral amphotericin B for the prevention of Candida bloodstream infection in critically ill children. Pediatr Crit Care Med 2006;7(2):115–8.

30. Blanco JD, Jorgensen JH, Castaneda YS, et al. Ceftazidime levels in human breast milk. Antimicrob Agents Chemother 1983;23(3):479–80.

31. Kafetzis DA, Lazarides CV, Siafas CA, et al. Transfer of cefotaxime in human milk and from mother to foetus. J Antimicrob Chemother 1980;6(Suppl A):135–41.

32. Kafetzis DA, Siafas CA, Georgakopoulos PA, et al. Passage of cephalosporins and amoxicillin into the breast milk. Acta Paediatr Scand 1981;70(3):285–8.

33. Matsuda S. Transfer of antibiotics into maternal milk. Biol Res Pregnancy Perinatol 1984;5(2):57–60.

34. Shyu WC, Shah VR, Campbell DA, et al. Excretion of cefprozil into human breast milk. Antimicrob Agents Chemother 1992;36(5):938–41.

35. Yoshioka H, Cho K, Takimoto M, et al. Transfer of cefazolin into human milk. J Pediatr 1979;94(1):151–2.

36. Bourget P, Quinquis-Desmaris V, Fernandez H. Ceftriaxone distribution and protein binding between maternal blood and milk postpartum. Ann Pharmacother 1993;27(3):294–7.

37. Harmon T, Burkhart G, Applebaum H. Perforated pseudomembranous colitis in the breast-fed infant. J Pediatr Surg 1992;27(6):744–6.

38. Lumbiganon P, Pengsaa K, Sookpranee T. Ciprofloxacin in neonates and its possible adverse effect on the teeth. Pediatr Infect Dis J 1991;10(8):619–20.

39. Giamarellou H, Kolokythas E, Petrikkos G, et al. Pharmacokinetics of three newer quinolones in pregnant and lactating women. Am J Med 1989;87(5A):49S–51S.

40. Passmore CM, McElnay JC, Rainey EA, et al. Metronidazole excretion in human milk and its effect on the suckling neonate. Br J Clin Pharmacol 1988;26(1):45–51.

41. de Sa Del Fiol F, Barberato-Filho S, de Cassia Bergamaschi C, et al. Antibiotics and breastfeeding. Chemotherapy 2016;61(3):134–43.

42. Chung AM, Reed MD, Blumer JL. Antibiotics and breast-feeding: a critical review of the literature. Paediatr Drugs 2002;4(12):817–37.

43. Force RW. Fluconazole concentrations in breast milk. Pediatr Infect Dis J 1995;14(3):235–6.

44. Kaufman D, Boyle R, Hazen KC, et al. Fluconazole prophylaxis against fungal colonization and infection in preterm infants. N Engl J Med 2001;345(23):1660–6.

45. Jimenez E, Arroyo R, Cardenas N, et al. Mammary candidiasis: a medical condition without scientific evidence? PLoS One 2017;12(7):e0181071.

46. Boutroy MJ, Bianchetti G, Dubruc C, et al. To nurse when receiving acebutolol: is it dangerous for the neonate? Eur J Clin Pharmacol 1986;30(6):737–9.

47. Schimmel MS, Eidelman AI, Wilschanski MA, et al. Toxic effects of atenolol consumed during breast feeding. J Pediatr 1989;114(3):476–8.

48. Penny WJ, Lewis MJ. Nifedipine is excreted in human milk. Eur J Clin Pharmacol 1989;36(4):427–8.

49. Devlin RG, Duchin KL, Fleiss PM. Nadolol in human serum and breast milk. Br J Clin Pharmacol 1981;12(3):393–6.

50. Devlin RG, Fleiss PM. Captopril in human blood and breast milk. J Clin Pharmacol 1981;21(2):110–3.

51. Redman CW, Kelly JG, Cooper WD. The excretion of enalapril and enalaprilat in human breast milk. Eur J Clin Pharmacol 1990;38(1):99.

52. Miller ME, Cohn RD, Burghart PH. Hydrochlorothiazide disposition in a mother and her breast-fed infant. J Pediatr 1982;101(5):789–91.

53. Wisner KL, Perel JM, Findling RL. Antidepressant treatment during breast-feeding. Am J Psychiatry 1996;153(9):1132–7.

54. Bader TF, Newman K. Amitriptyline in human breast milk and the nursing infant's serum. Am J Psychiatry 1980;137(7):855–6.

55. Frey OR, Scheidt P, von Brenndorff AI. Adverse effects in a newborn infant breast-fed by a mother treated with doxepin. Ann Pharmacother 1999;33(6):690–3.

56. Stancer HC, Reed KL. Desipramine and 2-hydroxydesipramine in human breast milk and the nursing infant's serum. Am J Psychiatry 1986;143(12):1597–600.
57. Kimmel MC, Cox E, Schiller C, et al. Pharmacologic treatment of perinatal depression. Obstet Gynecol Clin North Am 2018;45(3):419–40.
58. Kristensen JH, Ilett KF, Hackett LP, et al. Distribution and excretion of fluoxetine and norfluoxetine in human milk. Br J Clin Pharmacol 1999;48(4):521–7.
59. Brent NB, Wisner KL. Fluoxetine and carbamazepine concentrations in a nursing mother/infant pair. Clin Pediatr 1998;37(1):41–4.
60. Hale TW, Shum S, Grossberg M. Fluoxetine toxicity in a breastfed infant. Clin Pediatr 2001;40(12):681–4.
61. Lester BM, Cucca J, Andreozzi L, et al. Possible association between fluoxetine hydrochloride and colic in an infant. J Am Acad Child Adolesc Psychiatry 1993; 32(6):1253–5.
62. Taddio A, Ito S, Koren G. Excretion of fluoxetine and its metabolite, norfluoxetine, in human breast milk. J Clin Pharmacol 1996;36(1):42–7.
63. Rampono J, Kristensen JH, Hackett LP, et al. Citalopram and demethylcitalopram in human milk; distribution, excretion and effects in breast fed infants. Br J Clin Pharmacol 2000;50(3):263–8.
64. Rampono J, Hackett LP, Kristensen JH, et al. Transfer of escitalopram and its metabolite demethylescitalopram into breastmilk. Br J Clin Pharmacol 2006; 62(3):316–22.
65. Chambers CD, Johnson KA, Dick LM, et al. Birth outcomes in pregnant women taking fluoxetine. N Engl J Med 1996;335(14):1010–5.
66. Spencer MJ. Fluoxetine hydrochloride (Prozac) toxicity in a neonate. Pediatrics 1993;92(5):721–2.
67. Stiskal JA, Kulin N, Koren G, et al. Neonatal paroxetine withdrawal syndrome. Arch Dis Child Fetal Neonatal Ed 2001;84(2):F134–5.
68. Yoshida K, Smith B, Craggs M, et al. Neuroleptic drugs in breast-milk: a study of pharmacokinetics and of possible adverse effects in breast-fed infants. Psychol Med 1998;28(1):81–91.
69. Ohkubo T, Shimoyama R, Sugawara K. Measurement of haloperidol in human breast milk by high-performance liquid chromatography. J Pharm Sci 1992; 81(9):947–9.
70. Stewart RB, Karas B, Springer PK. Haloperidol excretion in human milk. Am J Psychiatry 1980;137(7):849–50.
71. Whalley LJ, Blain PG, Prime JK. Haloperidol secreted in breast milk. Br Med J (Clin Res Ed) 1981;282(6278):1746–7.
72. Nordeng H, Gjerdalen G, Brede WR, et al. Transfer of aripiprazole to breast milk: a case report. J Clin Psychopharmacol 2014;34(2):272–5.
73. Mendhekar DN, Sunder KR, Andrade C. Aripiprazole use in a pregnant schizoaffective woman. Bipolar Disord 2006;8(3):299–300.
74. Hill RC, McIvor RJ, Wojnar-Horton RE, et al. Risperidone distribution and excretion into human milk: case report and estimated infant exposure during breastfeeding. J Clin Psychopharmacol 2000;20(2):285–6.
75. Ilett KF, Hackett LP, Kristensen JH, et al. Transfer of risperidone and 9-hydroxyrisperidone into human milk. Ann Pharmacother 2004;38(2):273–6.
76. Croke S, Buist A, Hackett LP, et al. Olanzapine excretion in human breast milk: estimation of infant exposure. Int J Neuropsychopharmacol 2002;5(3):243–7.
77. Gardiner SJ, Kristensen JH, Begg EJ, et al. Transfer of olanzapine into breast milk, calculation of infant drug dose, and effect on breast-fed infants. Am J Psychiatry 2003;160(8):1428–31.

78. Kirchheiner J, Berghofer A, Bolk-Weischedel D. Healthy outcome under olanzapine treatment in a pregnant woman. Pharmacopsychiatry 2000;33(2):78–80.

79. Dev VKP. The side effects and safety of clozapine. Rev Contemp Pharmacother 1995;(6):197–208.

80. Pistilli B, Bellettini G, Giovannetti E, et al. Chemotherapy, targeted agents, anti-emetics and growth-factors in human milk: how should we counsel cancer patients about breastfeeding? Cancer Treat Rev 2013;39(3):207–11.

81. Griffin SJ, Milla M, Baker TE, et al. Transfer of carboplatin and paclitaxel into breast milk. J Hum Lact 2012;28(4):457–9.

82. Johns DG, Rutherford LD, Leighton PC, et al. Secretion of methotrexate into human milk. Am J Obstet Gynecol 1972;112(7):978–80.

83. Baker T, Datta P, Rewers-Felkins K, et al. High-dose methotrexate treatment in a breastfeeding mother with placenta accreta: a case report. Breastfeed Med 2018;13(6):450–2.

84. Fierro ME, Datta P, Rewers-Felkins K, et al. Cyclophosphamide use in multiple sclerosis: levels detected in human milk. Breastfeed Med 2018. https://doi.org/10.1089/bfm.2018.0137.

85. Ross E, Robinson SE, Amato C, et al. Therapeutic monoclonal antibodies in human breast milk: a case study. Melanoma Res 2014;24(2):177–80.

86. Begg EJ, Malpas TJ, Hackett LP, et al. Distribution of R- and S-methadone into human milk during multiple, medium to high oral dosing. Br J Clin Pharmacol 2001;52(6):681–5.

Principles of Pharmacokinetics in the Pregnant Woman and Fetus

Robert M. Ward, MD[a],*, Michael W. Varner, MD[b]

KEYWORDS

- Pharmacokinetics • Perinatal pharmacology • Fetal pharmacology
- Developmental pharmacology • Maternal/fetal drug transfer

KEY POINTS

- Pharmacokinetics of the maternal/placenta/fetal unit change dramatically during pregnancy.
- Drug metabolism as well as drug transporters can alter the amount of drug reaching the fetus.
- Differences in maternal and fetal pharmacokinetics change the fetal/maternal drug concentrations at birth.
- Many aspects of maternal and fetal drug therapy need additional study.

INTRODUCTION

In 1962, prenatal exposure to thalidomide was identified as the cause of a severe congenital multiple malformation syndrome.[1–4] This was the first time that exposure to a maternal medication had been shown to directly injure the fetus. Since that time, every effort has been made to avoid exposure of the fetus to medications, especially in the first trimester during the critical period of organogenesis. Despite these efforts, there are occasions when fetal exposure to medications may be necessary in order to maintain maternal health, creating a challenging risk-benefit continuum. For example, the anticonvulsant phenytoin is a known teratogen responsible for a cluster of structural anomalies collectively known as the fetal hydantoin syndrome.[5,6] Fetal pharmacology studies subsequently confirmed that phenytoin is able to cross the placenta to reach the fetus during the period of organogenesis, suggesting a direct

Disclosure Statement: No authors have financial interest in any products mentioned in this article or with a maker of a competing product.
[a] Pediatrics, Pediatric Clinical Pharmacology, University of Utah, University of Utah School of Medicine, 295 Chipeta Way, Salt Lake City, UT 84108, USA; [b] Department of Obstetrics and Gynecology, University of Utah, 30 North 1900 East, Room 2B 200, Salt Lake City, UT 84132, USA
* Corresponding author.
E-mail address: Robert.ward@hsc.utah.edu

effect on fetal development.[7–9] And yet most prenatal exposures do not result in fetal injury. The sporadic occurrence of structural malformations associated with prenatal phenytoin exposure suggested for the first time that congenital malformation syndromes are more complex than simple in utero exposure. It is now clear that genetic factors are involved; specifically, in this instance, the inheritance of a genetic variant of epoxide hydrolase, the enzyme responsible for phenytoin metabolism, which causes the activity of the enzyme to be reduced to less than 30% of normal.[10] Not only can prenatal exposure to phenytoin (and other medications) result in structural malformations, but also in neurodevelopmental delay that may only become apparent later in life.[9]

Advances in perinatal diagnostics and fetal ultrasound during the 1980s allowed for the prenatal identification of conditions previously only recognized after birth. This included not only structural malformations, but also functional disorders such as supraventricular tachycardia and androgenization of a female fetus because of congenital adrenal hyperplasia. Some of these disorders can be prevented and/or treated by achieving an adequate concentration of a given drug within the fetus. As such, deliberate exposure of the fetus to medications can also have a therapeutic objective.

Our understanding of perinatal physiology has increased significantly starting in the 1990s and perinatologists have become more accepting of clinical interventions.[11] There are now numerous examples of the use of maternal drug administration to treat both fetal-related and pregnancy-related disorders, some of which are listed below.

i. Supraventricular tachycardia and other fetal dysrhythmias can be recognized and precisely diagnosed using fetal cardiac ultrasound and can be treated with a variety of anti-arrhythmic medications, usually administered to the mother but sometimes administered directly to the fetus via intra-amniotic injection.[12,13]

ii. Women pregnant with a female fetus after having delivered a child with androgenizing congenital adrenal hyperplasia can be treated with maternal corticosteroids to suppress the fetal adrenal glands, thereby reducing the production of endogenous fetal androgens and preventing masculinization of the external genitalia.[14] In this way, fetal treatment can either prevent the congenital syndrome altogether or at least minimize the need for extensive postnatal surgical procedures.

iii. Recent studies suggest that some cases of recurrent spontaneous preterm birth (SPTB) can be prevented with progesterone supplementation during pregnancy.[15]

iv. Judicious use of maternal halogenated corticosteroids can be used to reduce morbidities associated with prematurity, such as respiratory distress syndrome (RDS), intraventricular hemorrhage (IVH), and necrotizing enterocolitis (NEC).[16]

v. Bacterial infections, such as early-onset neonatal group B streptococcal infection, and vertical transmission of HIV have both been dramatically reduced through intrapartum administration of antimicrobial medications.[17]

Taken together, these clinical situations created a role for drug therapy to directly benefit the fetus and a need to better understand the pharmacokinetic changes in both the mother and the fetus during pregnancy. Over the past few decades, the field of perinatal pharmacology has evolved into a clinically important discipline. It has increased our understanding of the dynamic changes in physiology that occur during pregnancy and their effect on drug transport, metabolism, and degradation in the mother, placenta, and fetus.[18] Although the underlying physiologic changes that accompany pregnancy remain much the same as that outlined by Mirkin in 1973,[19] much has been learned about the patterns of pharmacokinetics that occur at the maternal-fetal interface, which has helped to better understand maternal-fetal drug transfer and inform fetal drug therapy.[20]

The goal of fetal drug therapy is to deliver an effective and nontoxic unbound drug concentration to the site of action within the fetoplacental unit. To achieve this, the clinician must understand the numerous pharmacokinetic changes that accompany the different stages of pregnancy and that may affect the drug concentration reaching the proposed site of action. **Fig. 1** lists the various steps involved in the therapeutic process by which medications are administered to the mother, transported across the placenta, and act on the fetus. Interference or dysregulation of any one of these steps may adversely affect drug delivery and fetal therapy. Changes in maternal body composition, physiology, and the activity of cytochrome P450 (CYP) enzymes that affect pharmacokinetics in pregnancy are summarized in **Tables 1** and **2** and in **Fig. 2** and are discussed in detail below.

CHANGES IN THE MOTHER THAT AFFECT PHARMACOKINETICS
Drug Absorption

Enteral drug absorption is reduced in pregnancy because both gastric emptying and gastrointestinal motility are slowed owing to high levels of circulating progesterone.[21] Both a reduction in intrinsic contractility and pressure from the enlarging uterus contribute to the slowing of gastrointestinal transit time.

Drug Distribution

Intravascular volume begins to expand early in pregnancy and continues to do so to term, by which time plasma volume has increased by 50%.[22] This expansion of the volume of distribution of polar drugs and those with a large molecular weight that remain primarily within the circulation reduces circulating drug concentrations. This dilutional effect is partially offset by a decrease in circulating protein concentration, which increases the bioavailability of unbound (biologically active) drug. At the same

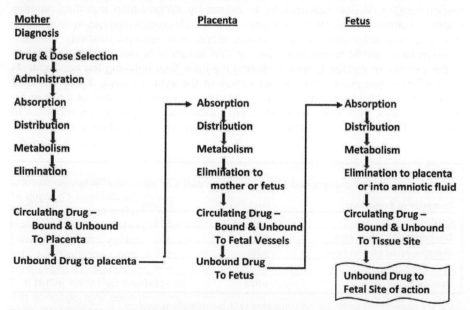

Fig. 1. Therapeutic process. Steps in the processing and transport of drugs from the mother to the proposed site of action in the fetus are shown.

Table 1
Changes in maternal body composition that affect pharmacokinetics by trimester of pregnancy

Trimester of Pregnancy	First (%)	Second (%)	Third (%)
Total body weight	+6	+16	+23
Total fat mass	+11	+16	+32
Total body water	+11	+27	+41
Plasma volume	+7	+42	+50
Red blood cell volume	+4	+20	+28
Hematocrit	−3	−8	−14
α-1 acid glycoprotein	−1	−22	−19

Data are represented as % change compared with nonpregnant women.
Data from Ke AB, Rostami-Hodjegan A, Zhao P, et al. Pharmacometrics in pregnancy: an unmet need. Ann Rev Pharmacol Toxicol 2014;54:53.

time, uterine perfusion increases from 2% of cardiac output per minute before pregnancy to 17% during pregnancy, thereby presenting more drug to the placenta and fetus.[23]

Drug Metabolism

Pregnancy-related changes in the activity of maternal phase I microsomal CYP enzymes are complex and variable, with some increasing and others decreasing during pregnancy (see **Fig. 2**).[22] CYP enzymes are essential for the metabolism of many medications, primarily in the liver. Although this class has more than 50 enzymes, 6 of them metabolize 90% of drugs, with the 2 most significant enzymes being CYP3A4 and CYP2D6. Uridyl glucuronosyltransferase 1A1, a phase II enzyme responsible for bilirubin conjugation, increases by midgestation and then remains stable.[22] Further complicating our ability to accurately predict changes in drug metabolism during pregnancy is that hepatic blood flow remains relatively constant whereas total cardiac output increases by 33% at term. The net effect is a reduction of the percent of cardiac output perfusing the liver, thus reducing the hepatic first-pass effect in pregnancy. This is not simply of theoretic concern. **Table 3** shows some of the medications that are metabolized or conjugated by each of these enzymatic pathways, all of which have altered metabolism in pregnancy. It is important to note that CYP3A4, which metabolizes more drugs than any other CYP enzyme,

Table 2
Maternal physiologic changes that affect pharmacokinetics by trimester of pregnancy

Trimester of Pregnancy	First (%)	Second (%)	Third (%)
Cardiac output	+18	+28	+33
Glomerular filtration rate	+19	+37	+40
Effective renal plasma flow	+38	+48	+31
Creatinine clearance	+28	+58	+26
Uterine blood flow	+923	+1567	+2721

Data are represented as % change compared with nonpregnant women.
Data from Ke AB, Rostami-Hodjegan A, Zhao P, et al. Pharmacometrics in pregnancy: an unmet need. Ann Rev Pharmacol Toxicol 2014;54:53.

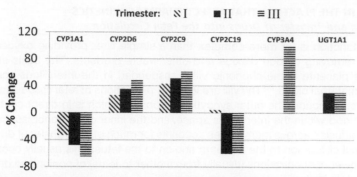

Fig. 2. Changes in the activity of maternal cytochrome p450 enzymes by trimester of pregnancy. Data are represented as % change compared with nonpregnant women. UGT1A1, uridyl glucuronosyltransferase 1A1. (*Data from* Ke AB, Rostami-Hodjegan A, Zhao P, et al. Pharmacometrics in pregnancy: an unmet need. Ann Rev Pharmacol Toxicol 2014; 54:53. Table 1.)

demonstrates a doubling in its level of activity by the end of pregnancy. Further complicating the situation, CYP3A4 is inhibited by macrolide antibiotics, imidazole antifungals, and many of the antiretroviral medications used to treat HIV. The reduction in activity of CYP2C19 in the latter half of pregnancy (see **Fig. 2**) may influence the efficacy of anticonvulsant medications as well as proton pump inhibitors and the antiplatelet medication, clopidogrel.

Drug Elimination

With an increase in cardiac output, renal plasma flow, and creatinine clearance (**Table 2**), the clearance of drugs that are renally excreted will usually increase in pregnancy. For this reason, many practitioners may compensation for this increased clearance by increasing the dose or shortening the dosing intervals of medications during pregnancy; however, the reduced protein binding in pregnancy may exaggerate the effects of medications at concentrations usually considered subtherapeutic. Data from studies on digoxin in pregnancy and the puerperium clearly illustrate the effect of renal function on drug clearance. In 1 study, digoxin, which is cleared primarily by renal excretion, was measured in 5 women with rheumatic heart disease at the end of an uncomplicated pregnancy and again 1 month postpartum.[24] Maternal digoxin concentrations increased from 0.6 ± 0.1 ng/mL at delivery to 1.1 ± 0.2 ng/mL 1 month later, indicating a decrease of almost 50% in drug clearance after delivery.

Table 3	
Representative drugs metabolized by cytochrome P450 enzymes	
Enzyme	**Drugs**
CYP1A1/2	Caffeine, aflatoxin B1, acetaminophen
CYP2D6	Codeine, hydrocodone, flecainide, propranolol, carvedilol, fluoxetine
CYP2C9	Phenytoin, warfarin, tolbutamide
CYP2C19	Omeprazole, pantoprazole, phenobarbital, diazepam, propranolol, clopidogrel, citalopram, bupropion
CYP3A4	Fentanyl, midazolam, cyclosporin, tacrolimus, carbamazepine, progesterone
UGT1A1	Bilirubin, irinotecan

Abbreviation: UGT1A1, uridyl glucuronosyltransferase 1A1.

CHANGES IN THE PLACENTA THAT AFFECT PHARMACOKINETICS
Absorption and Transfer of Drugs into the Fetal Circulation

Placental function is far more complex than a simple filter providing oxygen to the fetus and removing carbon dioxide and other waste products. The basic structural unit of the placenta is the chorionic villus suspended in the intervillous space and bathed in maternal blood.[25] The villi are vascular projections of fetal tissue surrounded by 2 layers of chorion: the outer syncytiotrophoblast, which is in direct contact with maternal blood within the intervillous space, and the inner cytotrophoblast cell layer.

Simple diffusion across membranes accounts for much of the transfer of drugs from the maternal circulation to the placenta and on to the fetus. This usually occurs from higher to lower concentrations (usually from mother to fetus) of nonionized drugs that are not protein bound.

The anatomy and function of the placenta changes throughout gestation, and this affects the ability of drugs to diffuse across to the fetus. Soon after the blastocyst implants into the uterine wall, the outer cells of the trophoblast layer immediately adjacent to the uterine epithelium fuse into multinucleated cells, the syncytiotrophoblast, which is in direct contact with the maternal blood.[25,26] Lacunae develop within the syncytiotrophoblast that enlarge to become the intervillous spaces. Maternal spiral arteries connect to the intervillous space to establish the uteroplacental blood flow. Fetal vessels extend into the intervillous space in chorionic villi, which initially are several cells thick. During pregnancy, both chorionic layers thin out from a thickness of 50 to 100 μM at 8 to 10 weeks of pregnancy to 4 to 5 μM at term. The immature structure of the early placenta helps to shield the fetus from potentially harmful xenobiotics during the period of organogenesis.[26] The fetoplacental circulation is reversed from that in newborns and adults with fetal arteries carrying deoxygenated blood from the fetus into the umbilical arteries, which flow into the chorionic arteries and capillaries within the placenta. There, gas exchange occurs before the oxygenated blood returns to the fetus through chorionic capillaries that flow into the umbilical vein.

It is important to note that only nonionized, nonprotein bound drugs diffuse passively into the fetal blood. The extent of ionization is determined by the chemical nature of the drug, its ionization constant (pK_a or pK_b), and the pH of its environment according to the Henderson-Hasselbach equation as refined by Stewart.[27] The fetal circulation is more acidic than the maternal circulation. This pH difference increases ionization of organic bases in the fetal circulation, which in turn increases their concentration on the fetal side of the placenta.

Several transporter proteins in the syncytiotrophoblast play a prominent role in the ability of drugs to move across the placenta and into and out of the fetal circulation (**Fig. 3**). Specific transporters may be bidirectional in their activity or unidirectional either toward or away from the fetus. These play a critical role in protecting the fetus from drug-related injury.[28] Indeed, genetic polymorphisms in placental transporter genes, especially those that reduce the efflux transporter p-glycoprotein, may increase the risk of drug-induced adverse effects.[29] Other methods of drug transport, such as pinocytosis and phagocytosis, play more minor roles in maternal/fetal drug exchange across the placenta.

Drug Distribution

By term, the placenta has grown to 500 g with a diameter of 15 to 20 cm and a thickness of 2 to 3 cm.[30] It can hold a volume of almost a liter of blood, mostly in the intervillous space, into which drugs may distribute as they diffuse out of the maternal circulation toward the fetus.

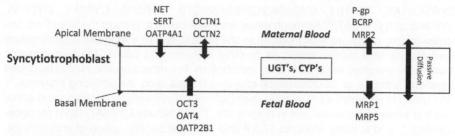

Fig. 3. Drug transport within the syncytiotrophoblast. The major transporter proteins within the syncytiotrophoblast responsible for the movement of drugs into and out of the fetal circulation are shown. BCRP, breast cancer resistance protein; CYP's, cytochrome P450's; MRP, multidrug resistance-associated protein; NET, norepinephrine transporter; OAT4, organic acid transporter 4; OATP2B1, organic anion-associated polypeptide 2B1; OATP4A1, organic anion-associated polypeptide 4A1; OCT3, organic cation transporter 3; OCTN1 and 2, organic acid/carnitine transporters; P-gp, P-glycoprotein; SERT, serotonin transporter; UGTs, uridine diphosphate glucuronosyl-transferases. (*Adapted from* Rubinchik-Stern M, Eyal S. Drug interactions at the human placenta: what is the evidence? Front Pharmacol 2012. https://doi.org/10.3389/fphar.2012.00126.)

Drug Metabolism

The placenta contains several CYP enzymes that are active early in fetal development. These include CYP 1A1, 1A2, 1B1, 2C, 2D6, 2E1, 2F1, 3A4, 5, 7, and 4B1.[31] By term, CYP2D6 and 1A2 are no longer detectable in the placenta. Several of these enzymes are essential in the maintenance of pregnancy by metabolizing endogenous compounds, such as steroids, that may otherwise activate parturition.[18] Activity of most of these CYPs are highest early in gestation and decrease toward term.[32]

CHANGES IN THE FETUS THAT AFFECT PHARMACOKINETICS
Drug Absorption

Absorption of drugs by the fetus is usually through the blood returning from the placenta through the umbilical vein. Transcutaneous and oral absorption by the fetus are possible, but have received limited study. With the buildup of the vernix caseosa, a lipid barrier forms on the surface of the skin preventing penetration by many polar compounds and water. Recent studies have shown that vernix is composed of 80% water, 10% proteins, and 10% lipids.[33] Vernix components have been shown to be actively involved in host defense, exhibiting antifungal and antimicrobial activity.[34] The lipid component of vernix are comprised of an estimated 54 different lipid mediators (21 oxylipins, 23 sphingolipids, and 10 endocannabinoids) all with functions yet to be fully explained.

Drug Distribution

Drug distribution within the fetus is influenced primarily by its body composition. Early in gestation, the fetus is 94% water with 0.5% fat.[35] By full term, its water content has decreased to 76% and fat content has increased to 12% to 16%. Clearly, the distribution to tissues of polar as well as lipophilic compounds will vary significantly based solely on body composition related to the stage of gestation.

Drug Metabolism

Fetal drug metabolizing enzyme activity varies markedly during pregnancy. Older studies reported high level of activity of several enzymes early in pregnancy, including

CYP1A1/1A2, CYP1B1, CYP2C8/2C9/2C18/2C19, CYP2D6, CYP2E1, CYP3A4, CYP3A5, and CYP3A7.[36] Although these enzymes can help protect the fetus from potential toxins, many are also involved in the metabolism of endogenous compounds essential for fetal development. As in older children and adults, the liver contains most of the enzymes involved in drug metabolism. In a recent review, Hines described 3 general patterns of developmental changes in fetal drug metabolizing enzymes.[32] One group of enzymes demonstrate their highest activity early in gestation and either stay the same or decrease later in pregnancy. These include CYP3A7, flavin monooxygenase 1, and sulfotransferases 1A3/4 and 1E1. The second group of enzymes express their activity at a relatively constant level from fetal development into adulthood, and include CYP3A5, sulfotransferase 1A1, and CYP2C19 (although the latter does show a moderate increase during the first year of life). The third and largest group of enzymes begin with little or no activity in the fetus and later increase to adult activity. These include CYP1A2, CYP2C9, CYP2D6, CYP2E1, CYP3A4, flavin monoxygenase3, and sulfotransferase 2A1. The time course for the increase in activity is highly variable, ranging from 2 to 3 weeks to many years, an interval that is, particularly relevant to pediatric therapeutics.

The placental barrier

There seems to be both an anatomic and physiologic barrier to fetal drug exposure early in gestation. There is clear anatomic separation of the maternal and fetal circulations during the early stages of placental development, and there is variable activity of critical CYP's and macromolecule transporters within the fetoplacental unit during this same time period. This is well illustrated by the developmental differences in fetal gentamicin concentrations during continuous infusions in midpregnancy compared with full term (**Fig. 4**).[37,38] In both of these studies, gentamicin was infused continuously to the pregnant woman and each time point represents 1 pair of simultaneous maternal and umbilical plasma concentrations of gentamicin. The time course and extent of the passage of gentamicin from the mother to the fetus during continued maternal drug infusion to maintain a constant maternal concentration is shown.

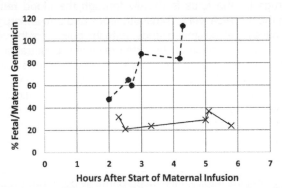

Fig. 4. Difference in maternal/fetal gentamicin concentrations early and late in gestation. Continuous maternal infusion of gentamicin at 18 to 23 weeks' gestation (*solid line and X*) compared with maternal gentamicin infusion at full term (*solid circles and dashed line*). (*Data from* Kauffman RE, Azarnoff DL, Morris JA. Placental transfer and fetal urinary excretion of gentamicin - comparison between an animal model and the human fetus. In: Morselli PL, Garattini S, Sereni F, editors. Basic and therapeutic aspects of perinatal pharmacology. New York: Raven Press; 1975. p. 75–82; and Daubenfeld O, Modde H, Hirsch HA. Transfer of gentamicin to the foetus and the amniotic fluid during a steady state in the mother. Arch Gynakol 1974;217(3):333–40.)

Despite infusion for almost 6 hours, the fetal concentration at 18 to 23 weeks of gestation remains less than 40% of the maternal concentration. In contrast, at term, fetal concentrations reach 100% of maternal concentrations within 5 hours.

INTERPRETATION OF MATERNAL/UMBILICAL DRUG CONCENTRATIONS AT BIRTH

Many studies have used the ratio of drug concentrations in maternal and umbilical blood samples to determine how much drug is being transferred to the fetus. However, this can be misleading. Because of differences in the pattern of clearance from the maternal circulation, passage across the placenta, and clearance within the fetus, this ratio can vary widely depending on the time interval at which the last dose was administered to the mother.[20] This can be illustrated by plotting pairs of maternal/fetal drug concentrations from several mothers and newborns according to the time after the last maternal dose. Using data from studies of the maternal and umbilical cord blood concentrations of the antibiotic cephaloridine drawn at the time of birth, **Fig. 5** shows how the umbilical/maternal ratio can vary widely from 0.35 to 1.92 depending on how long it takes for delivery after the last maternal dose. It also illustrates the marked difference in the pattern of change in drug concentrations between the fetus and mother. These variations in maternal and fetal kinetic patterns mean that single sets of maternal and umbilical blood drug concentrations cannot be relied on to accurately reflect the extent of maternal to fetal drug transfer.

Specific Examples of Fetal Drug Therapy

Antenatal corticosteroids to reduce neonatal lung disease in premature newborns
Pioneering work led by Professor Graham (Mont) Liggins from New Zealand illustrates the importance of pharmacokinetics within the fetoplacental unit. While using direct fetal infusions of corticotropin, dexamethasone, or cortisol to induce preterm delivery in sheep, Liggins[39,40] noted improved aeration of the lungs at a stage in gestation when newborn lambs almost always developed RDS with progressive atelectasis. This improvement in RDS was confirmed in sheep and rabbits and, combined with

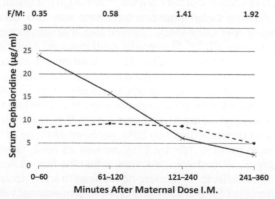

Fig. 5. Effect of dose interval on the concentration of drug within the maternal and fetal circulation. The ratio of distribution of drugs across the placental barrier varies with the time interval from the last dose. This graph illustrates the concentrations of cephaloridine in the maternal circulation (*X*) and the fetal/umbilical circulation (*solid circles*) at birth at varying times after the last maternal dose given intramuscularly (I.M.). The ratio of fetal to maternal concentrations (F/M) are shown. (*Data from* Stewart KS, Shafi M, Andrews J, et al. Distribution of parenteral ampicillin and cephalosporins in late pregnancy. J Obstet Gynaecol Br Commonw 1973;80:902–08. Data in Table II and Figure 3.)

the observations by Naeye and colleagues[41] of smaller adrenal glands in newborns dying from RDS, suggested that a corticosteroid deficiency or depletion may be causally related to the development of RDS. As an obstetrician familiar with the clinical sequelae of RDS, Liggins began a clinical trial of antenatal glucocorticoid treatment of mothers in preterm labor at 24 to 36 weeks' gestation. Maternal treatment used a compound formulation of a halogenated corticosteroid derived from prednisolone known as betamethasone, a stereoisomer of dexamethasone with the same structure and molecular weight but a different spatial orientation of the 16-methyl group. This formulation of betamethasone (Celestone) was a combination of 6 mg of the immediate release phosphate salt and 6 mg of the poorly soluble, slowly released acetate salt. The intramuscular (i.m.) injection was repeated once 24 hours later if the mother had not delivered. The success of this transplacental therapy can be explained by the pharmacokinetics of betamethasone and dexamethasone and how they cross the human placenta. The placenta protects the fetus from increased maternal cortisol concentrations through the activity of 11-β hydroxysteroid dehydrogenase type 2, which inactivates cortisol to cortisone.[42] In contrast, the synthetic halogenated structural isomers, betamethasone and dexamethasone, are minimally inactivated by 11-β hydroxysteroid dehydrogenase type 2 and pass through the placenta largely unchanged.

The original study[16] was blinded and controlled, with the control group receiving 6 mg cortisol, a minimal dosage. Of 117 betamethasone and 96 control mothers enrolled, 94 betamethasone and 78 control subjects continued pregnancy for at least 24 hours, which was considered the minimal time for induction of an effect on surfactant release/synthesis, and which also allowed for 2 doses of steroids to be administered. In the betamethasone-treated group, the frequency of RDS progressively decreased with increasing time to delivery up to 7 days, from 24.0% for delivery at less than 24 hours to 10% for delivery at 24 to 48 hours and 3.6% at 2 to 7 days. Although RDS was reduced significantly overall from 24.0% to 4.3%, the significant reduction was confined to infants delivering at 26 to 32 weeks' gestation (69.6% to 11.8%). In the most premature newborns, no IVH was seen in the betamethasone-treated group, but was seen in 4 of the controls.[16] Although not statistically significant, this reduction in IVH with betamethasone treatment was later confirmed in larger studies.[43,44] Despite 2 NIH Consensus Conferences that supported treatment with betamethasone to reduce RDS,[45,46] prenatal corticosteroid treatment was slow to gain acceptance. This might have related to the then-recent memory of long-term problems associated with attempts to prolong pregnancy using diethylstilbestrol leading to cancer in the children and young adults exposed in utero.[47,48] Such intervention has now become "standard of care" for impending preterm birth less than 34 weeks. A recent Cochrane review carried out a meta-analysis of 30 studies confirming that antenatal steroids reduced perinatal death by 28%, neonatal death by 31%, RDS by 34%, moderate/severe RDS by 41%, IVH by 12%, as well as NEC, need for mechanical ventilation, and early-onset systemic infections within the first 48 hours after birth.[44]

Given these beneficial effects, what more do we need to know about antenatal treatment with corticosteroids? Here are some unanswered questions: What is the optimal dose? Is the current dosage of 2 doses of 12 mg of betamethasone acetate and phosphate administered 24 hours apart the optimal treatment? The initial study by Liggins and Howie[16] did not include a dose-ranging study or variation of the interval between doses. Although 12 mg doses administered 24 hours apart is effective, some authors recommend completing the betamethasone treatment in a shorter time interval, such as 12 hours.[49] With the 24 hour treatment course with betamethasone, Liggins and Howie[16] noted adrenal suppression in the mothers for around 72 hours and other studies have shown a suppression of neonatal cortisol secretion for several days after birth.[50] A lower betamethasone dosage might be equally effective as the Liggins' protocol, but produce less suppression of the hypothalamic-pituitary-adrenal axis. Studies by Jobe and colleagues[51] have shown that a single dose of the slowly released betamethasone acetate is more effective than 2 doses of the rapidly released betamethasone phosphate. In another study in sheep, an even lower dose of betamethasone acetate improved lung function.[52] Similar studies in humans may provide similar benefits of antenatal corticosteroids with less hypothalamic-pituitary-adrenal suppression.

Such questions are not uncommon when discussing drug treatment. If the initial dosage tested is effective and relatively safe, additional studies may be difficult to conduct to attempt to reduce the dose or change the dosing interval. This is especially the case in obstetrics and pediatrics, whereby drug studies are time-consuming and expensive with few sites prepared to carry them out. It is nonetheless important to understand the extent of the initial studies of a drug and whether alternate doses, dose intervals, and formulations have been adequately explored and tested.

If 1 course (2 doses totaling 24 mg) of antenatal corticosteroids is good, can repeated courses sustain or even amplify the improvement? The effectiveness of betamethasone decreases in most studies by 7 days after the initiation of treatment, so some obstetricians began to repeat the 24 mg dosage on a weekly basis. If the pregnancy continued, repeated administration was continued for several weeks up to 11 times. In 1999, a retrospective review published by Banks and colleagues[53] suggested that repeated courses of antenatal corticosteroids increased perinatal mortality, reduced fetal growth, and prolonged adrenal suppression. This was followed in 2000 by an NIH Consensus Conference recommending that only a single course of antenatal corticosteroids be administered unless repeated courses were part of an investigative protocol.[46] Like all retrospective studies, the study by Banks and colleagues[53] was susceptible to confounding effects that might not be known and could not be controlled for. Several prospective randomized studies of repeated courses of antenatal corticosteroids followed. A meta-analysis in 2017 of 30 studies, including 9 with repeated courses of antenatal corticosteroids, concluded that both single and repeated doses of antenatal corticosteroids reduced perinatal death, neonatal death, RDS, moderate/severe RDS, IVH, NEC, need for mechanical ventilation, and infections within 48 hours of birth.[44] No serious adverse events were reported.

Although it is clear that fetuses can respond favorably to antenatal corticosteroids, the stages of lung development when that response occurs was not initially clear. Liggins and Howie found a reduction in RDS in fetuses who received antenatal corticosteroids and delivered at 26 to 32 weeks of gestation.[16] The benefit for the most immature preterm newborns (<26 weeks) was initially uncertain. However, more recent studies have shown reductions in RDS and mortality also at gestations of less than 25 weeks.[54,55] The upper limit of gestational age at which fetuses could respond to antenatal corticosteroids has expanded as well and now includes late preterm fetuses (gestational age 34–37 weeks), a group who are known to have increased respiratory morbidities compared with full term newborns. In 1 prospective randomized trial, antenatal corticosteroid treatment of late preterm deliveries reduced surfactant use, transient tachypnea, and bronchopulmonary dysplasia without increasing neonatal sepsis.[56] The reduction was modest (14.4% versus 11.6%) and hypoglycemia was increased in the betamethasone-treated group. Other recent studies support antenatal corticosteroid treatment before elective cesarean section at term to reduce respiratory morbidity.[57]

Multiple studies have followed the initial 1972 report from Liggins and Howie, and all support single course treatment of mothers in preterm labor to improve neonatal outcomes. The importance of controlled trials in perinatal medicine to improve pregnancy outcomes has had other far reaching and often unanticipated consequences, I including a major contribution to the development of the Cochrane systematic reviews.[58–60] Questions still remain regarding antenatal corticosteroid treatment that deserve continued study to determine the minimal effective dosage, optimal interval between doses, whether adverse effects of repeated maternal treatment harm a specific population or are safe, and whether there are upper and lower limits of gestational age at which benefits no longer occur. Long-term follow-up studies of people exposed in utero to antenatal corticosteroids to investigate growth, cardiovascular health, and neurologic outcomes should continue as this population ages.

Progesterone to prevent preterm birth, the intersection of pharmacogenomics and pharmacokinetics

The decrease in recurrent SPTB with progesterone supplementation has significantly reduced morbidity associated with prematurity and raised several possible explanations. After several small studies, a large prospective, randomized trial suggested that 17-hydroxyprogesterone caproate (17OHPC) reduced the recurrence of SPTB in singleton pregnancies at high risk of this event by virtue of a prior SPTB over a broad range of gestations, and resulted in a reduction in NEC, IVH, and need for supplemental oxygen.[15] The possible explanation for this effect involves pharmacokinetics and pharmacogenomics.[61]

One study of the pharmacokinetics of 17OHPC in singleton pregnancies was extended after delivery with continued sampling up to 28 days postpartum.[61] Women were treated weekly with 17OHPC 250 mg i.m. formulated in oil starting in the early second trimester. At birth, the umbilical to maternal plasma concentrations averaged 0.2, and the umbilical concentrations did not change with the time after the last maternal dose. The concentrations of 17OHPC varied inversely with body mass index, which may indicate a need for weight-based dosage adjustment. Clearance was faster in African American women; unfortunately, the CYP3A4 genotype, which is responsible for metabolism of 17OHPC was not determined in this cohort. Interestingly, the disposition half-life of 17OHPC was 18 ± 6 days, which led to progressive accumulation of drug with weekly injections.[61]

In another study, supplementation of women with twin pregnancies with 17OHPC allowed evaluation of both the pharmacokinetics and potential mechanism of action.[62] Concentrations of 17OHPC were inversely correlated with gestation at delivery, with lower concentrations at more advanced gestations, the opposite of what would be expected. Circulating C-reactive protein concentrations were increased in pregnancies with the highest concentrations of 17OHPC, but it did not reach statistical significance. The authors of this study speculated that the rise in C-reactive protein was related to the underlying mechanisms of parturition rather than to treatment with 17OHPC. This study along with many subsequent publications showed no lengthening of gestation with 17OHPC supplementation in the setting of multiple gestations (twins or triplets) or for women with a shortened cervical length.[63]

Roughly two-thirds of high-risk women with singleton pregnancies who receive 17OHPC supplementation do not respond and will go on to have a recurrent SPTB.[64] Although a pharmacokinetic explanation is possible, Manuck and colleagues[65] used DNA from the original study by Meis and colleagues[15] to look more closely at progesterone receptors A and B. Because of variation in allele frequency by race, the samples were stratified by self-reported race into African American and

White/Hispanic. Several gene response interactions were observed which differed by race/ethnicity. Some haplotypes identified women with an underlying risk of SPTB, others identified women with a favorable response to 17OHPC, whereas other genotypes were associated with an increased risk of SPTB in women who received 17OHPC supplementation.[65] Thus, successful prevention of SPTB with 17OHPC treatment is not simple pharmacokinetics, but a complex interplay between pharmacogenetics and pharmacokinetics.

In women without a history of SPTB but who are found in the midtrimester to have a short cervix on transvaginal ultrasound, supplementation with vaginal progesterone is currently recommended by the American College of Obstetricians and Gynecologists.[66] This is not a US Food and Drug Administration recommended intervention. Although some evidence exists to suggest that vaginal progesterone may be superior to intramuscular 17OHPC,[67] the American College of Obstetricians and Gynecologists has not yet endorsed the primary use of vaginal progesterone for prevention of recurrent SPTB. The pharmacokinetics of vaginal progesterone for SPTB prevention has not been adequately studied.

SUMMARY

Pregnancy profoundly alters a woman's physiology. When combined with the progressive impact of the developing fetus and placenta, these changes result in multiple alterations in drug absorption, distribution, metabolism, and elimination. As outlined earlier in this article, these changes emphasize the pharmacologic complexity of pregnancy. They also emphasize the dangers of extrapolating pharmacologic expectations from nonpregnant populations to pregnant women and their fetuses. Although concerns about fetal safety have historically limited pharmacokinetic studies during pregnancy, it is important to recognize that many medications are clinically indicated for various maternal or fetal conditions. Recommendations for the use of medications in pregnancy should be based on the prevailing evidence, including short-term and long-term outcome data.

REFERENCES

1. Taussig HB. Thalidomide – a lesson in remote effects of drugs. Am J Dis Child 1962;104:111–3.
2. Taussig HB. The thalidomide syndrome. Sci Am 1962;207:29–35.
3. Taussig HB. Thalidomide and phocomelia. Pediatrics 1962;30:654–9.
4. Lenz W, Knapp K. Thalidomide embryopathy. Arch Environ Health 1962;5:100–5.
5. Hanson JW, Myrianthopoulos NC, Harvey MA, et al. Risks to the offspring of women treated with hydantoin anticonvulsants, with emphasis on the fetal hydantoin syndrome. J Pediatr 1976;89:662–8.
6. Hanson JW, Smith DW. Fetal hydantoin syndrome. Lancet 1976;1:692.
7. Mirkin BL. Placental transfer and neonatal elimination of diphenylhydantoin. Am J Obstet Gynecol 1971;109:930–3.
8. Mirkin BL. Diphenylhydantoin: placental transport, fetal localization, neonatal metabolism, and possible teratogenic effects. J Pediatr 1971;78:329–37.
9. Diav-Citrin O. Prenatal exposures associated with neurodevelopmental delay and disabilities. Dev Disabil Res Rev 2011;17:71–84.
10. Buehler BA, Delimont D, van Waes M, et al. Prenatal prediction of risk of the fetal hydantoin syndrome. N Engl J Med 1990;322:1567–72.
11. Ward RM. Maternal drug therapy for fetal disorders. Semin Perinatol 1992;16: 12–20.

12. Steinfeld L, Rappaport HL, Rossbach HC, et al. Diagnosis of fetal arrhythmias using echocardiographic and Doppler techniques. J Am Coll Cardiol 1986;8: 1425–33.

13. Alsaied T, Baskar S, Fares M, et al. First-line antiarrhythmic transplacental treatment for fetal tachyarrhythmia: a systematic review and meta-analysis. J Am Heart Assoc 2017;6 [pii:e007164].

14. Nimkarn S, New MI. Congenital adrenal hyperplasia due to 21-hydroxylase deficiency: a paradigm for prenatal diagnosis and treatment. Ann N Y Acad Sci 2010; 1192:5–11.

15. Meis PJ, Klebanoff M, Thom E, et al. Prevention of recurrent preterm delivery by 17 alpha-hydroxyprogesterone caproate. N Engl J Med 2003;348:2379–85.

16. Liggins GC, Howie RN. A controlled trial of antepartum glucocorticoid treatment for prevention of the respiratory distress syndrome in premature infants. Pediatrics 1972;50:515–25.

17. Benitz WE, Gould JB, Druzin ML. Antimicrobial prevention of early-onset group B streptococcal sepsis: estimates of risk reduction based on a critical literature review. Pediatrics 1999;103:e78, 71-13.

18. Mahmood I, Burckart GJ, Ward RM. Perinatal pharmacology and maternal/fetal dosing. In: Mahmood I, Burckart GJ, editors. Fundamentals of pediatric drug dosing. Cham (Switzerland): Springer International; 2016. p. 127–46.

19. Mirkin BL. Maternal and fetal distribution of drugs in pregnancy. Clin Pharmacol Ther 1973;14:643–7.

20. Ward RM. Pharmacological treatment of the fetus. Clinical pharmaco-kinetic considerations. Clin Pharmacokinet 1995;28:343–50.

21. Wald A, Van Thiel DH, Hoechstetter L, et al. Effect of pregnancy on gastrointestinal transit. Dig Dis Sci 1982;27:1015–8.

22. Ke AB, Rostami-Hodjegan A, Zhao P, et al. Pharmacometrics in pregnancy: an unmet need. Annu Rev Pharmacol Toxicol 2014;54:53–69.

23. Frederiksen MC. Physiologic changes in pregnancy and their effect on drug disposition. Semin Perinatol 2001;25:120–3.

24. Rogers MC, Willerson JT, Goldblatt A, et al. Serum digoxin concentrations in the human fetus, neonate and infant. N Engl J Med 1972;287:1010–3.

25. Gude NM, Roberts CT, Kalionis B, et al. Growth and function of the normal human placenta. Thromb Res 2004;114:397–407.

26. Al-Enazy S, Ali S, Albekairi N, et al. Placental control of drug delivery. Adv Drug Deliv Rev 2017;116:63–72.

27. Kurtz I, Kraut J, Ornekian V, et al. Acid-base analysis: a critique of the Stewart and bicarbonate-centered approaches. Am J Physiol Renal Physiol 2008;294: F1009–31.

28. Iqbal M, Audette MC, Petropoulos S, et al. Placental drug transporters and their role in fetal protection. Placenta 2012;33:137–42.

29. Daud AN, Bergman JE, Bakker MK, et al. Pharmacogenetics of drug-induced birth defects: the role of polymorphisms of placental transporter proteins. Pharmacogenomics 2014;15:1029–41.

30. Rubinchik-Stern M, Eyal S. Drug interactions at the human placenta: what is the evidence? Front Pharmacol 2012;3:126.

31. Pasanen M. The expression and regulation of drug metabolism in human placenta. Adv Drug Deliv Rev 1999;38:81–97.

32. Hines RN. Developmental expression of drug metabolizing enzymes: impact on disposition in neonates and young children. Int J Pharm 2013;452:3–7.

33. Checa A, Holm T, Sjodin MO, et al. Lipid mediator profile in vernix caseosa reflects skin barrier development. Sci Rep 2015;5:15740.
34. Tollin M, Bergsson G, Kai-Larsen Y, et al. Vernix caseosa as a multi-component defence system based on polypeptides, lipids and their interactions. Cell Mol Life Sci 2005;62:2390–9.
35. Friis-Hansen B. Body water compartments in children: changes during growth and related changes in body composition. Pediatrics 1961;28:169–81.
36. Hakkola J, Pelkonen O, Pasanen M, et al. Xenobiotic-metabolizing cytochrome P450 enzymes in the human feto-placental unit: role in intrauterine toxicity. Crit Rev Toxicol 1998;28:35–72.
37. Kauffman RE, Azarnoff DL, Morris JA. Placental transfer and fetal urinary excretion of gentamicin - comparison between an animal model and the human fetus. In: Morselli PL, Garattini S, Sereni F, editors. Basic and therapeutic aspects of perinatal pharmacology. New York: Raven Press; 1975. p. 75–82.
38. Daubenfeld O, Modde H, Hirsch HA. Transfer of gentamicin to the foetus and the amniotic fluid during a steady state in the mother. Arch Gynakol 1974;217:333–40.
39. Liggins GC. Premature delivery of foetal lambs infused with glucocorticoids. J Endocrinol 1969;45:515–23.
40. Liggins GC. Premature parturition after infusion of corticotrophin or cortisol into foetal lambs. J Endocrinol 1968;42:323–9.
41. Naeye RL, Harcke HT Jr, Blanc WA. Adrenal gland structure and the development of hyaline membrane disease. Pediatrics 1971;47:650–7.
42. Benediktsson R, Calder AA, Edwards CR, et al. Placental 11 beta-hydroxysteroid dehydrogenase: a key regulator of fetal glucocorticoid exposure. Clin Endocrinol (Oxf) 1997;46:161–6.
43. Canterino JC, Verma U, Visintainer PF, et al. Antenatal steroids and neonatal periventricular leukomalacia. Obstet Gynecol 2001;97:135–9.
44. Roberts D, Brown J, Medley N, et al. Antenatal corticosteroids for accelerating fetal lung maturation for women at risk of preterm birth. Cochrane Database Syst Rev 2017;(3):CD004454.
45. Effect of corticosteroids for fetal maturation on perinatal outcomes. NIH consensus development panel on the effect of corticosteroids for fetal maturation on perinatal outcomes. JAMA 1995;273:413–8.
46. Antenatal corticosteroids revisited: repeat courses - National Institutes of Health Consensus Development Conference Statement, August 17-18, 2000. Obstet Gynecol 2001;98:144–50.
47. Herbst AL, Ulfelder H, Poskanzer DC. Adenocarcinoma of the vagina. Association of maternal stilbestrol therapy with tumor appearance in young women. N Engl J Med 1971;284:878–81.
48. Reed CE, Fenton SE. Exposure to diethylstilbestrol during sensitive life stages: a legacy of heritable health effects. Birth Defects Res C Embryo Today 2013;99:134–46.
49. Romejko-Wolniewicz E, Teliga-Czajkowska J, Czajkowski K. Antenatal steroids: can we optimize the dose? Curr Opin Obstet Gynecol 2014;26:77–82.
50. Nykanen P, Raivio T, Heinonen K, et al. Circulating glucocorticoid bioactivity and serum cortisol concentrations in premature infants: the influence of exogenous glucocorticoids and clinical factors. Eur J Endocrinol 2007;156:577–83.
51. Jobe AH, Nitsos I, Pillow JJ, et al. Betamethasone dose and formulation for induced lung maturation in fetal sheep. Am J Obstet Gynecol 2009;201:611.e1-7.

52. Schmidt AF, Kemp MW, Rittenschober-Bohm J, et al. Low-dose betamethasone-acetate for fetal lung maturation in preterm sheep. Am J Obstet Gynecol 2018; 218:132.e1-9.

53. Banks BA, Cnaan A, Morgan MA, et al. Multiple courses of antenatal corticosteroids and outcome of premature neonates. North American Thyrotropin-Releasing Hormone Study Group. Am J Obstet Gynecol 1999;181:709–17.

54. Travers CP, Clark RH, Spitzer AR, et al. Exposure to any antenatal corticosteroids and outcomes in preterm infants by gestational age: prospective cohort study. BMJ 2017;356:j1039.

55. Deshmukh M, Patole S. Antenatal corticosteroids in impending preterm deliveries before 25 weeks' gestation. Arch Dis Child Fetal Neonatal Ed 2018;103:F173–6.

56. Gyamfi-Bannerman C, Thom EA, Blackwell SC, et al. Antenatal betamethasone for women at risk for late preterm delivery. N Engl J Med 2016;374:1311–20.

57. Nada AM, Shafeek MM, El Maraghy MA, et al. Antenatal corticosteroid administration before elective caesarean section at term to prevent neonatal respiratory morbidity: a randomized controlled trial. Eur J Obstet Gynecol Reprod Biol 2016; 199:88–91.

58. Grant A, Chalmers I. Register of randomised controlled trials in perinatal medicine. Lancet 1981;1:100.

59. Chalmers I. Adrian Grant's pioneering use of evidence synthesis in perinatal medicine, 1980-1992. Reprod Health 2018;15:79.

60. Clarke M, Chalmers I. Reflections on the history of systematic reviews. BMJ Evid Based Med 2018;23:121–2.

61. Caritis SN, Sharma S, Venkataramanan R, et al. Pharmacology and placental transport of 17-hydroxyprogesterone caproate in singleton gestation. Am J Obstet Gynecol 2012;207:398.e1-8.

62. Caritis SN, Simhan HN, Zhao Y, et al. Relationship between 17-hydroxyprogesterone caproate concentrations and gestational age at delivery in twin gestation. Am J Obstet Gynecol 2012;207:396.e1-8.

63. Caritis SN, Feghali MN, Grobman WA, et al. What we have learned about the role of 17-alpha-hydroxyprogesterone caproate in the prevention of preterm birth. Semin Perinatol 2016;40:273–80.

64. Manuck TA, Stoddard GJ, Fry RC, et al. Nonresponse to 17-alpha hydroxyprogesterone caproate for recurrent spontaneous preterm birth prevention: clinical prediction and generation of a risk scoring system. Am J Obstet Gynecol 2016; 215:622.e1-8.

65. Manuck TA, Lai Y, Meis PJ, et al. Progesterone receptor polymorphisms and clinical response to 17-alpha-hydroxyprogesterone caproate. Am J Obstet Gynecol 2011;205:135.e1-9.

66. American College of Obstetricians and Gynecologists. Practice bulletin no. 130: prediction and prevention of preterm birth. Obstet Gynecol 2012;120:964–73.

67. Maher MA, Abdelaziz A, Ellaithy M, et al. Prevention of preterm birth: a randomized trial of vaginal compared with intramuscular progesterone. Acta Obstet Gynecol Scand 2013;92:215–22.

Challenges in Designing Clinical Trials to Test New Drugs in the Pregnant Woman and Fetus

Mark A. Turner, BSc, PhD, MRCP (UK), MRCPCH, DRCOG[a],*,
Louise Kenny, PhD, MRCOG[b], Zarko Alfirevic, MD, FRCOG[a]

KEYWORDS

- Pregnancy • Drug development • Clinical pharmacology • Ethics
- Public private partnership

KEY POINTS

- The development of new drugs to treat maternal and fetal conditions can be improved using approaches that are succeeding in other marginalized therapeutic areas.
- Improved information about the risks and benefits of interventions during pregnancy is needed to facilitate study design and review by ethics boards, regulators, funders, and potential participants of studies.
- It is important to ensure that the design and conduct of in vitro, ex vivo, and clinical studies are compatible with the needs of drug development programs.
- Collaboration in effective geographic and methodological, pan-stakeholder public-private partnerships, with global coordination, is essential to overcome the problems that arise during research about new drugs in pregnancy.

INTRODUCTION

The paucity of information about drugs used in pregnancy and the need for new drugs have been described elsewhere.[1–7] The marked lack of information to support prescribing drugs for pregnant women who present with intercurrent illness, specific conditions of pregnancy, or fetal conditions reflects several problems: science, trial recruitment, ethics, legal factors, and more. This review examines some specific challenges that

Disclosure Statement: No disclosures.
[a] Institute of Translational Medicine, University of Liverpool a member of Liverpool Health Partners, Centre for Women's Health Research, Liverpool Women's Hospital, Crown Street, Liverpool L8 7SS, UK; [b] Vice Chancellor's Office, University of Liverpool a member of Liverpool Health Partners, Centre for Women's Health Research, Liverpool Women's Hospital, Crown Street, Liverpool L8 7SS, UK
* Corresponding author. Centre for Women's Health Research, Liverpool Women's Hospital, Crown Street, Liverpool L8 7SS, UK
E-mail address: mark.turner@liverpool.ac.uk

arise from taking a comprehensive approach to these interconnected problems (**Table 1**). The authors outline actions that can be taken by individual drug development programs and actions that are required from the whole materno-fetal community.

CHALLENGES

Profound changes in maternal physiology fundamentally alter pharmacokinetics (PK) and pharmacodynamics, often in an unpredictable fashion. There are 3 discrete and intimately dependent units comprising the mother, the fetus, and the placenta. The placenta, once thought to be a passive filter between the maternal and fetal compartments, is in fact a highly complex organ rich in transporters. The human placenta remains relatively understudied, particularly in early healthy pregnancy. Comparative placentology has yet to identify an ideal animal model.[8] Although humans share a hemochorial placental structure with the other higher-order mammal and some rodents, there are some important differences that preclude robust extrapolation. For this reason, there has been much interest in evaluating transplacental transport using the ex vivo placental cotyledon model (for a review, see Ref.[9]).

A significant challenge is that the current regulatory environment somewhat ironically does not require drug research in pregnancy while at the same time allowing off-label use in this population.

Models

If experimental models are to make a meaningful contribution to drug development, then research needs to follow best practice.[10–12] Research should be reproducible within and between laboratories (https://www.nature.com/collections/wjsrmrdnsm#features). The promotion of reproducibility includes paying attention to validation (are the data precise and reproducible) and qualification (do the data do something useful in a specific context of use).[13]

Table 1
Overview of strategies and challenges (other than funding)

Strategy	Challenges (Other than Funding)	Solution
Models		
• Placental transfer • Impact on fetus (teratogenesis)	Identification Validation and qualification Animals Application of existing PBPK models	Science targeted at drug development Understanding of regulatory issues Understanding of relevance Dissemination of existing knowledge
Novel approaches to regulatory issues	Consensus, combined with working understanding of diversity	Precompetitive regulatory agreement, taking account of uncertainty
Funded registries	Design, including real world data Design: specific times/specific drugs	Focused methodologies Data quality Data standards Possible, but need some work Setup and run
Maternity investigation plan	Concept Adoption Enforcement (requirement)	Describe Educate Advocate
Involvement and engagement	Communication Partnership	Contacts and trust developed through honest broker third parties

There are some examples of work toward validation of placental models. Myllynen and colleagues[14] assessed 4 model compounds using the dual-perfused placental cotyledon model in 2 laboratories. Conings and colleagues[15] identified several quality control measures for the same model in a single laboratory. However, this work needs to be extended so that these and other models are sufficiently rigorous to inform drug development. Standardized approaches are being developed by an international human placental testing platform (PlaNet).[16] The importance of careful attention to validation during academic research is demonstrated by Prinz and colleagues,[17] who examined 67 attempts to reproduce literature findings in a single large Pharma company. In 43 cases (65%), the in-house findings of an experienced and well-resourced laboratory were not consistent with the literature so that most of therapeutic suggestions from the literature were "false positives."[17]

Regulatory issues

The Food and Drug Administration (FDA) issued an updated draft guidance about drug development during pregnancy in 2018.[18] Ethical criteria over a range of stages in clinical drug development covering maternal and fetal indications have been suggested.[19] Although many of these scientists aim to influence their peers through grant applications and publications, academic investigators who want to promote drug development need to gather more information than is needed for a publication. It is also important to influence decision-makers, such as industry, regulators, health services, and the agencies that reimburse costs. Addressing regulatory issues requires an awareness of the information needed by each decision-maker and linking of in vitro studies to clinical studies. Careful planning avoids wasted effort and will derisk drug development.[20,21]

Studies that will be submitted to regulatory agencies need to meet relevant guidelines, such as the "Guidance on non-clinical safety studies for the conduct of human clinical trials and marketing authorization for pharmaceuticals M3 (R2)" (http://www.ich.org/fileadmin/Public_Web_Site/ICH_Products/Guidelines/Multidisciplinary/M3_R2/Step4/M3_R2__Guideline.pdf).

Data sharing can facilitate drug development. Data should be collected in such a way that it can be added to generalizable pools, such as physiologically based pharmacokinetic (PBPK) models through standardized definitions and data standards.[22] Making the most of existing data allows extrapolation or modeling to help design trials.[18] Although extrapolation from animal models of pregnancy is challenging, well-defined physiologic models using published human data can underpin pharmacokinetic studies.[22,23]

There is a perception, with respect to study of drugs in pregnancy, that "a single FDA regulator may be in a position to derail a study, even one that has been approved by the IRB (institutional review board) and survived scrutiny from internal or external legal counsel, because of different interpretations about legally (or perhaps institutionally) acceptable levels of risk."[24] This perception may relate to the different perspectives of risk that institutions have due to legal constraints or from experience. Alternatively, it may reflect unnecessarily conservative attitudes to risk within an institution. In either case, it is important to pool experience and promote understanding of multiple perspectives so that shared expectations can be developed. Public private partnerships can contribute to shared understanding, preferably when they address issues that are relevant to all precompetitive projects.

Legal

Pertinent legal issues include different interpretations of the law, nonlegal constraints on decision making, such as finance or reputational issues, and ambiguities in legal and regulatory texts.[24] Ambiguities related to the definition of "minimal harm" and "prospect of direct benefit" are particularly troublesome. In legal argument, the lack of evidence about likelihood of fetal harm or benefit leads to uncertainty, which promotes a conservative interpretation of the law and regulations. Difficulties arising from legal uncertainty within jurisdictions is further compounded by the differing legal status of the fetus versus the mother internationally. In some jurisdictions, the fetus has a greater degree of legal protection than in others, which makes judgment about the risk-benefit ratio complex and ambiguous across multiple jurisdictions. The risk of liability is important, but is not specific to maternity research. The specific problems for liability in pregnancy arise from (a) the "long-tail problem," for example, diethylstilboestrol; (b) the magnitudes of potential effects, for example, thalidomide. This discourages pharmaceutical companies from accepting the risks arising from use of their products in pregnant women. Compensation from harm arising during clinical trials varies between countries, and this can increase reluctance for US companies (that do not need to provide this compensation) to conduct research in other countries.[24]

Although some of these problems cannot be resolved directly, action by the materno-fetal community on some points will be beneficial:

i. Taking account of influences on legal perspectives (law, widely accepted guidelines) in addition to family, clinical, regulatory, and commercial perspectives
ii. Shared understanding of terms, such as minimal harm and direct benefit, as they apply in pregnancy, including different stages of pregnancy
iii. More information about harms and benefits that can inform judgments
iv. Precedents for successful management of risk and liability (including insuring clinical trials) with a focus on the rationale for these successes and relevant legal arguments used
v. Many adverse fetal outcomes are rare (death, disability, and so forth), and therefore, observational cohort studies and clinical trials need to be very large

Registries

Clinical trials provide limited information during the development of new drugs. Accordingly, it is important to set up registries for women and their offspring who are exposed to new drugs. The concept of registries of drug exposure during pregnancy has been described, including ethical aspects.[25] Observational studies of drug safety have been conducted during pregnancy,[26] but high-quality studies of adequate size are rare. The assessment of potential adverse drug reactions can be challenging. Tools such as the Naranjo score do not take account of pregnancy so that population-specific tools need to be developed and validated. As an example, pediatric-specific tools have been developed.[27–29]

Registries can also provide information to support the design of clinical trials. Considerable methodological challenges need to be addressed. One challenge relates to data quality and the ability to share data across similar studies and reuse data for a different purpose than initially intended. Core outcome sets have been promoted as 1 way to meet this challenge but do not address the challenge completely.[30] Data standards are a useful approach to standardize data collection and allow legitimate variation in the selection of outcomes.[31] Registries should not be drug based but need to be participant based or even population based. Registries are expensive, and costs need to be shared between the stakeholders who will benefit from them.

Maternity investigation plan

This suggestion[1] relates to a pregnancy analogue to the Paediatric Investigation Plan (PIP) in Europe[32] and to the Pediatric Study Plan in the United States.[33] There are 2 aspects to a PIP: content and importance. The *content* of a Maternity Investigation Plan is relatively easy to state, based on FDA guidelines (FDA 2018), taking account of the different uses of drugs in pregnancy, such as maternal concurrent illness, maternal pregnancy-related complications, and fetal indications.[19] The *importance* of the PIP stems from its status as a legal requirement for all drug development programs that are relevant to pediatrics.

Senior members of the European Medicines Agency have written: "Regulators should require comprehensive information regarding safety and efficacy of medicines in pregnancy and apply a much more systematically balanced and all-encompassing approach regarding the inclusion and follow-up of pregnant women in well-designed clinical trials and postauthorization, rather than excluding them systematically from clinical trials."[34] However, regulators can only implement the law and a change in practice by regulators requires a change in law. Examples of the changes in legal mandate required to change regulatory practice are the long process that led to the current requirements for pediatric studies in the United States and the PIP in Europe. In the United States, impetus for legislative efforts related to pregnancy may come from a task force established by The 21st Century Cures Act, the Task Force on Research Specific to Pregnant Women and Lactating Women (PRGLAC). PRGLAC reported to the Secretary of Health and Human Services in September 2018 about gaps in knowledge and research on safe and effective therapies for pregnant and lactating women and made specific suggestions for changes in US legislation and policy (https://www.nichd.nih.gov/About/Advisory/PRGLAC, see later discussion). Challenges of development plans include discordant approaches across jurisdictions. In other therapeutic areas, these can be addressed in discussions between regulators.[35]

Involvement and engagement

Identification of research needs and the design and conduct of trials need to involve potential participants and their families.[36–40] Specifically, women indicate that their informed choices must be based on information about the risks related to the study. A sensitive approach must take into account their needs and perspectives in the specific context that the trial addresses. Because pregnancy encompasses a vast range of physiologic, emotional, and pathologic states, each trial team needs to undertake preparatory work about the information needs, and communication preferences, of potential participants.

FUNDING

Globally, the allocation of resources to the development of new drugs is controversial, and pharmaceutical companies currently have many reasons to avoid investing in pregnancy research.[24,41] As noted in the legal section of this review, disadvantage risks are highly visible (legal liability, and so forth) and compare unfavorably to any potential financial benefits. Information about the burden of disease is available but needs to be presented more effectively to decision-makers in companies, government, and public funders. Widespread off-label or off-evidence use also undermines incentives to drug development. Fisk and Atun[3] outlined the issues relating to commercial drug development in 2008. The situation has not changed in the past decade, except that even fewer drugs are under commercial development. The health economic considerations related to the development of new drugs for pregnant women have been described.[42]

Broader pharmaceutical policy may offer some solutions relating to early-phase push (such as public funding for research that does not depend on subsequent profits) and late-phase pull mechanisms (such as legal and regulatory facilitation, reimbursement advantages, prizes, or predictable reimbursement through insurance-like models). The example of antibiotics illustrates the strengths and weaknesses of these approaches and the need for global coordination and oversight.[43] The costs and benefits of each approach need to be considered carefully.[44] Efficient research requires incentives for academic investigators and "hidden" contributors to drug development, such as the sites that host research. Relevant actions are summarized in **Table 2**. Individual researchers and sponsors will not be able to gather all the information that is required to change the funding environment: another potential task for public-private partnerships.

ETHICS

The ethics of research involving pregnant women may seem straightforward. For example, a 1994 report by the US Institute of Medicine recommended that "pregnant women be presumed to be eligible for participation in clinical studies."[45] International ethical guidance also promotes appropriate research that recruits pregnant women (CIOMS 2016; https://cioms.ch/wp-content/uploads/2017/01/WEB-CIOMS-EthicalGuidelines.pdf). On the other hand, a systematic review of ethical issues that arise during research about vaccines that recruits pregnant women found 60 separate issues.[46] Experience indicates that the clear, international consensus statements are often not reflected in daily research practice and attitudes to research.[47]

Some of the complexity arises from different frameworks for reviewing research. Emanuel and Grady[48] identify 4 paradigms for research review: researcher paternalism; regulatory protectionism; participant access; and community participation.[48] Among ethical and legal reviewers, "regulatory protectionism" appears to be the dominant paradigm.[49] Many clinicians work with the "participant access" paradigm. "Community participation" is less well developed among the materno-fetal community than among other populations, such as seen with human immunodeficiency virus. Within drug development programs, it is important to recognize the paradigm that reviewers are using so that data and justifications can be presented appropriately. The choice of paradigm is not easy to change and will require influence across the materno-fetal community. No matter which paradigm is used, the core task is to gather sufficient data to allow skilled judgments about tradeoffs in trial design (see later discussion for comments on making skilled judgments). Appropriate trade-offs about trial design require information that academic researchers do not usually gather when developing new drugs.

Pregnant women are seen as vulnerable. A review of the concept of vulnerability with respect to pregnant women in research argued that vulnerability can manifest

Table 2
Funding challenges and solutions

Challenges	Solution	
Describing costs and benefits	Targeted gathering of information	Public-private
Comparing options	Develop methodologies for comparisons	partnerships
Building a market for research	Relevant incentives for all contributors to the research process	
Building a market for drugs	Access to new medicines, improve implementation of new interventions	
Comparing moral arguments to economic arguments	Policy advocacy	
Political awareness	Coordinated campaign free from conflicts of interest	

in 4 ways: (i) informed consent, (ii) susceptibility to coercion, (iii) higher exposure to risk due to lack of knowledge, (iv) vulnerability of the fetus.[50] Each of these may be due to lack of information that women can use to make decisions.

Women with a sick fetus may be at particular risk of "therapeutic misconception" (a bias toward wanting to help their fetus), so information needs to be presented in a way that reflects their specific cognitive and emotional condition.[51] For example, some women who had participated in the ORACLE trial of antibiotics for preterm, prolonged rupture of membranes were told of possible adverse results from exposure to co-amoxiclav.[52] Even several years after they were recruited, many felt guilt about their participation, whereas others remained happy with their involvement.

On the basis of personal experience and the widespread unwillingness of institutions to support investigation of medicinal products in pregnant women, the authors speculate that the risk of "therapeutic misconception" among families is mirrored by a risk of "ethical misconception" among ethical and legal reviewers. This "ethical misconception" may arise when the possibility of adverse outcomes clouds the ability of reviewers to focus on the possibility that research drugs under evaluation may provide significant benefit globally to pregnant women. Therapeutic misconception can be managed by context-specific information for families. Similarly, ethical misconceptions can be addressed with context-specific information for reviewers. Facilitating dialogue between researcher, ethics committees, and family advocates involves clear presentation of information and explicit justification of the clinical reasoning used in the situation that drives the research.

The authors believe that a clear view about how to address many of these ethical issues is available, but needs to be more widely propagated. They suggest the following actions:

1. Improved presentation and uptake of the international consensus that research about new drugs used during pregnancy is appropriate and necessary
2. Clearer guidance about when and how to apply international consensus
   a. When standards can be used, and when judgments are appropriate
   b. Acceptance of diversity in practice, such as the need in countries, such as the United States, for biological fathers to give consent for some research during pregnancy; these countries cannot expect biological fathers to be required to give consent in other countries
3. Reducing uncertainty about safety by freely sharing information about the magnitude and nature of risks in a way that allows comparison with potential benefits
4. Sharing experience about how to handle ethical issues through case studies and formal research into communication, family perspectives, and other key ethical concerns

Public-private partnerships that work across multiple drug development programs would be well placed to take these actions.

FETUS AND NEONATE

The central, and unique, problem for research in pregnancy is the need to account for the interests of 2 (or more) participants: the mother and her offspring. The balance between maternal and fetal interests is difficult to consider, both emotionally and cognitively, unless you have experienced it as a parent or a caregiver. However, families and clinicians do this regularly in clinical practice. Many people approach the situation with a natural inclination to avoid harm to a fetus. However, in many clinical situations it is impossible to avoid harm: the harm has already occurred. Pregnant women and fetuses are not excluded from clinical care because they may be "vulnerable." This needs to be the starting point for the design and review of research about new drugs for pregnant women or the fetus. The conversation about research should not be made more difficult than the usual conversation related to the clinical problem that drives the research.

These principles need careful application given the wide range of potential treatments. Some treatments may be highly innovative, and it may be difficult to assess safely in any population, examples being gene therapy and nanoparticle-targeted delivery of therapeutics. A patient-centered view is possible and can guide researchers.[53] Some of the uncertainty can be managed by careful surveillance with registries. A key question is who owns the risk? That is, who owns the adverse human outcomes and the benefits that actually happen? Who will suffer or benefit? The authors contend that well-informed families are best positioned to inform discussions about benefits and risks. The views of families should be the basis for judgments by ethics committees, regulators, and other decision-makers. Long-term uncertainty is part and parcel of clinical care and is an important driver for research.

A key issue is how to assess benefits and harms. Currently, there is no consensus about when and how to follow up high-risk neonates. The balance between harms and benefits is complicated by the evolution of outcomes; outcomes at discharge are frequently discordant with outcomes at 5 years' corrected gestational age.[54,55] It is often not possible to provide accurate information about risks and benefits at the start of the study, or even midway through it.[56] These uncertainties are not the result of research. These uncertainties are the clinical reality that families and clinicians deal with daily. Each study needs a plan for follow-up that takes account of outcomes that are predictable from the pharmacology of the new drug as well as outcomes that are unexpected. This requires significant investment. Adaptive licensing may play a role in addressing these uncertainties during the evaluation of new drugs.[57] The neonatal community is grappling with these issues so that collaboration between the communities is essential.

SOLUTIONS

Activities in single programs and for the community are summarized and compared in **Fig. 1**. These activities cannot be done in isolation. A systems approach is needed to address "all the layers of the onion," which is illustrated in **Fig. 2**.

Steps for Single Programs

Programs and individual trials should involve a broad study team with all relevant disciplines and include potential participants (or their advocates). Steps toward designing clinical trials are summarized in **Box 1**. Aspects that are specific to pregnancy include the following:

1. Identify which data are needed for design and review of the trial. For example, FDA review of a clinical program or study requires information about nonclinical safety, a case series if the drug has been used off-label, information about epidemiology, and information that supports efficacy. This information needs to be gathered prospectively in a manner that informs decisions about clinical studies and in a form that can be submitted to regulatory agencies.
2. Identify information about the context that is needed to inform trial design and review. This includes information about the ethical, legal, and social features of the specific condition and population under study.

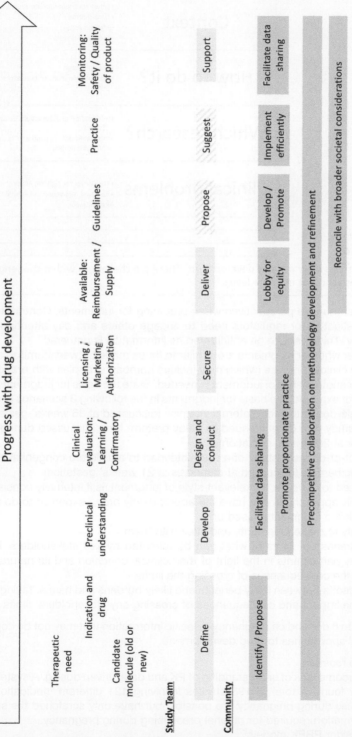

Fig. 1. A comparison between the contributions of study teams and the community to drug development in pregnancy. Hatched areas indicate where there are potential conflicts of interest.

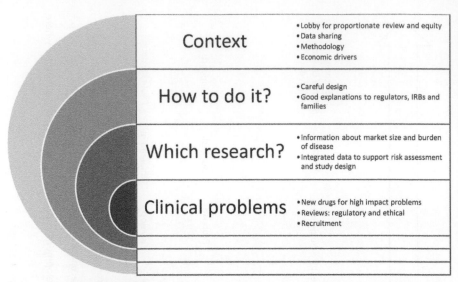

Fig. 2. A systems view of drug development. There are challenges within challenges: progress requires action at multiple levels.

3. Consider multiple perspectives when preparing for judgments. Contributors such as investigators or regulators need to engage others and pay attention to what they say. This needs to be anticipated as information is gathered.
4. Consider whether judgments are similar to those made between families and clinicians in clinical practice (which may include comparing apples with oranges),[56] or whether another style of judgment is needed. State the basis for judgments that are used. For example, the basis for judgments in the following 3 scenarios is different:
   i. Single-dose study of maternal vitamins (discussed at 36 weeks' gestation)
   ii. PK study of a drug intended to delay preterm birth (discussed during preterm labor at 26 weeks' gestation)
   iii. Proof-of-concept study of a drug intended to ameliorate congenital diaphragmatic hernias (discussed at diagnosis at 21 weeks' gestation)
5. IRBs need to consider the relevant style of judgment (is it internally consistent and societally appropriate) and have the appropriately broad expertise to do so.
6. Make skilled judgments based on
   i. Ability to make judgments and stick with them
   ii. Awareness of limits of what can be tolerated by key stakeholders, including study participants in the light of their clinical condition and its natural history, and the consequences of crossing the limits
   iii. Tradeoffs between likely benefits and likely burdens and harms, taking account of the impact and consequences of crossing any stakeholders' limits

Steps 1 to 6 depend on pregnancy-specific information that may not be collected in "standard" approaches to drug development.

7. Dosage regimen
   a. Overcome lack of understanding of PK and data-driven dosing. A systematic review found a total of 198 studies involving 121 different medications.[58] PK studies during pregnancy are possible but have only scratched the surface of information required for rational prescribing during pregnancy.
   b. Consider PBPK models[22]

Box 1
Steps for individual clinical drug development program (see text for pregnancy-specific details)

Generate information needed for judgments about the design of the program/study
  Identify which judgments are needed:
  • Study design by sponsor and investigators
  • By families approached about recruitment
  • Review by ethics and regulators
  Identify information about the context that is needed to inform trial design and review
  Consider how to minimize harm while optimizing likelihood of identifying a reliable signal
  for efficacy (or the lack of an effect): what is the factual basis for tradeoffs?
  Consider multiple perspectives when preparing for judgments

Identify options for key design features
  Eligibility
  Outcomes: identify clinically important or validated/qualified surrogate
  Interventions: nature and dosage
  Invasiveness of assessments
  Harms from the trial
  Direct benefit or not
  Minimal harm or not: justifications, not assertions

Judgments about safety and efficacy: using information to select between options
  Consider whether judgments are similar to judgments made between families and clinicians
  in clinical practice
  Consider precedents and guidelines taking account of the context, the intervention, and
  similarity to the current situation

Plan
  Preparedness of clinical studies, including site-level feasibility
  Consider studies that test procedures and assumptions about recruitment (in silico Modeling
  and simulation, in vivo trial simulation, pilot trials)

Dosage regimen
  Overcome lack of understanding of PK

Trial supplies
  Active pharmaceutical ingredient
  Excipients and formulations

Approvals

Recruitment

---

8. Trial supplies

Excipients (nonactive components of the pharmaceutical preparation) are important. In other populations, excipient selection can be based on whether a substance is "generally regarded as safe," but this is not a safe approach during pregnancy.[59] Nanoparticles and other novel excipients need dedicated assessment if they are to be used during pregnancy.

9. Recruitment

As noted above, recruitment should be based on a trial-specific and patient-centered approach to education about trial features. A patient-centred approach, tailored to each trial and tested for each trial, is especially important for discussions about safety.[60]

10. Developing, agreeing, and adhering to core data sets and shared outcomes that will promote comparison of data arising from multiple trials and better facilitate individual patient data meta-analyses.

Community

Many of the challenges that arise during the evaluation of new drugs used during pregnancy can only be addressed by a community made up of multiple disciplines and perspectives. The actions needed to promote maternal and neonatal health care in low- and middle-income countries have been described (**Table 3**).[61]

Materno-fetal investigators are trying to build a community through the Global Obstetrics Network (http://www.globalobstetricsnetwork.org), and this academic initiative is an ideal basis for the development of a private public partnership that includes PlaNet.[16]

Table 3
Steps for the materno-fetal community

Steps	Actions
General	
Recognize the stakeholders as a community	Open and transparent recognition of the value of many perspectives Integrate multiple perspectives into a tractable vision and mission, and community of practice
Build a coalition	Develop formal and informal groups in appropriate geographic and methodological settings, with global coordination
Policy development (context specific)	Prioritize and form appropriate, pan-stakeholder groups
Specific	
Identify therapeutic needs	Epidemiology, burden, ethical, legal, and social contexts
Facilitate data sharing (before and after licensing)	Data standards Governance for data sharing Facilities for data sharing
Promote proportional review (legal, ethical, and regulatory)	Identify key features of important clinical situations that should guide the design and review of programs and individual studies, including consistent interpretation of regulatory and legal texts, and identification of useful precedents
Precompetitive collaboration on methodology development and refinement	Prioritize and form appropriate, pan-stakeholder groups
Lobby for equity between pregnancy and other populations	Resources for medicines Access to medicines
Develop and promote guidelines for research design, review, and conduct	Prioritize and form appropriate, pan-stakeholder groups
Implement innovations efficiently	Develop effective links with relevant communities and use good implementation science/knowledge exchange strategies
Reconcile with broader societal considerations	Recognize competing priorities and make a strong case for drug development in pregnancy

The materno-fetal community refers to all groups and individuals that contribute to the design, review, implementation, and use of research about drugs used to treat maternal or fetal conditions during pregnancy.

The report by PRGLAC includes some recommendations that can form the basis for influencing policies (https://www.nichd.nih.gov/sites/default/files/2018-08/TaskForce_MeetingSummary4.pdf), including

- Remove pregnant women as an example of a vulnerable population in the Common Rule and FDA regulations
- Provide more resources for research (funding, human, infrastructure)
- Ensure that only 1 parental signature is required for research during pregnancy
- Implement a liability-mitigation strategy for conducting research and evaluating new therapeutic products in pregnant women and lactating women
- Drive discovery and development for new therapies in high-priority conditions
- Develop programs to study off-patent products used during pregnancy, similar to the programs for products used in children
- Proactive approach to the inclusion of pregnant women in research
- Leverage established and support new infrastructures/collaborations to perform research in pregnant women and lactating women

The US community needs to influence Congress to pass the necessary legislation. Advances in the United States are an opportunity for the materno-fetal community outside the United States to promote these ideas.

Comparisons with Other Communities

In pediatrics, significant investment has been made through legislation, policy, and infrastructure over several decades[3,7] based on leadership from each stakeholder focused on the needs of the community. The International Neonatal Consortium is a precompetitive public-private partnership that has published several documents that clarify neonatal drug development.[62–65] Efficient public-private partnerships need to be well targeted with professional management of expectations and high-quality facilitation.[66] The clinical community and its learned societies need to promote regulatory, legal, and ethical changes.[67]

Additional investment in pediatric research infrastructure includes the setup of FDA-funded research networks led by the Institute for Advanced Clinical Trials (-https://www.iactc.org) and the Duke Clinical Research Institute (https://dcri.org/global-pediatric-clinical-trials-network/) in 2017 and the European Innovative Medicine Initiative 2/European Federation of Pharmaceutical and Industries Association–cofunded network Conect4Children (https://conect4children.org) that was initiated in 2018.

The authors note that there has been progress in other aspects of women's health when appropriate investment has been made in "multipronged" approaches, including attention to study design, communication, and policy initiatives.[68] Another example comes from the neglected disease community.[69]

SUMMARY

This review has addressed the challenges that arise when testing new and existing drugs that could be used during pregnancy. The authors have emphasized a multileveled approach needed to overcome these challenges.

Individual drug development programs need to gather a body of scientific and clinical information with drug development in mind. Drug development benefits from the structure provided by regulatory pathways, even if a regulatory filing is not an objective of a programme of research. Additional information is needed to support the judgments about benefits and risks related to trials made by study teams, sponsors, regulators, ethicists, and, above all, families who will decide whether to participate in a trial. Because this additional information has not emerged from research to date, researchers and the community need to develop strategies for information gathering that will supplement their current approaches.

Over the past decade, there have been many calls for the materno-fetal community to develop new drugs for pregnant women and fetuses. To do this, the community must develop a global public-private partnership and identify actions to take together. The mother and fetus, true drug orphans of the twenty-first century, urgently need us to deliver on these action plans.

Best Practices

What is the current practice for designing clinical trials to test new drugs in the pregnant woman and fetus?

1. Inconsistent, isolated approaches that are hampered by disproportionate concerns about safety

2. Legal frameworks that hinder important research

What changes in current practice are likely to improve outcomes?

1. Recognize and implement the international consensus that research about new drugs used during pregnancy is appropriate and necessary

2. Use approaches to the development of new drugs for maternal and fetal conditions that are succeeding in other marginalized therapeutic areas, including approaches to liability, insurance, consent; use of registries to support study planning

3. Embed participant involvement in all stages of drug development, so that research questions are relevant to families and risk is identified and presented appropriately

4. Take a systematic approach to drug development through a "maternity investigation plan" that is analogous to the PIP or pediatric study plan

5. Improve the evidence base about the risks and benefits of interventions during pregnancy and use new, and existing, information to facilitate study design and review by ethics boards, regulators, funders, and potential participants of studies

6. Promote proportionate review of research studies by considering the context for each study: the condition that is being researched and the clinical setting in which recruitment will take place

7. Ensure that the design and conduct of in vitro, ex vivo, and clinical studies are compatible with the needs of drug development programs

8. Collaborate in effective geographic and methodological, pan-stakeholder public-private partnerships, with global coordination

9. Change the legal framework to promote well-justified research that meets important needs of pregnant women and fetuses

10. Fund research that will improve pregnancy outcomes for women and their offspring

11. Recognize that vulnerability during pregnancy often stems from lack of access to high-quality research about drugs used during pregnancy; other aspects of vulnerability are context dependent and need to dealt with on a case-by-case basis rather than with blanket bans on research

12. Work in public-private partnerships

13. Remove pregnant women as an example of a vulnerable population in the US Common Rule and FDA regulations

14. Ensure that only 1 parental signature is required for research during pregnancy

15. Implement a liability-mitigation strategy for conducting research and evaluating new therapeutic products in pregnant women and lactating women

16. Drive discovery and development for new therapies in high-priority conditions

17. Develop programs to study off-patent products used during pregnancy, similar to the programs for products used in children

18. Leverage established and support new infrastructures/collaborations to perform research in pregnant women and lactating women

REFERENCES

1. Chappell LC, David AL. Improving the pipeline for developing and testing pharmacological treatments in pregnancy. PLoS Med 2016;13:e1002161.
2. Committee on Ethics. ACOG committee opinion no. 646: ethical considerations for including women as research participants. Obstet Gynecol 2015;126:e100–7.
3. Fisk NM, Atun R. Market failure and the poverty of new drugs in maternal health. PLoS Med 2008;5:e22.
4. Foulkes MA, Grady C, Spong CY, et al. Clinical research enrolling pregnant women: a workshop summary. J Womens Health (Larchmt) 2011;20:1429–32.
5. David AL, Thornton S, Sutcliffe A, et al. Developing new pharmaceutical treatments for obstetric conditions. London: Royal College of Obstetricians and Gynaecologists; 2015.
6. Sheffield JS, Siegel D, Mirochnick M, et al. Designing drug trials: considerations for pregnant women. Clin Infect Dis 2014;59(Suppl 7):S437–44.
7. Thornton JG. Drug development and obstetrics: where are we right now? J Matern Fetal Neonatal Med 2009;22(Suppl 2):46–9.
8. Grigsby PL. Animal models to study placental development and function throughout normal and dysfunctional human pregnancy. Semin Reprod Med 2016;34:11–6.
9. Sastry BV. Techniques to study human placental transport. Adv Drug Deliv Rev 1999;38:17–39.
10. David AL. Maternal uterine artery VEGF gene therapy for treatment of intrauterine growth restriction. Placenta 2017;59(Suppl 1):S44–50.
11. Girardi G. Pravastatin to treat and prevent preeclampsia. Preclinical and clinical studies. J Reprod Immunol 2017;124:15–20.
12. Winterhager E, Gellhaus A. Transplacental nutrient transport mechanisms of intrauterine growth restriction in rodent models and humans. Front Physiol 2017;8:951.
13. Leptak C, Menetski JP, Wagner JA, et al. What evidence do we need for biomarker qualification? Sci Transl Med 2017;9 [pii:eaal4599].
14. Myllynen P, Mathiesen L, Weimer M, et al. Preliminary interlaboratory comparison of the ex vivo dual human placental perfusion system. Reprod Toxicol 2010;30:94–102.
15. Conings S, Amant F, Annaert P, et al. Integration and validation of the ex vivo human placenta perfusion model. J Pharmacol Toxicol Methods 2017;88:25–31.
16. Brownbill P, Chernyavsky I, Bottalico B, et al. An international network (PlaNet) to evaluate a human placental testing platform for chemicals safety testing in pregnancy. Reprod Toxicol 2016;64:191–202.
17. Prinz F, Schlange T, Asadullah K. Believe it or not: how much can we rely on published data on potential drug targets? Nat Rev Drug Discov 2011;10:712.

18. FDA. Pregnant women: scientific and ethical considerations for inclusion in clinical trials guidance for industry 2018. Available at: https://www.fda.gov/downloads/Drugs/GuidanceComplianceRegulatoryInformation/Guidances/UCM603873.pdf. Accessed March 14, 2019.

19. Chervenak FA, McCullough LB. An ethically justified framework for clinical investigation to benefit pregnant and fetal patients. Am J Bioeth 2011;11:39–49.

20. Macleod MR, Michie S, Roberts I, et al. Biomedical research: increasing value, reducing waste. Lancet 2014;383:101–4.

21. Dahlin JL, Inglese J, Walters MA. Mitigating risk in academic preclinical drug discovery. Nat Rev Drug Discov 2015;14:279–94.

22. Ke AB, Greupink R, Abduljalil K. Drug dosing in pregnant women: challenges and opportunities in using physiologically based pharmacokinetic modeling and simulations. CPT Pharmacometrics Syst Pharmacol 2018;7:103–10.

23. Korth-Bradley JM. Industry perspective of drug development for pregnant/breastfeeding women. Clin Pharmacol Ther 2016;100:19–21.

24. Mastroianni AC, Henry LM, Robinson D, et al. Research with pregnant women: new insights on legal decision-making. Hastings Cent Rep 2017;47:38–45.

25. Koren G. Ethical framework for observational studies of medicinal drug exposure in pregnancy. Teratology 2002;65:191–5.

26. de Oliveira-Filho AD, Vieira AES, da Silva RC, et al. Adverse drug reactions in high-risk pregnant women: a prospective study. Saudi Pharm J 2017;25:1073–7.

27. Bracken LE, Nunn AJ, Kirkham JJ, et al. Development of the liverpool adverse drug reaction avoidability assessment tool. PLoS One 2017;12:e0169393.

28. Du W, Lehr VT, Lieh-Lai M, et al. An algorithm to detect adverse drug reactions in the neonatal intensive care unit. J Clin Pharmacol 2013;53:87–95.

29. Gallagher RM, Kirkham JJ, Mason JR, et al. Development and inter-rater reliability of the Liverpool adverse drug reaction causality assessment tool. PLoS One 2011;6:e28096.

30. Duffy J, Rolph R, Gale C, et al. Core outcome sets in women's and newborn health: a systematic review. BJOG 2017;124:1481–9.

31. Costeloe K, Turner MA, Padula MA, et al. Sharing Data to Accelerate Medicine Development and Improve Neonatal Care: Data Standards and Harmonized Definitions. J Pediatr 2018 Dec;203:437-41.e1.

32. EMA. Paediatric investigation plans 2018. Available at: https://www.ema.europa.eu/en/human-regulatory/research-development/paediatric-medicines/paediatric-investigation-plans. Accessed March 14, 2019.

33. FDA. Pediatric study plans: content of and process for submitting initial pediatric study plans and amended initial pediatric study plans guidance for industry 2016. Available at: https://www.fda.gov/downloads/drugs/guidances/ucm360507.pdf. Accessed March 14, 2019.

34. Saint-Raymond A, de Vries CS. Medicine safety in pregnancy and ambitions for the EU medicine regulatory framework. Clin Pharmacol Ther 2016;100:21–3.

35. Sun H, Vesely R, Nelson RM, et al. Steps toward harmonization for clinical development of medicines in pediatric ulcerative colitis-a global scientific discussion, part 2: data extrapolation, trial design, and pharmacokinetics. J Pediatr Gastroenterol Nutr 2014;58:684–8.

36. Daly KA, Toth JA, Giebink GS. Pneumococcal conjugate vaccines as maternal and infant immunogens: challenges of maternal recruitment. Vaccine 2003;21:3473–8.

37. Kenyon S, Dixon-Woods M, Jackson CJ, et al. Participating in a trial in a critical situation: a qualitative study in pregnancy. Qual Saf Health Care 2006;15:98–101.

38. Mohanna K, Tunna K. Withholding consent to participate in clinical trials: decisions of pregnant women. Br J Obstet Gynaecol 1999;106:892–7.

39. Palmer S, Pudwell J, Smith GN, et al. Optimizing participation of pregnant women in clinical trials: factors influencing decisions about participation in medication and vaccine trials. J Obstet Gynaecol Can 2016;38:945–54.

40. Rodger MA, Makropoulos D, Walker M, et al. Participation of pregnant women in clinical trials: will they participate and why? Am J Perinatol 2003;20:69–76.

41. Razum O, Schaaber J, Nayar KR. Of silver bullets and red herrings: invited commentary to Fisk et al. Trop Med Int Health 2011;16:669–71.

42. Fisk NM, McKee M, Atun R. Relative and absolute addressability of global disease burden in maternal and perinatal health by investment in R&D. Trop Med Int Health 2011;16:662–8.

43. Simpkin VL, Renwick MJ, Kelly R, et al. Incentivising innovation in antibiotic drug discovery and development: progress, challenges and next steps. J Antibiot (Tokyo) 2017;70:1087–96.

44. Rex JH, Outterson K. Antibiotic reimbursement in a model delinked from sales: a benchmark-based worldwide approach. Lancet Infect Dis 2016;16:500–5.

45. Institute of Medicine. Women and health research: ethical and legal issues of including women in clinical studies. Washington, DC: The National Academies Press; 1994. p. 288p.

46. Beeler JA, Lambach P, Fulton TR, et al. A systematic review of ethical issues in vaccine studies involving pregnant women. Hum Vaccin Immunother 2016;12: 1952–9.

47. Saenz C, Cheah PY, van der Graaf R, et al. Ethics, regulation, and beyond: the landscape of research with pregnant women. Reprod Health 2017;14:173.

48. Emanuel EJ, Grady C. Four paradigms of clinical research and research oversight. Camb Q Healthc Ethics 2007;16:82–96.

49. Lyerly AD, Little MO, Faden R. The second wave: toward responsible inclusion of pregnant women in research. Int J Fem Approaches Bioeth 2008;1:5–22.

50. van der Zande ISE, van der Graaf R, Oudijk MA, et al. Vulnerability of pregnant women in clinical research. J Med Ethics 2017;43:657–63.

51. Sheppard MK. Vulnerability, therapeutic misconception and informed consent: is there a need for special treatment of pregnant women in fetus-regarding clinical trials? J Med Ethics 2016;42:127–31.

52. Tarrant C, Jackson C, Dixon-Woods M, et al. Consent revisited: the impact of return of results on participants' views and expectations about trial participation. Health Expect 2015;18:2042–53.

53. Sheppard M, Spencer RN, Ashcroft R, et al. Ethics and social acceptability of a proposed clinical trial using maternal gene therapy to treat severe early-onset fetal growth restriction. Ultrasound Obstet Gynecol 2016;47:484–91.

54. Marlow N. Is survival and neurodevelopmental impairment at 2 years of age the gold standard outcome for neonatal studies? Arch Dis Child Fetal Neonatal Ed 2015;100:F82–4.

55. Parekh SA, Field DJ, Johnson S, et al. Accounting for deaths in neonatal trials: is there a correct approach? Arch Dis Child Fetal Neonatal Ed 2015;100:F193–7.

56. Snowdon C, Brocklehurst P, Tasker RC, et al. "You have to keep your nerve on a DMC." Challenges for data monitoring committees in neonatal intensive care trials: qualitative accounts from the BRACELET Study. PLoS One 2018;13: e0201037.

57. Eichler HG, Baird LG, Barker R, et al. From adaptive licensing to adaptive pathways: delivering a flexible life-span approach to bring new drugs to patients. Clin Pharmacol Ther 2015;97:234–46.
58. Pariente G, Leibson T, Carls A, et al. Pregnancy-associated changes in pharmacokinetics: a systematic review. PLoS Med 2016;13:e1002160.
59. Finkelstein Y, Rezvani M, Garcia-Bournissen F, et al. Inactive pharmaceutical ingredients: implications for pregnancy. Can J Clin Pharmacol 2007;14:e17–28.
60. Goff SL, Youssef Y, Pekow PS, et al. Successful strategies for practice-based recruitment of racial and ethnic minority pregnant women in a randomized controlled trial: the IDEAS for a healthy baby study. J Racial Ethn Health Disparities 2016;3:731–7.
61. Sather M, Fajon AV, Zaentz R, et al. Global report on preterm birth and stillbirth (5 of 7): advocacy barriers and opportunities. BMC Pregnancy Childbirth 2010; 10(Suppl 1):S5.
62. Turner MA, Davis JM, McCune S, et al. The International Neonatal Consortium: collaborating to advance regulatory science for neonates. Pediatr Res 2016;80: 462–4.
63. Ward RM, Benjamin D, Barrett JS, et al. Safety, dosing, and pharmaceutical quality for studies that evaluate medicinal products (including biological products) in neonates. Pediatr Res 2017;81:692–711.
64. Davis JM, Baer GR, Portman R, et al. Enrollment of neonates in more than one clinical trial. Clin Ther 2017;39:1959–69.
65. Steinhorn R, Davis JM, Gopel W, et al. Chronic pulmonary insufficiency of prematurity: developing optimal endpoints for drug development. J Pediatr 2017;191: 15–21.e1.
66. Brumfield M. The Critical Path Institute: transforming competitors into collaborators. Nat Rev Drug Discov 2014;13:785–6.
67. White A. Accelerating the paradigm shift toward inclusion of pregnant women in drug research: ethical and regulatory considerations. Semin Perinatol 2015;39: 537–40.
68. Institute of Medicine. Women's Health research: progress, pitfalls, and promise. Washington, DC: The National Academies Press; 2010. p. 438p.
69. Trouiller P, Olliaro P, Torreele E, et al. Drug development for neglected diseases: a deficient market and a public-health policy failure. Lancet 2002;359:2188–94.

Moving?

Make sure your subscription moves with you!

To notify us of your new address, find your **Clinics Account Number** (located on your mailing label above your name), and contact customer service at:

Email: journalscustomerservice-usa@elsevier.com

800-654-2452 (subscribers in the U.S. & Canada)
314-447-8871 (subscribers outside of the U.S. & Canada)

Fax number: 314-447-8029

Elsevier Health Sciences Division
Subscription Customer Service
3251 Riverport Lane
Maryland Heights, MO 63043

*To ensure uninterrupted delivery of your subscription, please notify us at least 4 weeks in advance of move.

Printed and bound by CPI Group (UK) Ltd, Croydon, CR0 4YY

03/10/2024

01040401-0007